Palliative Care

Learning in Practice

Palliative Care
Learning in Practice

Edited by Janette Edwards and Elaine Stevens

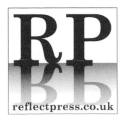

reflectpress.co.uk

In association with the
RCN Palliative Nursing Forum

The right of Janette Edwards, Elaine Stevens, Mary Bredin, Linda Kerr, Emma Ream and Norrie Sutherland to be identified as authors of this work has been asserted by them in accordance with the Copyright, Designs and Patents Act 1988.

First published in 2008

ISBN: 978 1 906052 16 4

British Library Cataloguing in Publication Data
A catalogue record for this book is available from the British Library

The authors and publisher have made every attempt to ensure the content of this book is up-to-date and accurate. However, health care knowledge and information is changing all the time so the reader is advised to double-check any information in this text on drug usage, treatment procedures, the use of equipment, etc. to confirm that it complies with the latest safety recommendations, standards of practice and legislation, as well as local Trust policies and procedures.

Production project management by Deer Park Productions, Tavistock, Devon

Typeset by TW Typesetting, Plymouth, Devon

Cover design by Oxmed

Printed and bound by Bell & Bain, Glasgow

Distributed by BEBC, Albion Close, Parkstone, Poole, Dorset BH12 3LL

www.reflectpress.co.uk

Published by Reflect Press Ltd
11 Attwyll Avenue
Exeter
Devon, EX2 5HN
UK
01392 204400

Contents

Author biographies

Mary Bredin, RGN, MA
Mary has spent a number of years developing an integrated approach for the management of breathlessness with colleagues at the Macmillan Practice Development Unit, Centre for Palliative Care Studies, Institute of Cancer Research. She is currently teaching about breathlessness, writing and studying for a post-graduate diploma in psychotherapeutic counselling.

Janette Edwards
Open learning writer and editor.

Linda Kerr, RGN, MN (cancer nursing), Dip. Health & Social Welfare, BSc, Dip. Massage Therapy, Specialist Practitioner in Palliative Care, Nurse Specialist/Training Officer in Palliative Care, Ayrshire & Arran Acute Hospitals NHS Trust.

Emma Ream, MSc, BSc(Hons), RGN
Lecturer/Research Fellow, Florence Nightingale School of Nursing and Midwifery, King's College London.

Emma has spent many years researching fatigue in chronic illness. Latterly she has been working with colleagues at King's College London to develop an educational/supportive programme for patients with cancer, 'Beating fatigue'.

Elaine Stevens, MSc (Palliative Care), Specialist practitioner in palliative care, PGCE (HE/FE), RGN, RNT

At the start of this project, Elaine was the Day Care co-ordinator at the Victoria Hospice, Kirkcaldy. She is currently Education Manager at the Ayrshire Hospice and a lecturer in palliative care at the University of the West of Scotland.

Norrie Sutherland, BSc (Health Studies), RGN, CMB, RHV, RNT, Cert. Ed. (Post initial), Certificate in Clinical Aromatherapy.

At the start of this project Norrie was Senior Lecturer at the Ayrshire Hospice. She has since retired and now works freelance on various palliative care projects.

Acknowledgements

The Author team would like to thank the critical readers:

Caroline Nicholson
Lecturer in Palliative Nursing
Centre for Cancer and Palliative Care Studies
Royal Marsden Hospital
Fulham Road
London
SW3 6JJ

Virginia Dunn
Senior Lecturer
Marie Curie Cancer Care
Bradford
West Yorkshire

Kay Rowe
Tenovus Oncology Nurse Specialist
Tenovus Cancer Information Centre
Velindre Hospital
Whitchurch
Cardiff
CF14 2TL

Mary Wells
Clinical Research Fellow in Cancer Nursing
Tayside University Hospitals NHS Trust
University of Dundee
Ninewells Hospital and Medical School
Dundee
DD1 9SY

Also, for his help on the topic of anaemia in the Fatigue chapter, we would like to thank Alastair Smith, Consultant Haematologist and

Honorary Clinical Senior Lecturer, Haematology Department, Southampton University Hospitals NHS Trust, Southampton SO14 0YG.

This resource was piloted within 11 general palliative care settings:

- Nottingham City Primary Care Trust
- Bradford Teaching Hospitals NHS Foundation Trust
- Westminster Primary Care Trust
- The Leeds Teaching Hospitals NHS Trust
- Erewash Primary Care Trust
- Craven, Harrogate and Rural District PCT and Harrogate Healthcare NHS Trust
- Erskine Mains Home, Erskine, Renfrewshire
- Yorkshire Wolds and Coast Primary Care Trust
- Hull and East Yorkshire Hospitals NHS Trust
- Eastern Hull Primary Care Trust and East Yorkshire Acute Trust
- Calderdale and Huddersfield NHS Foundation Trust.

We thank all the facilitators and participants for their hard work. One pilot site has successfully negotiated accreditation for the prior experiential learning process and the participants have been awarded 45 Scottish Degree level points for the learning undertaken.

Amendments to the book were made in response to the pilot participants' comments, the comments by the critical readers and in relation to maintaining currency.

The following Introduction, and the accompanying *Facilitator Guide* (available online at **www.reflectpress.co.uk/book.asp?id = 26**), are based on the guides created for the open learning pack *Realising Clinical Effectiveness and Clinical Governance through Clinical Supervision* (2000), which was developed in conjunction with the RCN Institute by Radcliffe Publishing Ltd (**www.radcliffe-oxford.com** website accessed 30/6/06). The authors and publisher are grateful to Radcliffe Publishing Ltd for permission to adapt the guides for use with this textbook.

The RCN Palliative Nursing Forum is also exceedingly grateful to Janssen Cilag, whose generous funding has allowed the production of such a valuable resource. Without this funding the project would not have been possible.

Acknowledgements for the use of copyright material

The editors, authors and publisher would like to thank the following people and organisations for permission to reproduce their material in this book. Every attempt has been made to seek permission for the copyright material that has been used. However, if we have inadvertently used copyright material without permission/acknowledgement we apologise and we will make the necessary correction at the first opportunity.

Figure 1.1 Palliative care follows curative care, World Health Organization, 1990: 16.

Figure 1.2 Palliative care and curative care work together, World Health Organization, 1990: 16.

Figure 1.3 The Sheffield model of palliative care (Ahmedzai, 2006) from **www.sheffield-palliative.org.uk/Healthcare/smodel.html** Reprinted with kind permission of the author.

Figure 1.4 The theory of unpleasant symptoms, from Lenz, E.R., Suppe, F., Gift, A.G., Pugh, L.C., and Milligan, R.A. (1995) Collaborative development of middle-range nursing theories: toward a theory of unpleasant symptoms, *Advancing in Nursing Science 17* (3) pp.1–13. Reprinted with permission of Lippincott William & Wilkins.

Figure 1.5 Effective and ineffective approaches to dealing with anger (Faulkner, 1998: 49) from Faulkner, A., (1998) 'Communication with patients, families and other professionals' in Fallon, M. and O'Neill, B. (editors) *ABC of Palliative Care*, London BMJ Books, pp.47–9, Reprinted with permission of Blackwell Publishing Ltd.

Figure 2.1 Dimensions of care in the supportive care model, from Davies, B., and Oberle, K. (1990) Dimensions of the supportive role of the nurse in palliative care, *Oncology Nursing Forum*, 17 (1) pp.87–94. Reprinted with permission of Oncology Nursing Forum c/o Copyright Clearance Center.

Figure 2.2 The ethical grid, from *Ethics: the heart of healthcare* (2nd edition) by Seedhouse, D. (1998) © John Wiley & Sons Limited. Reprinted with permission.

Figure 2.3 Reflective Cycle, from Marks-Maran D: *Reconstruction Nursing: Beyond Art and Science* 1997: 128 © 1997 Elsevier Limited. Reprinted with permission of Elsevier Limited.

Figures 5.2 Effects of breathlessness on quality of life (adapted), **Figure 5.3** Breathlessness assessment guide, page 1, **Figure 5.4** Breathlessness assessment guide page 2, **Figure 5.5** Breathlessness assessment guide page 3, **Figure 5.8** The breathlessness intervention (adapted) 5.31 Script of simple relaxation, from *A Breath of Fresh Air*, The Institute of Cancer Research. Reprinted with permission.

Figure 5.6 The integrative model of breathlessness (Corner *et al.* 1995: 6) Reproduced with permission of MA Healthcare Limited **http://www.ijpn.co.uk**

Figures 5.9 'Inhalation' side view, **5.10,** 'Exhalation' side view, **5.11** 'Inhalation' front view and **5.12** 'Exhalation' front view' from *The TAO of Natural Breathing* by Dennis Lewis. Reprinted with permission of Rodmell Press.

Figure 6.1 Winningham's Psychobiological-Entropy Model, from Winningham, M., Nail, L.M., Burke, M.B., Brophy, L., Cimprich, B., Jones, L.S., Pickard-Holley, S., Rhodes, V., St Pierre, B., Beck, S., Glass, E.C., Mock, V.L., Mooney, K.H., and Piper, B. (1994) Fatigue and the cancer experience: the state of the knowledge *Oncology Nursing Forum*, 21 (1) pp.23–36. Reprinted with permission of Oncology Nursing Forum c/o Copyright Clearance Center.

Figures 6.2a 'Piper fatigue scale page 1', **6.2b** 'Piper fatigue scale page 2, **6.2c** 'Piper fatigue scale page 3', and **6.5** 'Piper fatigue assessment guide' Copyright © Barbara. F. Piper. Reprinted with the kind permission of the author.

Figure 6.3 Brief fatigue inventory BFI© Reprinted with permission of Charles S. Cleeland, Ph.D., Pain Research Group.

Figure 6.4 FACT-F from Cella, D. 'The Functional Assessment of Cancer Therapy – Anemia (FACT-An) scale: a new tool for the assessment of outcomes in cancer and anemia and fatigue pp.13–19 (1997) in *Seminars in Hematology* 34 (3 Suppl 2) July. Reprinted with permission of Elsevier Limited.

Figure 6.6 Clinical assessment guide for fatigue and functioning, from *Cancer Symptom Management* by S. Groenwald, M. Frogge, M. Goodman and C. Yarbro. Copyright © Jones and Bartlett Publishers, Sudbury, MA **www.jbpub.com.** Reprinted with permission of Jones & Bartlett Publishers Inc.

Figure 6.7 Self-care strategies for the relief of fatigue, from Ream, E., and Richardson, A. (1999) 'From theory to practice: designing interventions to reduce fatigue in patients with cancer' *Oncology Nursing Forum*, 26 (8) pp.1295–1305. Reprinted with permission of Oncology Nursing Forum c/o Copyright Clearance Center.

Figure 7.1 Central nervous system, pathways and structures from 'Alongside the person in pain: holistic care and nursing practice' by Fordham, M. and Dunn, V (1994) Reprinted with permission of Elsevier Limited.

Figure 7.2 Factors affecting pain tolerance, adapted from Scottish Intercollegiate Guidelines Network (SIGN) 2000: 6. Reprinted with permission of SIGN.

Figure 7.5 'The Bourbonnais pain ruler' from Bourbonnais, F. (1981) 'Pain assessment of a tool for the nurse and the patient', *Journal of*

Advanced Nursing, 6 (4) pp.277–82 (p.279). Reprinted with permission of Blackwell Publishing Ltd.

Figure 7.6 Brief pain inventory (short form) page 1 BPI © Reprinted with permission of Charles S. Cleeland, Ph.D., Pain Research Group.

Figure 7.7 Brief pain inventory (short form) page 2 BPI © Reprinted by permission of Charles S. Cleeland, PhD., Pain Research Group.

Figure 7.10 'Adjuvant analgesics for neuropathic pain. If caused by cancer, use only if pain does not respond to the combined use of an NSAID and a strong opioid', from Twycross & Wilcock, 2001: 55, Figure 2.14. Reprinted with the kind permission of the author.

Figure 8.1 Delivering improved quality (Department of Health 1998: Introduction: 5) Crown copyright material is reproduced with the permission of the Controller of HMSO.

Figure 8.2 The audit cycle from Morrell, C. and Harvey, G. (1999) 'The clinical audit handbook: improving the quality of health care' Reprinted with permission of Elsevier Limited.

Figure 8.3 Standard No. 1: Symptom Management, SPA, 1996: 5. Reprinted with permission.

Introduction to This Textbook

This Introduction covers the following topics:
- The aims of this textbook
- Who is this textbook for?
- What's in the book?
- What is open learning?
- What is action learning?
- What is work-based learning?
- What is critical companionship?
- What is reflective practice?
- Can I get academic credit?
- What is professional accreditation?
- Working with others
- Planning your study
- Where are we starting from? Clarifying values
- Action planning
- References
- Further reading, useful websites and recommended sources of information and support.

WELCOME

Welcome to the RCN Palliative Nursing Forum's *Palliative Care: Learning in Practice* textbook. This book is based on models of open learning, action learning, work-based learning, critical companionship and reflective practice. It has been designed to be used as a flexible learning resource in a variety of situations with local support from colleagues, professional and practice development staff, managers and educators.

There are a variety of ways that you can work through the textbook with support from:

- a facilitator and a group of your colleagues in:
  - an action learning set
  - a working group
  - a discussion group
- a critical companion who works with you in a one-to-one situation.

You are likely to do the reading and some activities on your own and then engage in discussion with your action learning set/group or critical companion about your thoughts and any problems/issues the material has raised for you. Sometimes we suggest that you do the activities with your action learning set/group or critical companion. The concepts of action learning, action learning sets and critical companionship are discussed briefly in this Introduction and explained in full in the *Facilitator Guide*. Due to the emotional and sensitive nature of some of the study materials, we recommend that you find someone with whom you can discuss the emotional aspects of the learning experience.

You may already have been approached by someone in your organisation and invited to join an action learning set/group. If not, we suggest that you discuss with your manager the possibility of setting up a set/group in your clinical area or health care organisation. If this is not possible, we suggest that you ask an appropriate person to be your critical companion (see page xxvi Working with others).

THE AIMS OF THIS TEXTBOOK

This book aims to enable participants to:

- understand and explore patients' experiences of pain, breathlessness, fatigue, anxiety and depression;
- discuss the impact of this experience on the patient's quality of life;
- develop strategies/expertise to assess, implement and evaluate palliative care;
- develop a repertoire of interventions that can be used for individuals in their own specific context;
- address support mechanisms for patients, families, formal and informal carers;
- access, critique and use the evidence base for care;
- explore the ethical issues relevant to palliative care;
- further develop reflective skills within the context of lifelong learning;

- contribute to and participate in the improvement of multidisciplinary teamwork in palliative care;
- contribute to policy development for the structure and management of palliative care.

WHO IS THIS TEXTBOOK FOR?

This book is designed for qualified nurses working in any setting that has palliative care patients. It is not aimed at those working within a specialist palliative care service. Others who may find the book interesting or useful include members of multidisciplinary teams and allied health professionals such as physiotherapists and occupational therapists.

We have assumed that all participants working through this book are members of multidisciplinary or multiprofessional teams. We therefore often refer to 'your colleagues' or 'members of your team'. If you are in an isolated situation, you may find it helpful to refer to the members of your action learning (AL) set instead. Even if you are a member of a team, you will find it helpful to discuss issues raised by your work on this book with your AL set, as they will be able to view your situation from another perspective. We have also assumed that you will have contact with individuals and organisations that provide specialist palliative care.

WHAT'S IN THE BOOK?

This book has been prepared carefully. Each chapter includes most or all of the following features.

- An introduction to the topics covered in the chapter.
- Preparation – a section that lists the documents you need to obtain, or other preparatory tasks you need to perform before starting the chapter, or before starting a specific activity. Your facilitator can give you guidance on library resources, advice on getting articles, and on how to undertake a literature review. Your librarian may be able to show you how to perform online searches for relevant material.
- Learning outcomes – the skills or knowledge that you will gain or improve by working through the chapter.
- Several sections that contain information and advice on a particular topic.
- Activities – some will be questions that you can answer from your own experience, but some will ask you to search for information, talk to colleagues, discuss your ideas, plans, actions and their effects in your

AL set, or try out new skills and gain feedback from colleagues. Each activity is followed by a 'Feedback' section, which illustrates the kinds of information you may have found, experiences you may have had, or other situations that may have occurred while working though the activity. Some 'Feedback' sections give advice on how to take the activity further, or deal with any issues. When undertaking new activities within your practice as a lone practitioner, like, for example, using new assessment techniques or assessing symptoms you have never assessed before, you may find it helpful to enlist some extra support from your manager.

Note that some activities in the book ask you to interview patients. If it is likely that patients will be disturbed beyond what would be normally required for clinical management, you should seek approval from your organisation's ethics committee before starting such an activity. Discuss this with your manager if you are in any doubt.

- Examples, case studies and quotes – to help illustrate what you are learning.
- Useful websites – details of websites that contain useful and interesting information on topics covered in the chapter.
- Recommended sources of information – books and articles that contain useful insights on topics discussed in the chapter.
- References – full publication details of books and articles referred to in the text.

The chapters have been written in a straightforward, open learning style. They are designed to enable you to gain, improve and update your knowledge and skills, and to take on more responsibility for your own learning and development. This book includes the following chapters:

- **This Introduction** – designed to help you find your way round the book, become familiar with some of the terms that are used in the book, understand the ways in which you can work with others and start to plan your study. It also includes suggested further reading.
- **The *Facilitator Guide*** (available online at **www.reflectpress.co.uk/ book.asp?id = 26**) – designed to help your facilitator to find their way round the book, understand how they can help you by facilitating an AL set, working group or support/discussion group or as a critical companion in a one-to-one relationship with you. It also includes the glossary and an evaluation questionnaire.
- **Chapter 1 – Introduction to Palliative Care.** In Chapter 1 we provide an introduction to palliative care, including a brief history of the

hospice movement. We define what we mean by palliative care, introduce the concept of multidisciplinary palliative care teams, and consider the members of such teams. We also investigate the types of settings in which palliative care can be provided, and stress the importance of taking a holistic approach to palliative care.

- **Chapter 2 – Essential Concepts.** In Chapter 2 we introduce a variety of concepts that are essential to effective palliative care, including the importance of effective teamwork and effective communication. We consider a number of nursing models that may be used in palliative care, and various coping mechanisms that may be employed by patients and their families. We emphasise the importance of the ethical issues surrounding palliative care and introduce a model of reflective practice.

- **Chapter 3 – Generic Assessment in Palliative Care.** In Chapter 3 we stress the importance of a thorough and holistic assessment process, and identify factors that may hinder this process. We also emphasise the importance of patient involvement in assessment. We investigate the use of tools such as forms and questionnaires in performing a general (or screening) assessment.

- **Chapter 4 – Anxiety and Depression.** Chapter 4 is in two parts: Part 1 on Anxiety and Part 2 on Depression. In this chapter we explain what we mean by anxiety and depression, and identify likely causes, manifestations and predisposing factors. We review tools for performing focused assessments of anxiety or depression in patients receiving palliative care. We investigate the use of various pharmacological and non-pharmacological management strategies for anxiety and depression, focusing on the over-arching importance of improving the patient's quality of life.

- **Chapter 5 – Breathlessness.** In Chapter 5 we give a definition of breathlessness and investigate its causes and pathophysiology. We review the medical management of breathlessness and introduce an integrative model that emphasises the importance of considering the emotional impact of breathlessness. We consider the tools that are available for measuring breathlessness, and the nursing strategies that may be used to manage it with a view to improving the patient's quality of life.

- **Chapter 6 – Fatigue.** In Chapter 6 we define fatigue and investigate the impact of fatigue on the patient's quality of life. We review the symptoms of fatigue, cancer-related fatigue and anaemia-related fatigue, and investigate the causes of fatigue. We ask why there appear to be barriers between patients and health care professionals that prevent dialogue about fatigue, and look at how those barriers can be overcome. We also consider the assessment and management of fatigue.

- **Chapter 7 – Pain.** In Chapter 7 we define pain and introduce the concept of total pain. We review the prevalence of pain and investigate possible causes of pain. We consider the use of tools to assess pain and review a variety of strategies for managing pain, focusing primarily on a pharmacological approach and once again stressing that the overall aim of palliative care is to improve the patient's quality of life. Although parts of this chapter focus on cancer pain, most of it is also relevant to chronic non-cancer pain.

- **Chapter 8 – Quality Improvement.** In Chapter 8 we discuss the impact of clinical governance on palliative care. We investigate how the concepts of evidence-based practice and clinical audit can be applied to palliative care, and we guide you through the audit cycle, looking closely at setting standards.

Which chapters are useful to me?

The book can be worked through intensively as a whole over, say, six months or less intensively over a period of a year or so, according to your needs, responsibilities and priorities. Alternatively, it can be used in a modular way, where you 'dip in and out' of different areas as required. For example, you may want to start with pain management if you are reviewing your policies and practice in that area.

WHAT IS OPEN LEARNING?

Open learning is a method that is designed to be more flexible than other more traditional methods of learning. Instead of another individual providing you with a structure and process, you make decisions on:

- where you will do your learning;
- when you will do your learning;
- how you will do your learning;
- the order in which you work through the chapters in the book;
- which chapters you will undertake and the thoroughness you will adopt.

Open learning is self-managed and participant-centred. If you intend to use your employer's resources in any way, for example using the book in work-time, you will need to negotiate this with your manager.

WHAT IS ACTION LEARNING?

A continuous process of learning and reflection, supported by colleagues, with an intention of getting things done.

McGill and Beaty (2001: 11). Source: Neubauer, J. (2001) 'Action learning guide book' (draft), London: King's Fund Management College (unpublished work).

Action learning (AL) is an approach to individual and group development, traditionally used to develop managerial and organisational effectiveness. Over several months, people work in a small group (an action learning set) to tackle important organisational issues or problems and learn from their attempts to change things – in this case, to improve the practice of palliative care. Action learning comprises four elements.

- The person – everyone joins and takes part voluntarily.
- The problem – everyone brings and must 'own' a problem on which he or she wants to act. In this case, it would be an issue to do with the implementation of palliative care.
- The group or set – because we often need colleagues to help us tackle difficult problems. Action groups, or action learning sets as we call them here, meet to help each other think through the issues, create options, agree on action and learn from the effects of that action through providing a high level of challenge and support. Learning about how groups work is an added benefit. The colleagues in your set may be from your own organisation or from another organisation.
- The action and the learning – having analysed the problems, thought through the options and decided what to do, with the help of the set, individuals act to resolve their problems. They then evaluate the results of those actions and identify what further actions, if any, are necessary.

There is more about action learning and how action learning sets work in the *Facilitator Guide* that accompanies this book.

WHAT IS WORK-BASED LEARNING?

The following text is adapted from the discussion paper *Proposed framework for 'work-based learning' through collaborative partnerships* (McCormack and Manley, 2000). McCormack and Manley (2000) suggest that work-based learning is about:

- learning that is planned for the future;
- learning processes that are negotiated;
- learning processes that are an integral component of practice development and practitioner research frameworks;
- learning processes that are based in practice and supported by a variety of potential supervisory frameworks (for example, academic supervision, clinical supervision, mentorship, external facilitation, and appraisal);
- learning that can demonstrate personal and professional effectiveness;
- learning that demonstrates the development of practice and a commitment to career progression.

McCormack and Manley identify a large number of benefits of work-based learning to nursing staff, service users and service providers. You are likely to benefit, for example, from the fact that the approach focuses on everyday practice and enables you to engage in learning appropriate for your level of ability, your practice context and your individual goals. You may also find it helpful that work-based learning may provide a means of achieving academic credit for learning in practice, and may therefore provide an access route into further academic development, if that is what you are seeking.

WHAT IS CRITICAL COMPANIONSHIP?

> Critical companionship . . . is a metaphor for a helping relationship, in which the critical companion accompanies less experienced practitioners on their own, very personal, experiential learning journeys.
>
> (Titchen, 1998)

Critical companionship is particularly geared to helping participants, in a one-to-one relationship, to acquire professional craft knowledge or practical know-how of palliative care. Critical companions can be sought either inside or outside your clinical area.

If you choose this kind of support for your journey through this book, your critical companion helps you to develop the knowledge and skills of palliative care by engaging in some of the activities with you, observing you and asking you questions, giving you feedback, challenging and supporting you and helping you to develop a rationale for what you are doing. We make suggestions shortly about who your critical companion could be.

WHAT IS REFLECTIVE PRACTICE?

The definition of reflective practice as defined by Johns (1996) underpins this programme:

> A window for practitioners to look inside and know who they are as they strive towards understanding and realising the meaning of desirable work in their everyday practices. The practitioner must expose, confront and understand the contradictions within their practice between what is practised and what is desirable. It is the conflict of contradiction and the commitment to achieve desirable work that enables the practitioner to become empowered to take action to appropriately resolve these contradictions.
>
> (Johns, 1996)

To articulate this philosophy, components of the programme include, for example, the recording of significant experiences, the use of a model of structured reflection and the maintenance of a learning/reflective diary. Reflection is used throughout the book as a means of exploring approaches to palliative care and reflecting on the effectiveness of the participant's skills.

Keeping a learning/reflective diary

Your learning diary is somewhere for you to record incidents from practice. When you look back on an incident, you can write about:

- what happened;
- how you felt and how you thought others felt;
- what was good/bad about the incident;
- why you think it happened;
- why it went so well/badly;
- what you could have done to improve the situation;
- what you would do if a similar situation arose again.

In this way you can create new learning from practice.

Why should I keep a learning/reflective diary?

Keeping a learning diary is useful because it helps you to:

- recall events and the sequence in which they occurred;
- think about and perhaps question parts of practice which you usually take for granted;

- frame problems and identify possible solutions;
- tap your unconscious and make things which are usually hidden explicit;
- form a detailed account of your progress over time;
- evaluate your own learning;
- view your experiences within broader social, political, economic and health care contexts.

It will also assist you with theorising and reflecting, and in your personal development as a practitioner whatever your area of expertise or practice. It acts as an archive of your practice experiences and serves as a base for informing and developing your practice.

Getting started

First of all, a learning diary need not be a formal type of diary with days and dates in it. You could make an audiotape or videotape, or you could include paintings or poetry. If you decide to keep a written diary, don't be concerned if you find it difficult to get started. You will probably find that you have to write about several incidents before your personal style begins to emerge and you feel comfortable with the process.

Remember that you need to get started and 'have a go' before you can develop your own style. Don't be afraid of getting it wrong – there is no right way to keep a learning diary. Find the way that is right for you. Share your thoughts with your critical companion. You don't have to show them your diary, but you can discuss issues that it raises for you. Keeping a learning diary can be an extremely useful part of the learning process.

CAN I GET ACADEMIC CREDIT?

You may be able to gain academic credit for your work through the nationally-recognised Credit Accumulation and Transfer Scheme (CATS). These credits are available at a number of levels:

Level 1	Certificate level
Level 2	Diploma level
Level 3	Degree level
Level 4	Masters level.

Levels 1–4 are equivalent to Scottish Credit and Qualifications Framework (SCQF) Levels 7 (Certificate), 8 (Diploma) 9 and 10 (Ordinary and Honours Degree) and 11 (Masters).

This book can be studied from Level 2 to Level 4. If you are interested in gaining accreditation, we suggest that you contact a local higher education institution or university that delivers educational programmes for nurses and health care professionals. The institution may already have accredited this book, according to local criteria, or may be interested in doing so if your organisation enters into accreditation discussions with them. If not, then most institutions have a well-documented Accreditation of Prior Learning (APL) mechanism, and all higher education institutions offering nursing programmes are required to provide an APL mechanism for practitioners. We suggest that you explore this idea when you start making enquiries about getting your work accredited. As a rough guide to assessing the number of CATS points you could obtain, formal educational courses that award 20 CATS points suggest 200 hours of nominal study activity, while those that award 40 points expect around 400 hours of study. Below, we offer ways of demonstrating learning at the different levels. These could be discussed when you contact your local institution. You should be aware, however, that collected credits cannot automatically be traded in for a diploma or a degree without any consideration of any compulsory units or pathways that may have been determined by the institution.

If you do not wish to undertake assessments that would be required for academic accreditation, you may be interested in obtaining Royal College of Nursing Continuing Education Points (CEPs). These would be offered to participants who can demonstrate completion of the chapters. These points could be included in your portfolio to demonstrate your personal and professional growth. This would help you to meet the Nursing and Midwifery Council requirements for renewing your registration (see Nursing and Midwifery Council, 2006). However, you may decide that undertaking the whole book would be too much work for only receiving CEPs or maintaining registration. Perhaps this route is only appropriate if you undertake only one chapter. If you do more than one chapter, then CATS/APL routes are more appropriate. Even if you didn't want to apply for CEPs, the work you undertake on this programme could be included in your portfolio if evidence of reflection on the learning that has taken place is provided.

Suggested ways of demonstrating personal and professional growth

If you decide to take a non-academic route, but want to use your work in your portfolio development or to apply for RCN CEPs, you might choose to include:

- essays;
- case studies;
- care plans;
- critical, reflective and evaluative accounts of the activities you pursue in the book;
- a demonstration of your personal and professional growth;
- a Practice Profile.

You could include a reference from your manager stating your progress in the management of patients and their carers when undertaking palliative care.

You may also wish to record the amount of time it has taken you to complete each chapter in a table like that below.

	Hours of work
Chapter 1	
Chapter 2	
Chapter 3	
Chapter 4	
Chapter 5	
Chapter 6	
Chapter 7	
Chapter 8	
Total	

If you are not seeking academic accreditation, the length of time the book will take you will depend on your learning needs, the level of thoroughness you want to pursue or the time you have available. For example, if you are new to palliative care then you may decide to do Chapters 1 and 2 thoroughly including all the activities. This might take you some time as it is unlikely that you would want to move onto Chapters 3–8 until you have had an opportunity to develop and practise what you have learned in Chapters 1 and 2. However, if you are already experienced in palliative care, you may want to focus on a specific symptom, such as pain, so you would use Chapters 1 and 2 to refresh and consolidate your knowledge and skills, and do activities that help you to develop palliative care in your own clinical practice, before you moved on to Chapters 3–8.

WORKING WITH OTHERS

If you are working in an action learning set, you may be able to do many of the activities together. If you are working together like this, trust and confidentiality within the set are essential because it is likely that sensitive issues will be shared. One way of working together as a set through the book would be to work on each activity individually, and then to discuss your ideas before going on to look at the suggested answers or feedback. Another way might be to examine the reflective and learning processes that are going on in your set as you undertake the activities or critique and debate issues.

If you aren't working in an action learning set, it may still be possible for you to get practice at discussing and explaining. You can do this by setting up either a support/discussion group or working group with others who are using this book (see the *Facilitator Guide* for suggestions on how such groups could work), or by choosing a critical companion. A critical companion can be:

- a colleague at work;
- a practice development nurse;
- a practitioner with experience of/in palliative care.

A critical companion is someone who can:

- help you along the way;
- discuss the material with you;
- comment on your ideas;
- help you to evaluate yourself critically and acquire new knowledge about yourself and palliative care;
- give you constructive feedback;
- generally help make your studies come alive.

If you are setting up an action learning set/group and have found a facilitator or critical companion, we recommend that you suggest that they read through the *Facilitator Guide* to help them prepare for their role.

PLANNING YOUR STUDY

You will need to plan your study before you begin work on this book. Chapter 3 in Northedge (1990) and Chapter 5 in Rowntree (1991) (see the list of Further Reading, Study Skills, at the end of this Introduction for these references) suggest you can approach this by:

- arranging a place to study and getting together all the resources and equipment you need;
- planning your times for study and sticking to them;
- keeping a learning diary.

By planning out your work you will have regular targets to aim for and a sense of achievement as you reach them. It is also vital that you set your targets for completion. We'll look at this next.

Setting targets for completion

Your target date for completing the course will depend on:

- the date on which you intend to start the book;
- the number of hours you intend to do per week.

The whole book should take you around 200–300 hours to work through, depending on how many of the activities you undertake. So, if you intend to spend, say, seven hours a week, it should take you around 28–43 weeks to complete it. This is roughly equivalent to one academic year's learning. Make a note of your intended completion date. Alternatively, if you have a date by which you must complete the book, you can work out how many hours a week you must do to complete it in good time.

WHERE ARE WE STARTING FROM? CLARIFYING VALUES

Behaviour is greatly influenced by our beliefs and values. One of the underpinning aims of this book is to enable you to make your beliefs and values about your practice explicit. This will help you work as a member of a palliative care team and as a member of your action learning set. Clearly expressed values that are shared by your work colleagues and other action learning set members will help you to work together more effectively.

Below there is a values clarification exercise to help you identify your values and beliefs about palliative care. We suggest that you do this now and discuss it with your critical companion or action learning set/group when you have completed it. Compare similarities and differences between your values and beliefs and theirs. If there are major differences, discuss the reasons for them and ways in which you think that you will be able to work together effectively, despite your differences – or perhaps because of them. Keep in mind, though, that your own values and beliefs about palliative care may change as a result of your work on this book. Doing this exercise now gives you a recorded baseline, so that you can see where you are starting from. Make a note of the date you answered these questions. We suggest that you review and revisit the exercise as you work through this book, for comparison.

Values clarification exercise

Makes notes in response to the following statements:

1 I believe palliative care is:
2 I believe the purpose of palliative care in my ward, unit, community area or directorate is:
3 I believe effective palliative care can be achieved by:
4 I believe barriers to establishing effective palliative care are:
5 The things that I believe make palliative care a good idea are:
6 Other values and beliefs I hold about palliative care are:

(Adapted from Warfield and Manley, 1990)

ACTION PLANNING

This plan is different from the study plan that you have already considered. This plan is designed to help you carry out any action plans that you develop as you progress through this textbook. What follows is a template that you can use to record:

- your objective (for example, to understand and explore the patient's experience, to develop strategies/expertise to assess, implement and evaluate palliative care, to access, critique and use appropriately the evidence base for care, to further develop reflective skills within the context of lifelong learning);
- the timescale that you have to work to;
- the resources that are available to you;
- any support that you might need;
- a force-field analysis of your situation;

- a chart of the tasks that need to be performed to enable you to reach your objective;
- a list of the evaluation methods you will use to work out whether you have achieved your objective.

You will decide when you are ready to start action planning, but we will remind you in the chapters about starting and about reviewing and revising your plans.

You will need to have two copies of your completed template – one for use with your action learning set/group or critical companion, and one for use with your work colleagues, i.e. colleagues who are not participating in this book, but with whom you are working to improve the practice of palliative care.

If you are in a working group of colleagues (i.e. colleagues who are also participating in this book – see the *Facilitator Guide*), you will need to discuss with the other members how a balance is to be achieved between individual action planning and shared/jointly-owned action planning. If your group is doing this as part of a strategy development/review, you must link into the appropriate committee meetings or other groups within your organisation. This is a simple courtesy that may result in more support for your studies and activities. Your action planning may need to take account of organisational timescales and deadlines. If you will be using your employer's resources at all, such as, for example, work-time, you must clearly identify the benefits of your plan to the organisation.

Action plan

Date: _____

Objective: What do I/we need to achieve?

```
┌────────────────────────────────────────────────────────────┐
│                                                            │
│                                                            │
│                                                            │
│                                                            │
│                                                            │
└────────────────────────────────────────────────────────────┘
```

Timescale: When do I/we need to have achieved the objective?

```
┌────────────────────────────────────────────────────────────┐
│  Insert date:                                              │
│                                                            │
└────────────────────────────────────────────────────────────┘
```

Resources: What resources do I/we need to have available to achieve my/our objective? (Consider any resources that are already available to you.)

```
┌─────────────────────────────────────────────────────┐
│                                                     │
│                                                     │
│                                                     │
│                                                     │
│                                                     │
└─────────────────────────────────────────────────────┘
```

Support available: What support do I/we need to achieve my/our objective? (Consider any sources of support already available to you.)

```
┌─────────────────────────────────────────────────────┐
│                                                     │
│                                                     │
│                                                     │
│                                                     │
└─────────────────────────────────────────────────────┘
```

Force-field analysis: What factors may help or hinder the achievement of my/our objective?

1. Identify your desired outcome (your objective).
2. Group members identify factors that may help you to achieve your objective (driving forces).
3. Group members identify factors that may hinder you in achieving your objective (restraining forces).
4. Each member considers each force and gives it a value (for example, 0=not relevant/no force; 1=low force, 2=medium force, 3=high force).
5. Add up the score for each factor.
6. Factors with the most points need to receive the most attention.
7. Plan how to overcome the restraining forces and harness the driving forces to achieve your objective.

```
┌─────────────────────────────────────────────────────┐
│  Desired outcome                                    │
│                                                     │
│                                                     │
│                                                     │
└─────────────────────────────────────────────────────┘
```

Driving forces	Restraining forces

Chart: What tasks do I/we need to undertake to achieve my/our objective?

Task				
Start time				
Finish time				
Person responsible				
Person(s) providing support				

What methods will I/we use to evaluate the achievement of the objective? Who will validate this?

```



```

Date action plan agreed

```
Insert date:
```

Participants' signatures: _____

_____

_____

REFERENCES

Johns, C. (1996) 'Visualizing and realizing caring in practice through guided reflection'. *Journal of Advanced Nursing*, 24(6), pp.1135–43.

McCormack, B. and Manley, K. (2000) 'Proposed framework for "work-based learning" through collaborative partnerships' (unpublished work). Contact Kim Manley, Head of Practice Development at the RCN Institute, for details.

McGill, I. and Beaty, L. (2001) 'Action learning' (revised 2nd Ed.). London: Kogan Page.

Neubauer, J. (2001) *Action learning guide book* (draft). London: King's Fund Management College (unpublished work).

Nursing and Midwifery Council (2006) PREP handbook. London: NMC. Go to: **www.nmc-uk.org** and search for 'PREP handbook' – the NMC document search will indicate which is the latest version. Site accessed 13/5/08.

Scrivens, E. (1995) *Accreditation: protecting the professional or the consumer?* Buckingham: Open University Press.

Titchen, A. (1998) *A conceptual framework for facilitating learning in clinical practice*. Oxford: Royal College of Nursing/Centre for Professional Education Advancement.

Warfield, C. and Manley, K. (1990) 'Developing a new philosophy in the NDU'. *Nursing Standard*, 4(41), 4 July, pp.27–30.

USEFUL WEBSITES

www.cancerworld.org
Cancerworld – the online world of oncology. Site accessed 13/5/08.

www.cancerhelp.org.uk
CancerHelp UK is a free information service about cancer and cancer care for the general public, provided by Cancer Research UK. Site accessed 13/5/08.

www.crc.org.uk
Website of Cancer Research UK. Site accessed 13/5/08.

www.ejpc.eu.com
The *European Journal of Palliative Care* is the official journal of the European Association for Palliative Care (EAPC). Site accessed 13/5/08.

www.helpthehospices.org.uk
Help the Hospices is the national charity in the UK for the hospice movement. Site accessed 13/5/08.

www.ijpn.co.uk
The *International Journal of Palliative Nursing* is a world-renowned palliative care journal. Site accessed 13/5/08.

www.sagepub.co.uk/journalsProdDesc.nav?prodId = Journal201823
Palliative Medicine – the multiprofessional journal of the EAPC. Site accessed 13/5/08.

www.library.nhs.uk
The National Library for Health has a palliative and supportive care specialist library, accessible to all professionals. Site accessed 13/5/08.

www.ncpc.org.uk
The National Council for Palliative Care is an independent umbrella body dedicated to keeping you up to date on all areas of palliative care. Site accessed 13/5/08.

www.oncolink.upenn.edu
Oncolink – the link to University of Pennsylvania cancer centre with information for patients and health professionals. Site accessed 13/5/08.

www.pallcare.info
Palliative Care Matters is a website intended for health care professionals working in palliative care or related fields. Site accessed 13/5/08.

www.palliativecarescotland.org.uk
The Scottish Partnership for Palliative Care is the national umbrella and representative body for palliative care in Scotland. It is an independent body with charitable status which was set up in 1991 to promote the

extension and improvement of palliative care services throughout Scotland. Site accessed 13/5/08.

www.palliativedrugs.com
Provides 'essential, comprehensive and independent information for health professionals about the use of drugs in palliative care'. Site accessed 13/5/08.

www.elib.scot.nhs.uk/portal/elib/pages/index.aspx
The library is available to Scottish professionals through a free password system. Site accessed 13/5/08.

www.stoppain.org
Department of Pain Medicine and Palliative Care at Beth Israel Medical Centre. Site accessed 13/5/08.

FURTHER READING

The readings in this section are set out in the following categories:

- action learning;
- reflective practice;
- study skills.

Titles followed by O/P are out of print – but you may be able to find library copies.

Action learning

Carr, W. and Kemmis, S. (1986) *Becoming critical: education, knowledge and action research*. London: Falmer.

Kolb, D.A. (1984) *Experiential learning: experience as the source of learning and development*. Englewood Cliffs: Prentice-Hall. O/P

Pedler, M. (1997) *Action learning in practice* (3rd Ed.). Aldershot: Gower.

Associated with action learning

Gagne, R.M. (1985) *The conditions of learning and theory of instruction* (4th Ed.). New York: Holt, Rinehart and Winston. O/P

Jarvis, P. (1987) *Adult learning in the social context*. London: Croom Helm. O/P

Knowles, M., Holton, E. and Swanson, R. (2005) *The adult learner* (6th Ed.). Amsterdam: Elsevier.

Lovell, R.B. (1987) *Adult learning*. London: Routledge. O/P

Reflective practice

Andrew, M.E. (1996) 'Reflection as infiltration: learning in the experiential domain'. *Journal of Advanced Nursing*, 24(2), pp.391–9.

Atkins, S. and Murphy, K. (1995) 'Reflective practice'. *Nursing Standard*, 9(45), 2 August, pp.31–7.

Bailey, J. (1995) 'Reflective practice: implementing theory'. *Nursing Standard*, 9(46), 9 August, pp.29–31.

Bowles, N. (1995) 'Story telling: a search for meaning within nursing practice'. *Nurse Education Today*, 15(5), pp.365–9.

Bradshaw, A. (1994) 'Critical care'. *Nursing Times*, 90(40), 5 October, pp.28–31.

Burrows, D.E. (1995) 'The nurse teacher's role in the promotion of reflective practice'. *Nurse Education Today*, 15(5), pp.346–50.

Clarke, B., James, C. and Kelly, J. (1995) 'Reflective practice: reviewing the issues and refocusing the debate'. *International Journal of Nursing Studies*, 33(2), pp.171–80.

Dewing, J. (1990) 'Reflective practice'. *Senior Nurse*, 10(10), pp.26–8.

Durgahee, T. (1996) 'Promoting reflection in post-graduate nursing: a theoretical model'. *Nurse Education Today*, 16(6), pp.419–26.

Edwards, M. (1996) 'Patient-nurse relationships: using reflective practice'. *Nursing Standard*, 10(25), 13 March, pp.40–3.

Greenwood, J. (1993) 'Reflective practice: a critique of the work of Argyris and Schön'. *Journal of Advanced Nursing*, 18(8), pp.1183–7.

Hargreaves, J. (1997) 'Using patients: exploring the ethical dimension of reflective practice in nurse education'. *Journal of Advanced Nursing*, 25(2), pp.223–8.

Jarvis, P. (1992) 'Reflective practice and nursing'. *Nurse Education Today*, 12(3), pp.174–81.

Johns, C. (1991) 'The Burford Nursing Development Unit holistic model of nursing practice'. *Journal of Advanced Nursing*, 16(9), pp.1090–8.

Johns, C. (1996) 'The benefits of a reflective model of nursing'. *Nursing Times*, 92(27), 3 July, pp.39–41.

Lauder, W. (1994) 'Beyond reflection: practical wisdom and the practical syllogism'. *Nurse Education Today*, 14(2), pp.91–8.

Lumby, J. (1991) *Nursing: reflecting on an evolving practice*. Geelong: Deakin University Press. O/P

Marks-Maran, D. and Rose, P. (1997) *Reconstructing nursing: beyond art and science*. London: Baillière Tindall/RCN.

Morgan, S. (1996) 'Gods, daemons and banshees on the journey to the magic scroll: the use of myth as a framework for reflective practice in nurse education'. *Nurse Education Today*, 16(2), pp.144–8.

Newell, R. (1992) 'Anxiety, accuracy and reflection: the limits of professional development'. *Journal of Advanced Nursing*, 17(11), pp.1326–33.

Reid, B. (1993) ' "But we're doing it already!" Exploring a response to the concept of Reflective Practice in order to improve its facilitation'. *Nurse Education Today*, 13(4), pp.305–9.

Rich, A. and Parker, D.L. (1995) 'Reflection and critical incident analysis: ethical and moral implications of their use within nursing and midwifery education'. *Journal of Advanced Nursing*, 22(6), pp.1050–7.

Richardson, R. (1995) 'Humpty Dumpty: reflection and reflective nursing practice'. *Journal of Advanced Nursing*, 21(6), pp.1044–50.

Rolfe, G. (1994) 'Towards a new model of nursing research'. *Journal of Advanced Nursing*, 19(5), pp.969–75.

Wakefield, A. (2000) 'Nurses' responses to death and dying: a need for relentless self-care'. *International Journal of Palliative Nursing*, 6(5), pp.245–51.

Study skills

Britton, A. and Cousins, A. (1998) *Study skills: a guide for lifelong learners* (revised edition). London: Distance Learning Centre, South Bank University. O/P

Buzan, T. (2000) *Use your head* (revised edition). London: BBC Books.

Fairbairn, G.J. and Winch, C. (1996) *Reading, writing and reasoning: a guide for students* (2nd Ed.). Buckingham: Open University Press.

Marshall, L. and Rowland, F. (1998) *A guide to learning independently* (3rd Ed.). Buckingham: Open University Press. O/P

Mayon-White, B. (2007) *Study skills for managers* (2nd Ed.). Thousand Oaks: Sage.

Northedge, A. (2005) *The good study guide* (2nd Ed.). Milton Keynes: Open University Press.

Rowntree, D. (1991) *Teach yourself with open learning*. London: Kogan Page.

Rowntree, D. (1998) *Learn how to study: a realistic approach* (4th Ed.). London: Warner Books. O/P

RECOMMENDED SOURCES OF INFORMATION AND SUPPORT

Bereavement

CRUSE – Bereavement Care, 126 Sheen Road, Richmond TW9 1UR
Helpline: 0870 167 1677 (Mon–Fri, 9.30am–5pm) Scotland: 0131 229 6275
www.crusebereavementcare.org.uk Site accessed 13/5/08.

Cancer

CancerBACUP, 3 Bath Place, Rivington Street, London EC2A 3JR
Tel: 020 7696 9003 Fax: 020 7696 9002
www.cancerbackup.org.uk Site accessed 13/5/08.

Cancer Care Society, 11 The Cornmarket, Romsey, Hants. SO51 8GB
Tel: 01794 830300
www.cancercaresociety.org Site accessed 2/4/08

Irish Cancer Society, 43–45 Northumberland Road, Dublin 4, Ireland.
Tel: 01 2310 500 (International +353-1-2310500) Fax: 01 668 7599
   Helpline 1 800 200 700
www.cancer.ie Site accessed 13/5/08.

Macmillan Cancer Support, 89 Albert Embankment, London SE1 7UQ
Information line: 0808 808 2020
www.macmillan.org.uk Site accessed 13/5/08.

Marie Curie Cancer Centre, 89 Albert Embankment, London SE1 7TP
Tel: 020 7599 7777 Fax: 020 7599 7708
Scotland: 0131 456 3700 Wales: 01873 30 3000 Northern Ireland: 026
   9088 2060
www.mariecurie.org.uk Site accessed 13/5/08.

Non-cancer

Motor Neurone Disease Association, PO Box 246, Northampton, NN1
   2PR
Tel: 01604 250505 Fax: 01604 624726/638289
www.mndassociation.org Site accessed 13/5/08.

Scottish Motor Neurone Disease Association, 76 Firhill Road, Glasgow
   G20 7BA
Tel: 0141 945 1077 Fax: 0141 945 2578
www.scotmnd.org.uk Site accessed 13/5/08.

Heart Failure: British Heart Foundation, 14 Fitzhardinge Street, London
   W1H 6DH
Tel: 020 7935 0185 Heart Information Line: 08450 70 80 70
www.bhf.org.uk Site accessed 13/5/08.

Dementia: Alzheimer's Society, Gordon House, 10 Greencoat Place,
   London SW1P 1PH
Tel: 020 7306 0606 Fax 020 7306 0808
www.alzheimers.org.uk Site accessed 13/5/08.

COPD: The British Thoracic Society COPD Consortium, The British
   Thoracic Society, 17 Doughty Street, London WC1N 2PL
Tel: 020 7831 8778 Fax: 020 7831 8766
www.brit-thoracic.org.uk/ClinicalInformation/COPD/COPDConsor
   tiumPublications/tabid/165/Default.aspx Site accessed 13/5/08.

Stroke: The Stroke Association, Stroke Information Service, The Stroke Association, 240 City Road, London EC1V 2PR
Stroke helpline 0845 3033 100 (open Monday to Friday, 9am to 5pm)
www.stroke.org.uk/ Site accessed 13/5/08.

Carers

Carers UK, Head Office, 20–25 Glasshouse Yard, London EC1A 4JT
Tel: 020 7490 8818 Fax: 020 7490 8824 Scotland: 0141 221 9141
Wales: 029 2081 1370 Northern Ireland: 028 9043 9843
Freephone Carers' Line: 0808 808 7777 (Wed–Thurs 10am–12 noon, 2pm–4pm)
www.carersuk.org Site accessed 13/5/08.

CROSSROADS, Head Office, 10 Regent Place, Rugby, Warwickshire.
Tel: 0845 450350
www.crossroads.org.uk Site accessed 13/5/08.

Complementary therapies

British Complementary Medicine Association, PO Box 5122, Bourne-mouth BH8 0WG
Tel: 0845 345 5977 Fax: 0845 345 9978
www.bcma.co.uk Site accessed 13/5/08.
Encourages communication between existing organisations to establish codes of conduct and ethics.

The Prince's Foundation for Integrated Health, 33–41 Dallington Street, London EC1V 0BB
Tel: 020 3119 3100 Fax: 020 3119 3101
Has produced guidelines for the use of complementary therapies in palliative and supportive care.
www.fih.org.uk Site accessed 13/5/08.

Institute for Complementary and Natural Medicine, PO Box 194, London SE16 7QZ
Tel: 020 7237 5165
Provides information and maintains a register of practitioners.
www.i-c-m.org.uk Site accessed 13/5/08.

Research Council for Complementary Medicine, c/o 1 Harley Street, London W1G 9QD
www.rccm.org.uk Site accessed 13/5/08.

Hospices

Hospice Information Service, St Christopher's Hospice, 51–59 Lawrie Park Road, Sydenham, London SE26 6DZ

Tel: 0870 903 3 903 (calls charged at national call rates) or 020 7520 8232 between 9am and 5pm, Monday to Friday.
www.hospiceinformation.info Site accessed 13/5/08.

Help the Hospices, Hospice House, 34–44 Britannia Street, London WC1X 9JG
Phone and website details as above.

Chapter 1

Introduction to Palliative Care

Norrie Sutherland and Elaine Stevens

INTRODUCTION

A large number of patients with life-threatening illness are cared for in general hospitals, care homes, psychiatric units and in the community setting, and the nurse is often the carer who spends the most time with them. Nurses' knowledge of palliative care – the way in which they define it and the actions they take based on that knowledge – directly affect the quality of care they provide for the patient and the quality of the patient's life.

Nurses' attitudes also affect the care they provide, and the relationships they are able to develop with patients. It makes a considerable difference if you view someone as 'a living patient with a limited future' rather than as 'a dying patient'. In the latter case, nurses often focus on providing 'a peaceful death', rather than 'providing joy in living and setting realistic goals', which can only really be considered in the former case (Holmes *et al.*, 1997).

We have assumed that all participants working through this book are members of multidisciplinary or multiprofessional teams. We therefore often refer to 'your colleagues' or 'members of your team'. If you are in an isolated situation, you may find it helpful to refer to the members of your action learning (AL) set instead. Even if you are a member of a team, you will find it helpful to discuss issues raised by your work on this book with your AL set, as they will be able to view your situation from another perspective. We have also assumed that you will have contact with individuals and organisations that provide specialist palliative care.

If you have not already done so, we recommend that you read the Introduction to this textbook before you start work on this chapter. It contains lots of useful information, including details of how to plan your study, what we mean by action learning, and how to keep a learning (or reflective) diary. You don't need to read all of it in detail, but you should at least skim through it so that you know what sorts of topics it covers. You will then be able to find them when you need them.

In this chapter we will briefly review the history of palliative care and then look in more depth at what we mean by palliative care. We will investigate the general concept of palliative care teams, the individuals and professions that may make up those teams, and the many different settings in which palliative care may take place.

This book focuses on a holistic approach to palliative care, considering all aspects of the patient's life, including their family and/or carers. Holistic care also involves considering the patient's quality of life, and this will be different for each patient. In this book we use the term 'family' to mean those people who are important to the patient. This may include a patient's friends and carers, even if they are not related to the patient, if that is the patient's wish.

LEARNING OUTCOMES

When you have completed this chapter, you will be able to:
- briefly outline the history of palliative care;
- describe what is meant by palliative care;
- list the professions involved in delivering palliative care in your area;
- identify the members of the specialist palliative care team in your area;
- identify the types of setting in which palliative care may be delivered;
- explain the importance of holistic palliative care, with reference to a theory of unpleasant symptoms;
- explain why and how palliative care should involve caring for the patient's family and/or carers.

Preparation

In Activity 8, we ask you to talk to some patients about your care setting. Before you do this, discuss it with your manager and colleagues so that they are aware of what you are doing and why. If it is likely that patients will be disturbed beyond what would be normally required for clinical management, you should seek approval from your organisation's ethics committee before starting this activity.

THE HISTORY OF PALLIATIVE CARE

The history of palliative care begins in the first few centuries AD, with Christian institutions that welcomed ill and dying pilgrims. Hospices developed along pilgrim routes throughout the Middle Ages, caring for the sick and giving them friendship and food. In Britain, this came to an abrupt end with the Reformation (1531) when Henry VIII broke with the Church of Rome. The sick and dying were thrown out on the streets, and had to beg to survive. London organised the first system for poor relief through four institutions – Christ's Hospital for children (1552), St Bartholomew's and St Thomas Hospitals for the sick and Bridewell for the able-bodied destitute (1553). Other cities developed their own local schemes.

The early hospice movement arose in the nineteenth century. Hospice philosophy was based on philanthropy, religion and the care of the poor. In France, Jeanne Garnier founded an association of widows, Les Dames du Calvaire, which opened a hospice in Lyons in 1842. In 1879 Mary Aikenhead's order, The Irish Sisters of Charity, founded Our Lady's Hospice for the Dying in Dublin, Ireland.

In England the early hospices were located in London, as was the world's first modern hospice, St Christopher's at Sydenham, which opened in 1967. St Christopher's owes its existence almost entirely to the determination of Dame Cicely Saunders. She had trained as a nurse, studied philosophy and economics at Oxford and been employed as an almoner (medical social worker), before becoming the first modern doctor to dedicate her entire career to caring for those at the end of life with a diagnosis of cancer, because the treatment of pain and other symptoms was so poor.

St Christopher's and Dame Cicely Saunders proved to be an inspiration. Hospices opened in Manchester, Sheffield, Worthing and elsewhere. By the mid-1970s major cancer charities and the National Health Service (NHS) were taking a strong interest. A hospice movement had come into being which attracted the support of the wider public, of patients and families and of a growing number of volunteers and professionals who would dedicate themselves to its work.

Much of the information given above came from **www.helpthe hospices.org.uk/movement.html**. This webpage is no longer available, but if you are interested in the history of the hospice movement, you can find more information in Doyle *et al.*, 2004, in the foreword by Dame Cicely Saunders.

The form of care provided in hospices became known as palliative care, derived from the Latin word *pallum*, a cloak. It does not try to deal with the cause of the patient's illness, but rather it attempts only to relieve the symptoms. (This is a narrow definition of palliative care, and we will be looking at its meaning in more detail in the next section: 'What is palliative care?') In this book we will be considering the following symptoms:

- anxiety and depression (Chapter 4)
- breathlessness (Chapter 5)
- fatigue (Chapter 6)
- pain (Chapter 7).

As most health care professionals' practice involves some aspects of palliative care (sometimes called the palliative care approach), the phrase 'specialist palliative care' is often used to identify situations in which palliative care is a professional or organisation's prime focus, and where the senior medical and nursing staff have qualifications in aspects of managing palliative care patients.

Palliative care developed outside the mainstream of health care, and this has its drawbacks:

> The growth of specialist palliative care services has been mostly unplanned and uncoordinated by health authorities. Development has been largely in response to local pressure, enthusiasm and fund-raising activity, and remained mostly within the charitable, independent sector. Some development, mostly within the hospital setting, has been prompted by and within the NHS. This has led to a wide variety in models of service provision, distribution and funding across the country, with some areas, and therefore patients, being better served than others.
>
> Faull (1998: 2)

Activity 1: The history of palliative care

Investigate the history of a local hospice, or other provider of palliative care or specialist palliative care, with which your ward or clinical area has contact. Your manager, colleagues and members of your AL set may be able to help if you are not sure about local provision of palliative care.

Find out when the hospice (or other provider) was set up and why. Find out what sorts of patients are catered for. Brochures and other advertising leaflets are good sources of this sort of information, and many organisations have their own websites.

Find out what forms of contact exist between your clinical area and the provider of palliative care you are investigating. Find out if there is a contact person who would be willing to talk to you about the work done in their care setting, and arrange an appointment.

Discuss the history and purpose of their organisation with them – for example, was the organisation created initially as a specialist cancer care organisation? Ask them about staff numbers and responsibilities.

Find out how patients and professionals can access the services offered by the institution, and what barriers to access may exist.

Make brief notes on your conversation, and keep them with this book. You may like to keep your notes in your learning diary.

Feedback

This activity should have provided much useful information. You probably created or renewed a link with a specialist palliative care provider. This will help when you need to refer people on or, for example, if you need to provide information to a patient who may be reluctant to go into a hospice. You may have found that the organisation was initially created to care for patients with cancer, and then diversified to care for patients requiring palliative care for other reasons. This links back to Dame Cicely Saunders and the foundation of St Christopher's. If you search for books, articles and websites about palliative care, you will find that cancer care has had an enormous influence on the delivery, expectations and literature within palliative care.

If you would like further information about the work of the hospice movement, contact the Hospice Information Service:
The Hospice Information Service at St Christopher's Hospice,
51–59 Lawrie Park Road,
London
SE26 6DZ
Tel: +(44) (0)870 903 3 903
email: info@hospiceinformation.info
website: www.hospiceinformation.info/ (Site accessed 30/6/08)

As we mentioned earlier, St Christopher's, the world's first modern hospice, owes its existence almost entirely to the determination of Dame Cicely Saunders. In 1948, Dame Cicely Saunders was the social worker for David Tasma, a man who was dying of cancer. Through their many discussions, she came to believe that the care provided for the dying was wholly inadequate. After his death, she worked in a home for the dying, later qualifying as a nurse. She then undertook her medical education, becoming a researcher, after which she became the first doctor to specialise in terminal care. Many years after Tasma's death she used a bequest he had left her to start the trust for St Christopher's. Having spent some 40 years dedicated to the care of the terminally ill, Dame Cicely Saunders died in July 2005 in the hospice she created.

Activity 2: Your own personal history of palliative care

Why are you interested in palliative care? Make brief notes on how you became interested in palliative care, giving descriptions of incidents that made you feel that palliative care is important. If you want to write longer notes use separate sheets of paper, but keep them with this book or keep your notes in your learning diary.

Feedback

A probable answer is that, in your experience, you feel that not enough is being done for those who are dying to relieve their pain and suffering. Furthermore, palliative care offers you an opportunity to practise holistically. You may feel you have the potential to make a real difference to patients' quality of life, and working so closely/intimately with patients and their families can be very fulfilling.

Here are explanations of why some of the authors of this book became interested in palliative care.

I felt that in acute medicine there wasn't enough time for those who were not 'curable'. Doctors were embarrassed by their failure to cure, and at not being able to offer anything else. In community health there was isolation, and in mental health the staff had neither the knowledge nor the expertise to cope with physical illness.

Co-ordinator, palliative day care

I became interested in palliative care during my nurse training. When I was newly qualified, there was an incident involving a terminally ill patient that has stayed with me ever since. The emphasis appeared to be on saving life regardless of its futility, or its effect on the patient and the family. I decided then that I had to do something about this to improve the quality of life for patients and their families.

Nurse Specialist/Training Officer in Palliative Care

I was concerned about the way that seriously ill and dying patients were largely ignored in general wards, not encouraged to ask questions or to be participants in their care. I was (and still am!) convinced that by teaching nurses and doctors about palliative care then they would be in a stronger position to help patients and their families, and that they would also be able to pass on their knowledge and skills to their colleagues and other professionals.

Lecturer in palliative care

Attending to people who may be facing loss and change requires a great deal of sensitivity and compassion, and challenges our very humanity. For these reasons, I believe we are drawn to work in this area – maybe we also need to work out some of these issues for our own personal reasons.

Member of Macmillan Practice Development Unit

Activity 3: Your future

Now you have thought about how you became interested in palliative care, consider where you want to go from here. Think about where you want to be in a year, or five years, and make notes on the knowledge and skills that you think you will need. If you are interested in a particular type of job, and if your team or AL set includes someone who has knowledge of that job, ask them what sorts of knowledge and skills they think are important to perform it effectively.

Start off by identifying the knowledge and skills that you already have that are relevant to palliative care. For example, you may feel you have knowledge and skills in some of the following areas: clinical, education, practice development, management, patient contact.

If you want to think about five years ahead, but find it difficult to focus so far ahead, you may find it helpful to draw up a 'timeline' that identifies your aspirations for, say, a year, three years and five years from now. By breaking it down into smaller steps, you may find it easier to identify your goals for each time frame.

Knowledge and skills that I already have:

Knowledge and skills that I need:

Feedback

Most of us are unlikely to have long-term plans that include building a hospice, as Dame Cicely Saunders did, but whatever you choose to be or do, you know that you can improve the lives of patients who are not going to recover from illness.

WHAT IS PALLIATIVE CARE?

The World Health Organization's (WHO) definition (World Health Organization, 2002) of palliative care is given below.

WHO definition of palliative care

Palliative care improves the quality of life of patients and families who face life-threatening illness, by providing pain and symptom relief, spiritual and psychosocial support from diagnosis to the end of life and bereavement.

Palliative care:

- provides relief from pain and other distressing symptoms;
- affirms life and regards dying as a normal process;
- intends neither to hasten nor postpone death;
- integrates the psychological and spiritual aspects of patient care;
- offers a support system to help patients live as actively as possible until death;
- offers a support system to help the family cope during the patient's illness and in their own bereavement;
- uses a team approach to address the needs of patients and their families, including bereavement counselling, if indicated;
- will enhance quality of life, and may also positively influence the course of illness;
- is applicable early in the course of illness, in conjunction with other therapies that are intended to prolong life, such as chemotherapy or radiation therapy, and includes those investigations needed to better understand and manage distressing clinical complications.

In their research into general nurses' perceptions of palliative care, Holmes *et al.* (1997) suggested the following definition as a summary of the nurses' views:

Palliative care is solicitous care which assists the patient to prepare himself for death. The nurse does as much as possible for the patient in order to fulfil his wishes and make his life as comfortable as possible. Integration of the family into care is as important as the participation of inter-disciplinary services in promoting physical and psychological well-being, without disturbing the patient or wanting to prolong his life.

Holmes *et al.* (1997: 96)

One of the problems they identified with this definition was the concept of 'doing for'. By protecting the patient, and doing as much for them as they could, nurses could actually cause the patient to feel a loss of control over their life, which has a negative effect on the patient's self-esteem and on their quality of life.

Holmes *et al.* (1997) identified a further problem in the attitudes of the general nurses they interviewed. The nurses identified palliative care with little or no hope of improvement, suffering, an inability to accomplish tasks and imminent death. This passive attitude could lead to nurses becoming demotivated and depressed. This negative attitude affected the quality of care they provided, and the patient's quality of life. Holmes *et al.* (1997) suggest that nurses who have chosen to work with cancer patients may adopt a more positive attitude and also be highly motivated, and that this is reflected in the care they provide.

Holmes *et al.* (1997: 97) compared the nurses' view of palliative care for the 'dying patient', where they felt there was:

> nothing more to do except make the patient as comfortable as possible [so that his] misery is not prolonged.

with one of the basic tenets of palliative care, that the patient is:

> a living person until he dies, and he needs help to continue living his life in his own way, with purpose and fulfilment up to the end.
> St Christopher's Hospice (1974), cited in Holmes *et al.* (1997: 92)

Unfortunately, patients may also have negative views of palliative care. Prior and Poulton (1996: 89) cite an elderly patient who, when introduced to a specialist palliative care nurse, said:

> Ah yes, well that's that, I suppose I knew they weren't going to do anything more for me.

We would suggest that it is in your own interest and that of your patients to foster a positive attitude to palliative care. A positive attitude is the best basis for 'providing joy in living and setting realistic goals' (Holmes *et al.*, 1997: 95).

Activity 4: Your definition of palliative care

What is your own definition of palliative care? Make a few brief notes on this. If you have not already done it, you may find the values clarification exercise in the 'Introduction to this book' helpful.

Feedback

We believe that palliative care is not just about people with cancer, or those nearing death. We suggest that palliative care is about improving the quality of life of people who have a chronic condition from which they may not recover. It includes improving the quality of life of their family and encompasses their surroundings. It is based on a positive attitude toward the future and the development of a deep and honest relationship with patients and their families.

A palliative care philosophy encompasses the recognition of the patient, rather than the illness with a focus beyond the physical to include spiritual, emotional and social dimensions.

Davidson *et al.* (2003: 47)

The aims of palliative care are very different from those of curative care. Prior and Poulton (1996) identified these differences while attempting to develop palliative care speciality practices in acute general hospitals. They discovered that a major challenge was to find techniques to promote the palliative care philosophy in a curative environment. They suggest that palliative and curative ideologies differ in intention, goals and expected outcomes (Table 1.1).

Note that Prior and Poulton identify the importance of a team approach to palliative care. We will go on to look at this after Activity 5.

Concept	Curative	Palliative
Intention	Elimination of disease. Recovery and resuscitation from effects of disease. Preventing death.	Minimising the symptoms and dysfunctions associated with progressive disease. Allowing death.
Goals of care	Extending life. Remobilisation and rehabilitation. Promotion of full physical functioning. Family involvement tends to be minimal. Less emphasis on team approach to goal setting.	Quality of life. Maximising treatment benefits and minimising adverse effects. Patient and family-centred control. Mandatory interdisciplinary team approach to goal setting.
Expected outcomes	Patients discharged. Return to pre-disease functioning.	Comfortable death. Support and care for the bereaved.

Table 1.1 Comparison of curative and palliative ideology (adapted from Prior and Poulton 1996: 85)

Activity 5: Curative and/or palliative care?

Compare Prior and Poulton's (1996) models of curative and palliative ideologies with your own experience. Are the differences quite so cut and dried in your own experience? Make a few brief notes and then go on to discuss Prior and Poulton's models with your AL set.

Feedback

Although they may be quite different, the curative and palliative aspects often work together. A patient may be receiving active treatment for a disease, but may also be receiving palliation of his symptoms (which may have arisen from his disease or the treatment for it).

At one time it was thought that palliative care began when (unsuccessful) active treatment ended (see Figure 1.1). Now it is thought that they can work in partnership, but that the focus on palliative care increases as the focus on active treatment decreases (see Figure 1.2).

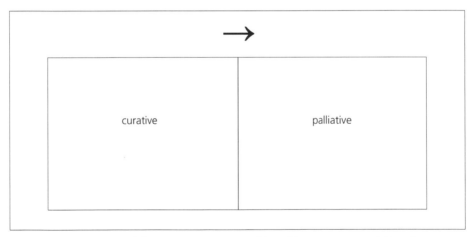

Figure 1.1 Palliative care follows curative care (World Health Organization, 1990: 16) **www.who.int** (site accessed 30/6/08).

Over the years some illness periods have increased, and the WHO model has been adapted to show how the palliative care model can be used throughout a longer illness period. The Sheffield model of palliative care (Figure 1.3) shows that whatever the length of a disease trajectory, there are distinct phases during the illness journey, and that care should focus on the treatments and support that are appropriate for that stage of the illness.

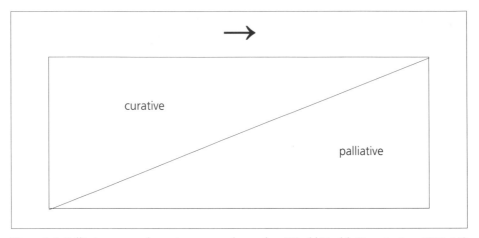

Figure 1.2 Palliative care and curative care work together (World Health Organization, 1990: 16) **www.who.int** (site accessed 30/6/08).

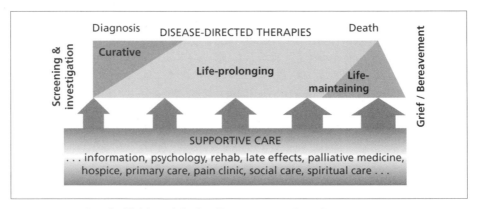

Figure 1.3 The Sheffield model of palliative care (Ahmedzai, 2006) **www. shef.ac.uk/medicine/research/sections/oncology/spcsg** (site accessed 13/5/08 – these pages are currently under development)

HOW IS PALLIATIVE CARE DELIVERED?

Palliative care is usually delivered through teamwork, as no single person would have all the skills and knowledge required to support a patient receiving palliative care. Furthermore, palliative care is delivered in a variety of settings, and sometimes at times and for periods requested by the patient, and so a well-organised team is often the best way of delivering care. A well-run team, including patients, their families and friends, in which all members are working towards the same goal – effective palliative care for each patient – is also good for morale. Good staff morale, providing support for the professional, can make your job more rewarding and enjoyable.

Who is in the palliative care team?

Firstly and most importantly, the patient and their family should be the centre of the palliative care team. The team may also include volunteers and professionals who provide specialist palliative care (i.e. whose main focus is palliative care), including any or all of the following:

- GP
- hospital nurses
- hospital doctors
- health visitors
- care assistants
- palliative care physician
- district nurse
- specialist palliative care nurse
- Marie Curie nurse
- practice nurse
- physiotherapist
- occupational therapist
- social worker

- practice counsellor
- clinical psychologist
- dietician
- home carer
- staff in residential accommodation
- people from voluntary organisations
- carers from private agencies
- volunteers
- spiritual advisor
- complementary therapist
- interpreter
- bereavement visitor.

Activity 6: Contact list

Do you know how to contact all the people listed above? Create a contact list for yourself, your patients and your colleagues so that everyone can easily find the contact details for all the volunteers and professionals who may be able to provide help in the specialist palliative care field.

Discuss this project with your manager, colleagues and AL set. They may have useful ideas of whom you can contact for information. Start by identifying who is available in your clinical area or organisation. You may, for example, have a hospital chaplain.

What resources are available outside your organisation? There may be a local specialist palliative care team whose members may be able to visit your clinical area if the need arises. They may also be able to suggest other individuals and organisations (professional and charitable) that may be able to provide help in your clinical area.

For each contact, obtain a name, address and phone number, plus a brief description of the services that they can provide. Place your contact list where all members of your team can get to it easily. (Don't forget that the patient is a member of the team.)

Feedback

A useful contact list like this may make a significant improvement in the quality of care that patients receive. It will mean that you, your patients and your colleagues will be aware of what resources are available, and provide the details that you need to contact those individuals and organisations. This should improve the quality of care received by patients not only while in your clinical area, but also elsewhere should they be able to leave your clinical area, as both you and they know what is available and who to ask for it.

WHERE IS PALLIATIVE CARE PROVIDED?

Palliative care may be provided at any of the following care settings:

- the patient's home;
- a hospital;
- a nursing home;
- a residential care home;
- a day-care unit, which may be
  - hospice day care;
  - a frail elderly day hospital;
  - an elderly mentally ill day hospital;
  - a psychiatric day hospital;
  - a residential care home;
  - a nursing home;
- specialist palliative care units in hospices/hospitals;
- palliative care beds in acute hospitals;
- community hospitals.

In a perfect world, palliative care would be provided wherever the patient needs it. Furthermore, palliative care may be provided in settings that might seem unlikely, such as maternity units, which may admit patients with life-threatening illnesses such as AIDS, multiple sclerosis and breast cancer. As we mentioned earlier, most health care professionals' work involves some aspects of palliative care – regardless of the setting in which they work.

Activity 7: Care settings

You may have already considered some of the settings in which you have worked in the past (Activity 2). Using the headings below, make a list of the last two or three settings in which you have worked, and the one in which you currently work, and make brief notes for each one of their strengths and weaknesses. Focus on factors that affect the quality of care provided to patients when identifying strengths and weaknesses.

Care setting: Strengths: Weaknesses:

Feedback

When you read through your list of strengths and weaknesses, you may find that items often refer to the people with whom you worked or work. This is a major reason why effective teamwork is important in palliative care. Dysfunctional teams, in which members disagree over what they're doing or why, or simply don't talk to each other at all, can spoil your working days, and this can have a negative impact on the quality of care you provide. We will look at the importance of effective teamwork in Chapter 2. While factors such as the availability of specialist equipment obviously affect the care that patients receive, the attitude of team members is just as important. A dedicated team in a non-specialist setting can provide good palliative care if they know what resources they can call on and how best to use them.

However, if there are environmental issues in your notes for your current workplace, discuss them with your manager, and also with the patient, if any change may affect them. You might have problems with some pieces of equipment, or room layout, or even the amount of light or heat in the rooms in which you work. Find out whether the situation can be improved. For example, a piece of equipment may be in a place that is difficult for you to reach, and it may be possible to have it moved to somewhere where you can more easily reach it.

The next activity asks you to discuss your current care setting with some patients. Discuss this with your manager and colleagues before starting the activity, so that they are aware of what you are doing and why.

Activity 8: The patient's view

Ask several of the patients in your current care setting if they would be prepared to discuss the care setting with you. Ask them the following questions, but try to guide them to talk about the environment if you can:

- What do you like about it here?
- What would you change if you could?
- What could be improved?

Feedback

You will probably find that the patients also talk about the people in the care setting, even if you keep guiding them back to environmental issues. Make notes on the environmental issues that patients report and on any solutions they suggest to problems. Discuss these issues with your manager and let the patients know the outcomes of your discussions. If there is anything you can do, or get done, to improve things, make sure that the patient knows that you are doing it as a result of talking to them. They will feel empowered if a change that they have suggested actually happens. Most importantly – make sure that you actually do what you say you are going to do!

A HOLISTIC APPROACH TO PALLIATIVE CARE

Holistic palliative care is concerned with the whole person and not just the physical aspects of disease and symptoms. It includes all aspects of the person:

- physical;
- psychological;
- social;
- spiritual;
- cultural.

It also includes the needs of the patient's family. Useful sources on holistic care include Doyle and Woodruff (2004) and Lugton and Kindlen (1999). The holistic approach is related to the theory of unpleasant symptoms, as proposed by Lenz *et al.* (1995), which we will look at next.

The theory of unpleasant symptoms

The theory of unpleasant symptoms (Lenz *et al.*, 1995) assumes that there are sufficient commonalities among symptoms to warrant a theory that is not limited to one symptom, but can explain and guide research and practice regarding an array of unpleasant symptoms (Lenz *et al.*, 1997). It proposes that some of the same factors may influence the experience of a number of different symptoms, and that consequently similar interventions may be effective in alleviating more than one symptom. The theory has three major components:

- **The symptoms** that the individual is experiencing. The theory asserts that although symptoms may occur alone, more often multiple symptoms are experienced simultaneously. For example, a patient who is breathless is often also fatigued. Furthermore, one symptom may impact upon another – depression may be more severe when the patient experiences poorly controlled pain (Chochinov, 2001).
- **The influencing factors** that give rise to or affect the nature of the symptom experience:
  - Physiologic factors – the patient's normally functioning bodily systems, any pathology (disease, infection) and the patient's energy level (nutrition and hydration).
  - Psychologic factors – the patient's mental state or mood, affective reaction to the illness, and degree of uncertainty and knowledge about the symptoms and their possible meaning.
  - Situational factors – aspects of the social and physical environment that may affect the individual's experience and reporting of symp-

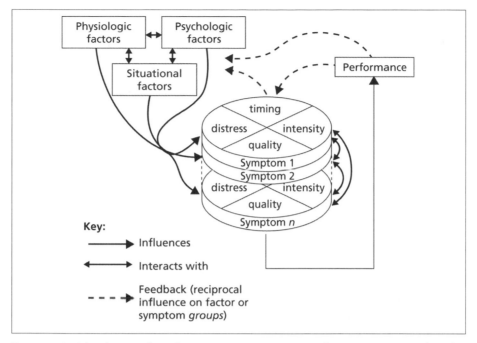

Figure 1.4 The theory of unpleasant symptoms (Lenz *et al.*, 1995: 8). Reproduced with permission from Lippincott William & Wilkins, the publishers of: Lenz, E.R., Suppe, F., Gift, A.G., Pugh, L.C. and Milligan, R.A. (1995) 'Collaborative development of middle-range nursing theories: toward a theory of unpleasant symptons', *Advances in Nursing Science*, 17(3), pp.1–13. **www.lww.com** (site accessed 30/6/08)

toms. Social considerations include employment status, marital and family status, social support, availability of and access to health care resources, and lifestyle behaviours such as diet and exercise.

- **The consequences** of the symptom experience – the outcome or effect of the symptom experience, including functional activities (physical activities, activities of daily living, social activities and interaction, work and other role-related tasks) and cognitive activities (concentrating, thinking and problem solving). Suffering is a major consequence of the symptom experience for many patients receiving palliative care.

As is illustrated in Figure 1.4, the patient's symptoms, influencing factors and performance are all inter-related. They all affect and are affected by one another. We will now go on to look at the following factors:

- physical;
- social;
- cultural.
- psychological;
- spiritual;

We will consider the needs of the patient's family in the next section, 'Caring for the carers', where we will also consider ways of caring for professional carers.

Physical factors

These include the patient's bodily systems, any disease or infection, and the patient's energy level. These are clearly linked with each other – if you are ill, the illness normally saps your energy levels. If you don't eat or drink properly, it usually takes longer to get better. But these physical factors may also affect other areas of your life. Patients who are experiencing severe symptoms that affect many parts of their lives, for example causing problems with sexual relationships and intimacy, may become anxious, depressed or angry. They may 'drive' their families and friends away and become isolated. By improving the patient's physical situation, you should achieve an overall increase in their quality of life.

Psychological factors

If a patient was exhibiting anxiety, an anxiolytic might be prescribed to manage the anxiety. However, it might do nothing about the root cause. Taking a holistic approach to the people you are caring for will give you an insight into the influencing factors. By being aware of the social aspects of this patient's life, you might know that he's worried about how his family will cope without him, or what's going to happen to his aviary. If his concerns about these issues can be allayed, through discussions with you, his family or others who might be able to help, his symptoms might be reduced to a level where it is not necessary to prescribe drugs for him. He may be able to recognise/validate his own management strategies or you may be able to teach him new ones, such as breathing exercises (see Chapter 5). Furthermore, research has shown (Strang, 1997) that pain is increased if patients have problems in other parts of their lives, and that using a holistic approach can reduce the amount of analgesia that is required.

Social factors

Pearce and Lugton (1999) identify four areas of social need:

- altered relationships/social isolation;
- ill health/disability of another family member;
- loss of work/role;
- financial problems.

Relationships within families inevitably change if one family member is terminally ill and requires palliative care. As illness progresses there will, for example, be changes in patients' normal patterns of intimacy and expressions of sexuality, which may distress patients and their partners.

If the patient is no longer able to maintain their role in the family, perhaps as breadwinner or main carer for the whole family, another member (or other members) may find it difficult to step into that role. It can also be problematic, for example, when the individuals in a parent-child relationship suddenly seem to switch roles.

Social isolation is often a problem if the patient can no longer get out and about, but this may be overcome if friends and family are willing to visit the patient. However, a further complication may be the over-protectiveness of the patient's main carer. Well-meaning loved ones may prevent people visiting, believing that visitors will tire the patient out. These are complex issues, but acknowledging that the loss is real can enable you to help the patient initiate management strategies.

If other family members are ill or disabled, the patient may already be anxious, and it may also mean that it will not be possible for them to be cared for at home. Loss of work will lead to a drop in income, which may cause the patient and their family financial difficulties. Loss of work also often leads to a loss of role/status. This in turn can cause anxiety and depression (Skilbeck *et al.*, 1997). Financial problems inevitably impact upon relationships within the family, often causing anxiety and depression. There may be concerns about the cost of care, mortgage repayments, utility bills, holidays, Christmas presents and so on.

Social needs are extremely complex and are interconnected with each other, and with needs in other areas of the patient's life.

Spiritual factors

Narayanasamy (2004) defines several common features of spirituality in ill people, which include:

- disorganisation and disruption;
- search for meaning;
- reliance on hope, inner strength and the love of others;
- reliance on other spiritual resources.

Patients in spiritual distress may be seeking meaning in what is happening to them and may be asking existential questions: Why me? Why this? Why now? They may explore feelings of guilt for former actions, be concerned about their own and others' futures and have thoughts about God and personal suffering (Bolmsjö, 2002).

Spiritual distress may be experienced by agnostics and atheists, as well as those who have religious faith. If your definition of spirituality is linked directly to religion, you may find it difficult to see how patients who have no faith, no belief in any kind of after-life, can be helped to see meaning in life, and we will look at these issues in Activity 9.

Most hospitals have a chaplain, or are able to provide chaplaincy services, and are able to provide somewhere for Christians of various denominations to pray. Difficulties may, however, arise when patients are followers of non-Christian faiths. Situations that may cause difficulties include:

- a lack of privacy in which to carry out the routines of their own religious practices (for example, no prayer room or place to spread a prayer mat);
- an inability to get down on their knees to pray;
- care being given by strangers instead of by the family;
- the use of alcohol in medicines and skin products;
- provision of foods which are not acceptable – meat in general, beef, pork, non-kosher items;
- the need for a blood transfusion where this is not acceptable in the patient's religion, for example the Jehovah's Witnesses;
- the need to celebrate certain festivals or holy days, or to fast at certain times of year;
- conflict between the patient's need for painkillers, the family's need for them not to be given, and the professional carer's desire to relieve the patient's pain.

This final example can be particularly problematic. Some religious groups believe that painkillers contaminate the spirit and have an effect on those who will remain after the patient dies. The patient's family may therefore not want the patient to receive painkillers. As long as levels of pain are low, the patient is often content not to receive painkillers as they are acting for the spiritual wellbeing of their family. However, if the pain becomes unbearable, the patients may ask the professional carers for painkillers and the professional carers will agree to the request. The family are then in conflict both with the patient and with the professional carers. This solution to a physical problem can unfortunately lead to a marked decrease in the patient's quality of life in the social, psychological and spiritual areas. The most effective way to deal with such difficulties is to negotiate with the patient and their family, to find the solution that is best for the patient.

Activity 9: Providing spiritual support

1. As we have mentioned, most hospitals have a chaplain or are able to provide chaplaincy services, and are able to provide somewhere for Christians of various denominations to pray. Find out what services are available in your organisation.

Once you have identified the services, discuss them with patients who use them. Find out what the patients think about the services they have used.

- What are the good aspects?
- What are the difficult aspects?
- What could be done to improve the services?

2. Is there a place in or near your clinical area where patients can go to pray that is not a consecrated Christian place of worship? If there is, discuss it with patients who use it. Ask them:

- what is good about it;
- what is difficult about it;
- what could be added or changed to improve it.

If there is no such place, identify what patients might need in such an area – the easiest way to do this would be to ask patients and their families, or non-Christian members of staff. Ask them what furnishings are necessary – chairs, tables, carpets, cushions, mats, etc. Followers of Islam might like a compass (particularly in a windowless room) so they can ascertain which way to face while praying.

3. Visit the following website: **www.humanism.org.uk** (Site accessed 30/6/08).

This website has been created by the British Humanist Association, which 'exists to support and represent people who seek to live good and responsible lives without religious or superstitious beliefs' (taken from the website). The site gives some interesting insights into the non-religious concept of spirituality. Find out what non-religious spiritual support your organisation can offer to those in spiritual distress.

Feedback

1 Now that you have asked patients for feedback on the services they have used, it is important that you act upon their comments. Discuss with your manager how it might be possible to improve the services, based on the patients' comments. This will probably involve discussions between your team or your manager and the chaplain or chaplaincy service.

2 Discuss any changes to the clinical area or identified space that the patients identify as being desirable with the rest of your team. Identify which of the changes are possible, and agree with your team how you are going to implement them.

If there is no specific place set aside, is there a side room that could be used temporarily? Discuss this with your manager and colleagues. For example, some nurses in a Glasgow hospital converted a small storeroom (which had previously housed broken furniture) to provide a comfortable relatives' area. If your clinical area has a storeroom full of broken furniture or wheel-less trolleys, you could ask the hospital management team for the use of the room. You could ask local businesses whether they would be prepared to supply paint or carpeting, or some comfortable seats.

3 Patients who are humanists, atheists or agnostics may need spiritual support through some other form of help or counselling. Some counselling psychologists specialise in existential philosophy, which is about making sense of human existence, and focuses on questions about freedom, the meaning of life and personal relationships. Your organisation, team or local specialist care team may include a therapist or counsellor who will be able to help patients.

Cultural factors

Britain is a multicultural society, embracing cultures from all over the world. Being multicultural is about different cultures co-existing, rather than one culture absorbing all others. Consequently, many people live in ways similar to the ways in which their families lived before they came to Britain. This is particularly true for the older members of families, as younger members often (although not always) give up traditional ways. Differences in culture need not be linked to differences in religion or skin colour.

When people who are used to the norms of another culture enter a hospital which expects everyone to share the culture of the region in which it is situated, difficulties may arise. Situations that may cause difficulties include:

- female patients needing to be seen only by female carers;
- female patients needing to be modestly dressed (for example, clothing that covers them completely, including coverings for the head and hair);
- a desire for appropriate eating utensils, for example, chopsticks;
- language difficulties, including medical language and body language, for example different interpretations of making eye contact (aggression, immodesty, truthfulness, trustworthiness);
- the patient's use of traditional medicines or reliance on traditional practitioners;
- responses or reactions to pain or death and dying – some cultures are very expressive and demonstrative, while others are not.

Leishman (2004) suggested that culture-sensitive care:

focuses on the similarities between cultures to provide appropriate healthcare based on individual values, beliefs and healthcare practices.

Leishman (2004: 33–4)

She goes on to identify culturally sensitive care as care that includes:

- valuing diversity;
- having the capacity for cultural assessment;
- being conscious of the dynamics inherent when cultures interact;
- having developed adaptations of service delivery that reflect an understanding of cultural diversity.

You may find it helpful to review the above model in relation to your practice to gain further understanding of others' behaviours and beliefs in the context of their cultures. If you can become more empathetic towards patients and their families, you will become better able to identify their cultural needs.

In negotiating with someone who has cultural needs that are in conflict with what you believe to be their best chances for a better quality of life, you need to listen, teach, compare and compromise.

- **Listen** – you will find out about patients' general beliefs as well as their beliefs about the biomedical causes of their illness.
- **Teach** – using language free of jargon and which patients can understand. Avoid authoritative language – say, 'We find that this treatment provides you with more comfort' rather than 'If you don't do/take this then I can't do anything else for you'.
- **Compare** – compare the outcomes of each treatment. For example, a patient may wish to go home to die, but the care staff may be concerned that he is not fit to travel. Going home will satisfy his cultural and religious needs. Since he is dying anyway, it may be better to support his wish to do this at home. What the care team thinks is best may not be significant in terms of belief to patients and their families.
- **Compromise** – starting from the Hippocratic concept of 'do no harm', attempt to combine and maximise the contribution of modern medical techniques and any form of traditional healing requested by the patient. Where it can do no harm, you should accept it. Where it is harmful, gently tell the patient that you cannot be involved in it and state your reasons (e.g. ethics, code of conduct).

If you cannot successfully negotiate with a patient, seek support and advice from your manager and supervisor. This will be easier in an institutional setting than in the community.

Activity 10: Holistic care

Think about the care you give to patients. On a separate sheet of paper, try to identify examples in your everyday interactions with patients where you have given holistic care. Try to give an example for each area of the patient's life:

- physical;
- psychological;
- social;
- spiritual;
- cultural;
- the needs of the patient's family.

For each example, explain how the patient benefited from your holistic approach.

Feedback

You may find it useful and interesting to discuss your answers to this activity with the members of your AL set.

For a real insight into the many ways in which people's lives are affected by illness, read the books by John Diamond, Ruth Picardie, Mitch Albom and Jean Dominique Bauby listed in the 'Recommended Sources of information' (Diamond, 1998; Picardie, 1998; Albom, 1997; Bauby, 1998). We will be looking at the importance of a holistic approach again in Chapter 3.

CARING FOR THE CARERS

In this section we will consider the importance of caring for those who care for the patient receiving palliative care, including both lay carers (often the patient's family and friends) and professional carers.

Lay carers – the patient's family and friends

> Much of the work of caring for people in the last year of their life is undertaken not by health professionals but by members of the patient's own family or their friends.
>
> (Bibby, 1999)

A crucial aspect of holistic care is involving the patients' families, including children as well as adult members. Be aware when dealing with carers that they are individuals too. Each person has their own unique blend of coping strategies, fears and experiences. Note too, that a study by Kissane *et al.* (1994) found that the way in which patients' spouses coped differed from the way in which the patients' children coped. Furthermore, carers may not only have differing needs, they may actually have competing needs. This calls for skilful judgement, and an ability to negotiate outcomes that benefit all the carers where possible. Exploring what each family member can do in this situation can help relieve some of the anxieties the carers are experiencing.

A patient's carers often experience physical, emotional, social and economic burdens as a result of the patient's illness. Research has shown that carers have significant unmet needs for support (Hodgson *et al.*, 1998; McIntyre, 1996). You can help carers by ensuring they receive:

- all the information they require – again, emphasising the importance of good communication;
- attention to their emotional strain – encourage them to talk about their own fears and anxieties;
- training for any behavioural coping strategies that the patient is using.

Information needs

We have already discussed the importance of communication, and mentioned that patients who feel they cannot discuss distressing issues often become anxious and distressed. The same is true for their carers. Lugton (1999) suggests that relatives often receive less information than patients, even though their anxiety is as great. Wilkes *et al.* (2000) found that the best way to support families, with a view to allowing them to effectively care for patients at home, was to satisfy their information needs. The family will want up-to-date information on the progress of the patient's disease. In the terminal phase they will need to know precisely what will happen, including the changes that will occur in the patient. This will help them to cope during this time (Doyle and Jeffrey, 2000). This may not be easy, as the changes may not be known, but the principle of openness is important.

This also applies to patients being cared for in settings other than the home, as the provision of sufficient information allows the family to take part in decisions about the patient's care, which dispels the anxieties caused by doubt and fear (Ramirez *et al.*, 1998).

You need to be proactive in seeking out relatives to ensure they have the information they need to cope with their situation. Edwards and Forster (1999) discovered that the elderly relatives they surveyed avoided contact with health care professionals to avoid having to discuss matters concerning them. If a patient has a number of relatives, it's a good idea to select one relative who is able to liaise between the staff and the family to allow them all to receive the information they require (Degner *et al.*, 1991).

Write the information down and revisit it frequently with the lay carers. The provision of information is an ongoing process and frequent reviews are necessary as the information will be processed at different levels. People take in information at different rates and this can be affected by worry and anxiety about their loved one's illness. Professionals need to check that the carers understood the last piece of information and have not forgotten it. You may find that you need to repeat it a few times. It's important to make sure that they have grasped the information, as you will probably need to give them more information in the future and you don't want to have to try and give them too much at one go.

The provision of information may be difficult if patients and carers are trying to protect each other by not being honest with each other. Collusion leads to mistrust and raised levels of anxiety in patients, families and professional carers (Buckman, 2000). Together with the other members of the care team, you should explore the reasons why the patient or family feel collusion is necessary and negotiate a way of resolving the issues involved.

Activity 11: Keeping carers informed

- What sorts of information do you provide for carers and how is it provided?

- Are you and the other members of your team proactive in giving information to carers?

Discuss these questions with the other members of your team, including patients and carers. Ask the carers what information they might want.

Identify what information needs are not being met, and how they might be met in the future.

Feedback

It is likely that information is provided to carers in a fairly *ad hoc* way. In the pressure of daily nursing, you probably only have time to answer questions when carers ask you directly and, sometimes, you may not have the time to discuss things as fully with them as you would like.

There may be leaflets available about the patient's illness, or about palliative care, which you could give to the carers to take away with them. Furthermore, you could provide carers with the details of local information sources including those which may help them address other needs, such as financial needs, and needs for home-help. This helps them to remain in control of their lives, promoting their psychological wellbeing and that of the patient. You could tell carers about:

- self-help groups;
- national and local carers' groups;
- Crossroads – they will help with care and can keep a patient company while a carer goes out;
- the Marie Curie Community Nursing Service;
- how to get a district nurse;
- complementary therapies;
- the Princess Royal Trust;
- spiritual support.

Be aware, however, that carers' needs may vary from day to day. Sometimes they may want detailed information, sometimes they may just want basic information about the patient's comfort (McIntyre, 1996). Often the greatest support comes from knowing that the patient is being well cared-for, and that their symptoms are being adequately controlled (McIntyre, 1996; Payne *et al.*, 1999). A major concern for carers is that their loved one is comfortable and receiving the best possible care. Particularly when care is primarily at home, the carer may experience great anxiety if they have concerns about how good the professional care is, or their ability to do the right thing. Therefore the information provided may also need to cover skills training, e.g. positioning, decision making about medication, mouth care, and so on.

Emotional support

In order to be able to cope with the patient's illness, the carers need to be able to face the reality of their own losses. You, therefore, need to provide care and support while investigating these anxieties to improve the carer's psychological wellbeing. Coming to terms with the loss of a loved one takes time, but the care team can support the family by ensuring they have the information they require, and by involving them in the patient's care, as we have already discussed.

Nurses are particularly well placed to offer emotional support to the family. Costello (1999) suggests that 'being there' for the family is one of the most valuable resources in hospital.

Changes to the roles played by members of the family can cause anxieties and family conflict. Family members may become angry with each other, and some of this anger may be misdirected at health care professionals. Figure 1.5 illustrates effective and ineffective approaches to dealing with anger.

Most carers tread a fine path between facing the reality of their situation and losing hope (Hinds, 1992). They often suffer distress caused by:

- the challenge of care giving;
- taking on additional roles;
- feelings of guilt at having to ask for help;
- refusal of help by family members;
- lack of formal help and information;
- patient's symptoms, e.g. cognitive impairment (Sherwood *et al.*, 2004).

If these problems are not addressed before the patient dies, the carer may be left with an exaggerated bereavement reaction (Doyle and Jeffrey, 2000).

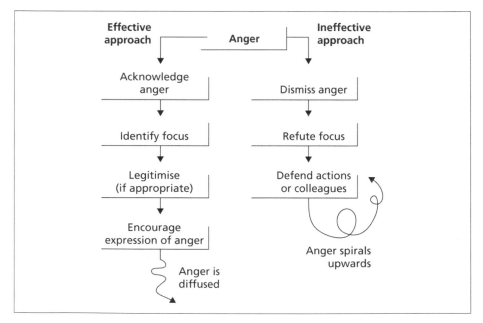

Figure 1.5 Effective and ineffective approaches to dealing with anger (Faulkner, 1998: 49). Reprinted from Faulkner, A. (1998) 'Communication with patients, families and other professionals', in Fallon, M. and O'Neill, B. (editors) *ABC of palliative care*, London: BMJ Books, pp.47–9, with permission from Blackwell Publishing Ltd. **www.blackwellpublishing.com/book.asp?ref=9781405130790&site=1** (site accessed 1/7/08)

After the patient's death

The care of the patient's family should continue after the patient's death. Doyle and Jeffrey (2000) suggest that as the primary heath care team will have been involved with the family during the patient's illness, it is ideally placed to provide support during the bereavement. However, not all community staff, for example, are equipped to provide bereavement support, nor may they have the time. In such situations, a team may assess whether formal support is necessary and, if it is, refer the family on to the appropriate services.

Failure to grieve normally is associated with an increased risk of physical and psychiatric illness and morbidity (Parkes, 2000; Maguire, 1995) and there are a number of risk factors that may indicate whether relatives are likely to suffer a severe bereavement reaction. These are described by Smith (1995).

- **A severe reaction to the loss.** The manifestation of severe distress, anger, yearning or self-reproach.
- **An ambivalent relationship.** Where the patient and carer had ambivalent feelings towards each other with unexpressed hostility or in situations when the relationship was highly dependent.
- **Circumstances surrounding the death.** Sudden deaths, where the carer has less than two weeks to adjust to the loss. Unnatural deaths like suicide or murder, or when confirmation of the death is uncertain because the body is never found.
- **Previously unresolved grief.** If a carer has previously unresolved grief about a loved one's death, when a subsequent death occurs it is much harder for them to adjust.
- **Multiple life crisis.** If the bereaved person has many additional problems or losses to cope with, this may inhibit normal grief resolution.
- **Personality factors.** People with a strong self-concept are usually better able to cope with crisis situations, including bereavement, by using their own coping mechanisms more appropriately.
- **Low socio-economic status.** Parkes and Weiss (1983) found this to be a factor in the early period, but found that grief resolution had returned to normal after two years.
- **Poor social support.** Those who have a close family and supportive friends cope better with bereavement. People who have recently moved house or whose family lives at a distance are more likely to be at risk. The carer's perception of the amount of support they receive may differ from the actual amount they receive, but their perception of support is at least as important as the actual support.

- **Age.** Young adults have more difficulty adjusting to their bereavement than older individuals.

Being aware of these risk factors can help you to assess the relatives for the possibility of a severe reaction to bereavement. You can then provide them with extra care, support and interventions as necessary, or refer them on to the appropriate services. Undertaking holistic assessment of families not only for their probable bereavement reaction (Ferrario *et al.*, 2004) but also to assess any other problems they might be encountering in coping with their situation (Maher and Hemming, 2005) is an integral part of palliative care.

Activity 12: Providing emotional support for carers

How does your team go about providing support for carers after a patient has died?

If this is not within your remit, what organisations can you suggest the carers contact for support? If you are unsure what services are available locally, contact your local palliative care team and local and national carers' support organisations to find out.

Discuss these issues with your team and AL set, and also discuss whether bereaved people need professional support. Is there a danger of 'medicalising' grief?

Feedback

You can provide emotional support to carers by talking to them, giving them the information they need and, above all, listening to them. You could suggest they contact local services such as a bereavement counsellor or patient/carer support group, or national groups such as CRUSE.

Grief is a normal process following bereavement, and rarely requires counselling or medical intervention. You can help the bereaved by giving them details of support sources, but it would be unrealistic to assume that everyone needs such a service. Grief and loss can be very strong, painful emotions, but most adults have coping strategies developed from earlier experiences of dealing with crises, which will enable them to cope with bereavement. Being supportive without creating dependency requires good communication skills and a belief in people's ability to cope (we look at coping strategies and the importance of effective communication in Chapter 2.)

For many nurses, involvement ends with the death of the patient. Not being involved in helping carers with their grief may leave nurses with unanswered questions, or 'unfinished business'.

Sharing coping strategies

Arrange for family members to be present if you teach the patient to use any behavioural coping strategies such as relaxation and visualisation. If possible, train them how to use them too, so they can take part in the experience with the patient. This is a fairly easy task when considering teaching abdominal breathing to a breathless patient, for example. Both patient and carer can use the method to calm themselves, and the patient will be less likely to suffer distress (and possibly trigger an attack) if they perceive that their carer is calm and not panicking. We look at abdominal breathing, visualisation and relaxation in Chapter 5.

Professional carers

> All carers need to care for themselves if they are to deliver a good standard of care to their patients.
>
> Bottrill and Kirkwood (1999: 186)

The stresses associated with caring for dying patients may be balanced out by the feelings of satisfaction with the quality of care provided (Ramirez *et al.*, 1998). These stresses, however, may be compounded by workplace stress caused by problems with colleagues, due, for example, to a lack of agreement over working practices and objectives. Professional carers need to take care of themselves because of their exposure to these stressors. Possible strategies include:

- in-service education;
- support provided by your organisation, including clinical supervision;
- taking care of yourself.

In-service education

In-service education helps to ensure that knowledge and skills are developed and sustained, and can also help nurses to understand how to deal with the everyday stresses they encounter. Topics you might find useful include:

- the use of reflective practice;
- professional relationships;
- ethical issues;
- how to handle personal issues that are raised as a result of working with palliative care patients;
- stress management techniques;
- assertiveness methods;
- self-awareness;

- team support mechanisms and effective teamwork;
- communication skills.

Support provided by your organisation

> Clinical directors and managers should ensure that systems for management and support are in place to meet the special needs which can be experienced among staff working in this field.
>
> Scottish Partnership for Palliative Care (1994: 18)

Ramirez *et al.* (1998) suggest that the provision of a confidential mental health service that allows discussion of both professional and personal issues may help the psychological wellbeing of professionals working within palliative care.

Clinical supervision

Clinical supervision is built into the professional roles of a number of professions allied to medicine, i.e. occupational therapists and social workers, and is not just the administrative tool used to supervise a worker's performance which some feared it might be. Clinical supervision is defined as:

> A formal process of professional support and learning which enables individual practitioners to develop knowledge and competence, assume responsibility for their own practice and enhance consumer protection in complex care.
>
> Department of Health (1993)

Wright and Giddens (1994) give a simpler definition to show the differences in the concept of supervision – they suggest supervision is:

> a meeting between two or more people who have a declared interest in examining a piece of work.
>
> Wright and Giddens (1994: 17)

Sloan (1998) suggests that effective clinical supervision relies on a supervisor who:

- is perceived by the supervisee to be able to develop supportive relationships;
- is actively supportive;
- is a role model;
- encourages discussion of personal limitations;

- has good listening skills;
- is able to provide literature.

Clinical supervision is believed to be the way forward for the professional support of nurses. The Nursing and Midwifery Council (NMC, 2006) advises that clinical supervision should enable nurses to:

- identify solutions to problems;
- increase their understanding of professional issues;
- improve standards of patient care;
- further their skills and knowledge;
- enhance their understanding of their own practice.

The NMC also believes that every nurse should have access to clinical supervision, which means the process must be implemented throughout the UK.

Clinical supervision can be undertaken one-to-one, or as a group using a facilitator. Clinical supervision is based on the use of reflective practice, which Cowe and Wilkes (1998) suggest has been shown to encourage:

- the discussion of experiences;
- the linking of practice to theory using the knowledge and experience of other colleagues;
- making the most of joint expertise in problem solving;
- the support of peers through sharing anxieties and stressors.

Taking care of yourself

Finally, away from the workplace, you can take care of yourself by relaxing, by doing exercise, or by doing less strenuous things such as reading, listening to music or having a hot relaxing bath.

> Taking care of yourself ensures a balance between giving and receiving.
>
> Bottrill and Kirkwood (1999: 187)

Activity 13: Support for professional carers

What forms of support are you able to rely on?

Find out what sorts of in-service training are available to you and identify which might be useful as a support mechanism. Find out how feasible it might be for you to enrol on a course or take up some other training/education opportunity. As you are already doing this course, you will probably want to consider workshops that last only a day or two rather than another lengthy course. Fortunately, many of the topics we have suggested, such as stress management techniques and assertiveness methods, are often taught at two-day workshops/seminars.

Investigate what support is offered by your organisation. If no system of clinical supervision exists, find out whether it might be possible to start one and, if so, how. You will need to find people who are interested in setting up the system with you.

Feedback

You will need to discuss these issues with your manager. Your manager will be a good source of information and you will also need to discuss the resource implications with them. The combination of your absence and the cost of the workshop may require some careful planning.

If there are appraisal/performance programmes or continuing professional development in place, there may be an ongoing implementation programme for clinical supervision – your manager should be able to tell you. Alternatively, your Occupational Health Department may be able to offer counselling.

If clinical supervision is unavailable, peer support/supervision is well worth considering. This is where you meet a colleague (or someone in a similar position but in a different organisation/Trust) at regular intervals to discuss and reflect upon experiences. This kind of support can be extremely important and of great value to nurses and it is therefore worth negotiating for protected time, although this may sometimes be extremely difficult.

Looking after each other is important too. As well as these formalised resources, it is important that you support your colleagues and feel you have support from them. You also need to know yourself and your own limits, and be aware of the effects and importance of your attitude to care.

SUMMARY

In this chapter we have introduced the concept of palliative care – its history and meaning. You have investigated a local specialist palliative care provider and created a contact list of individuals and organisations, both professional and charitable, that may be able to help you and your patients by providing 'hands-on' support or advice. We have reviewed the types of settings in which palliative care is delivered and you have considered your own setting and asked for feedback from patients. We have stressed the importance of a holistic view to palliative care – the 'whole person' approach – and suggested a variety of ways of caring for both formal and informal carers. Having completed this first chapter, you should be able to:

- briefly outline the history of palliative care;
- describe what is meant by palliative care;
- list the professions involved in delivering palliative care in your area;
- identify the members of the specialist palliative care team in your area;
- identify the types of setting in which palliative care may be delivered;
- explain the importance of holistic palliative care, with reference to a theory of unpleasant symptoms;
- explain why and how palliative care should involve caring for the patient's family and/or carers.

This chapter sets the groundwork for all the chapters that follow. The next two chapters, Chapter 2: 'Essential Concepts' and Chapter 3: 'Generic Assessment in Palliative Care', set the scene for the following five chapters. Chapters 4–7 focus on specific symptoms that may be experienced by a patient receiving palliative care and are (respectively): 'Anxiety and Depression', 'Breathlessness', 'Fatigue' and 'Pain'. In these chapters we consider what each symptom means for the patient, its causes and manifestations, and its assessment and treatment or palliation. The final chapter, 'Quality Improvement', looks at the evaluation and continuous improvement of care.

USEFUL WEBSITES

www.eolc-observatory.net
'Our team of social scientists at Lancaster collaborates with colleagues all around the world in an effort to provide research evidence to impact on the development of hospice and palliative care.' (Taken from the website, accessed 13/5/08.)

www.helpthehospices.org.uk
This is the homepage of Help the Hospices, the national charity for the hospice movement. Accessed 13/5/08.

www.hospiceinformation.info
This is the homepage of the Hospices Information Service: 'providing information on hospices and palliative care services for both professionals and the public. Through publications, research and professional links, the service encourages networking and provides a worldwide resource for all those engaged in palliative care.' (Taken from the website, accessed 13/5/08.)

www.ingentaconnect.com/content/0969-9260
The website for the journal *Progress in Palliative Care*. Accessed 13/5/08.

www.shef.ac.uk/medicine/research/sections/oncology/spcsg
The Academic Unit of Supportive Care (AUSC) at the University of
Sheffield, UK and the Trent Palliative Care Centre (TPCC) together
form the Sheffield Palliative Care Studies Group (SPCSG). SPCSG has
built up an international reputation for the quality of its research,
education, information and clinical practice development in the fields of
supportive and palliative care. (Site accessed 13/5/08.) These pages are
currently under development.

RECOMMENDED SOURCES OF INFORMATION

Some of these are short paperbacks and some are weighty textbooks. We
don't expect you to read the textbooks from cover to cover, but rather
to focus on the topics that interest you, or on the topic you are working
on in this book, as you move from chapter to chapter. Titles followed by
O/P are out of print – but you may be able to find library copies.

On spirituality

Bradshaw, A. (1997) 'Teaching spiritual care to nurses'. *International
Journal of Palliative Nursing*, 3(1), pp.51–7.
Cobb, M. and Robshaw, V. (1998) *The spiritual challenge of health care.*
Edinburgh: Churchill Livingstone.
Milligan, S. (2004) 'Perceptions of spiritual care among nurses undertak-
ing post registration education'. *International Journal of Palliative
Nursing*, 10(4), pp.164–6.

On the patient's experience

Albom, M. (1997) *Tuesdays with Morrie.* New York: Doubleday.
Bauby, J.D. (1998) *The diving bell and the butterfly.* London: Fourth
Estate.
Diamond, J. (1998) C: *because cowards get cancer too.* London: Vermilion.
O/P
Picardie, R. (1998) *Before I say goodbye.* London: Penguin.

On holistic care

Maher, D. and Hemming, L. (2005) 'Understanding patient and family:
holistic assessment in palliative care'. *British Journal of Community
Nursing*, 10(7), pp.318–22.
Morse, J.M. and Johnson, J.L. (editors) (1991) *The illness experience.*
Newbury Park: Sage. O/P
Oberle, K. and Davies, B. (1990) 'Dimensions of the supportive role of
the nurse in palliative care'. *Oncology Nursing Forum*, 17(1), pp.87–94.

On palliative care

Doyle, D., Hanks, G., Cherney N.I. and Calman, K. (editors) (2005) *Oxford textbook of palliative medicine* (3rd Ed.). Oxford: Oxford University Press.

Fallon, M. and O'Neill, B. (editors) (2006) *ABC of palliative care* (2nd Ed.). Malden: Blackwell Publishing.

Faull, C., Carter, Y. and Woof, R. (editors) (2005) *Handbook of palliative care* (2nd Ed.). Malden: Blackwell Publishing.

Lugton, J. and Kindlen, M. (editors) (2004) *Palliative care: the nursing role* (2nd Ed.). Edinburgh: Elsevier Churchill Livingstone.

Payne, S., Seymour, J. and Ingleton, C. (editors) (2004) *Palliative care nursing: principles and evidence for practice*. Maidenhead: Open University Press.

On psychosocial issues

Oliviere, D., Hargreaves, R. and Monroe, B. (1998) *Good practices in palliative care: a psychosocial perspective*. Aldershot: Arena.

Sheldon, F. (1997) *Psychosocial palliative care: good practice in the care of the dying and bereaved*. Cheltenham: Nelson Thornes.

On supporting lay carers

Davies, B., Reimer, J. and Martens, N. (1990) 'Families in supportive care, part 1: the transition of fading away: the nature of the transition'. *Journal of Palliative Care*, 6(3), pp.12–20.

Nicholls, E. (2003) 'An outcomes focus in carers assessment and review: value and challenges'. *British Journal of Social Work*, 33(1), pp.31–47.

Reimer, J., Davies, B. and Martens, N. (1991) 'Palliative care: the nurse's role in helping families through the transition of "fading away"'. *Cancer Nursing*, 14(6), pp.321–7.

You may also find the following journals useful and interesting:
Progress in Palliative Care
European Journal of Palliative Care
International Journal of Palliative Nursing
Journal of Palliative Care
Cancer Nursing

REFERENCES

Ahmedzai, S. (2006) Sheffield model of palliative care, Sheffield Palliative Care Studies Group. **www.shef.ac.uk/medicine/research/sections/oncology/spcsg** (accessed 13/5/08).

Ajemian, I. (1996) 'The interdisciplinary team', in Doyle, D., Hanks, G. and MacDonald, N. (editors) *Oxford textbook of palliative medicine*. Oxford: Oxford University Press, pp. 17–28.

Albom, M. (1997) *Tuesdays with Morrie*. New York: Doubleday.

Bauby, J.D. (1998) *The diving bell and the butterfly*. London: Fourth Estate.

Bibby, A. (1999) *Hospice without walls: the story of west Cumbria's remarkable hospice at home service*. London: Calouste Gulbenkian Foundation.

Bolmsjö, I. (2002) 'Meeting the existential needs in palliative care – who, when and why'. *Journal of Palliative Care*, 18(3), Fall, pp.185–91.

Bottrill, B. and Kirkwood, I. (1999) 'Complementary therapies', in Lugton, J. and Kindlen, M. (editors) *Palliative care: the nursing role*. Edinburgh: Churchill Livingstone, pp.163–91.

Buckman, R. (2000) 'Communication in palliative care', in Dickenson, D., Johnson, M. and Katz, J.S. (editors) *Death, dying and bereavement* (2nd Ed.). Buckingham: Open University/Sage Publications.

Chochinov, H.M. (2001) 'Depression in cancer patients'. *Oncology*, 2(8), pp.499–505.

Costello, J. (1999) 'Anticipatory grief: coping with the impending death of a partner'. *International Journal of Palliative Nursing*, 5(5), pp.223–31.

Cowe, F. and Wilkes, C. (1998) 'Clinical supervision for specialist nurses'. *Professional Nurse*, 13(5), pp.284–7.

Davidson, P., Daly, J., Paull, G., Jarvis, R., Wild, T., Cockburn, J., Dunford, M. and Dracup, K. (2003) 'Cardiorespiratory nurses' perceptions of palliative care in nonmalignant disease: data for the development of clinical practice'. *American Journal of Critical Care*, 12(1), pp.45–53.

Degner, L.F., Gow, C.M. and Thompson, L.A. (1991) 'Critical nursing behaviors in care for the dying'. *Cancer Nursing*, 14(5), pp.246–53.

Department of Health (1993) *A vision for the future: the nursing, midwifery and health visiting contribution to health and health care*. London: DoH.

Diamond, J. (1998) C: *because cowards get cancer too*. London: Vermilion. O/P

Doyle, D. and Jeffrey, D. (2000) *Palliative care in the home*. Oxford: Oxford University Press.

Doyle, D. and Woodruff, R. (2004) *The International Association of Hospice and Palliative Care manual of palliative care*. Houston: IAHPC.

Doyle, D., Hanks, G., Cherney, N.I. and Calman, K. (2004) *The Oxford textbook of palliative medicine* (3rd Ed.). Oxford: Oxford University Press. Foreword by Dame Cicely Saunders pp.i–xi.

Edwards, H. and Forster, E. (1999) 'Avoidance of issues in family caregiving'. *Contemporary Nurse*, 8(2), pp.5–13.

Faulkner, A. (1998) 'Communication with patients, families and other professionals', in Fallon, M. and O'Neill, B. (editors) *ABC of palliative care*. London: BMJ Books, pp.47–9.

Faull, C. (1998) 'The history and principles of palliative care', in Faull, C., Carter, Y. and Woof, R. (editors) *Handbook of palliative care*. Oxford: Blackwell Science, pp.1–12.

Ferrario, S.R., Cardillo, V., Vicario, F., Balzarini, E. and Zotti, A.M. (2004) 'Advanced cancer at home: caregiving and bereavement'. *Palliative Medicine*, 18, pp.129–36.

Hinds, C. (1992) 'Suffering: a relatively unexplored phenomenon among family caregivers of non institutionalized patients with cancer'. *Journal of Advanced Nursing*, 17(8), pp.918–25.

Hodgson, C., Higginson, I. and Jeffreys, P. (1998) *Carers' checklist: an outcome measure for people with dementia and their carers*. London: Mental Health Foundation.

Holmes, S., Pope, S. and Lamond, D. (1997) 'General nurses' perceptions of palliative care'. *International Journal of Palliative Nursing*, 3(2), pp.92–9.

Kissane, D.W., Block, S., Burns, W.I., McKenzies, D. and Posterino, M. (1994) 'Psychological morbidity in the families of patients with cancer'. *Psycho-Oncology*, 3(1), pp.47–56.

Leishman, J. (2004) 'Perspectives of cultural competence in healthcare'. *Nursing Standard*, 19(11), pp.33–8.

Lenz, E.R., Pugh, L.C., Milligan, R.A., Gift, A. and Suppe, F. (1997) 'The middle-range theory of unpleasant symptoms: an update'. *Advances in Nursing Science*, 19(3), pp.14–27.

Lenz, E.R., Suppe, F., Gift, A.G., Pugh, L.C., and Milligan, R.A. (1995) 'Collaborative development of middle-range nursing theories: toward a theory of unpleasant symptoms'. *Advances in Nursing Science*, 17(3), pp.1–13

Lugton, J. (1999) 'Support processes in palliative care', in Lugton, J. and Kindlen, M. (editors) *Palliative care: the nursing role*. Edinburgh: Churchill Livingstone, pp.89–113.

Lugton, J. and Kindlen, M. (editors) (1999) *Palliative care: the nursing role*. Edinburgh: Churchill Livingstone.

Maguire, P. (1995) 'Assessing the bereaved'. *Palliative Care Today*, 4(2), pp.18–20.

Maher, D. and Hemming, L. (2005) 'Understanding Patient and Family: Holistic Assessment in Palliative Care'. *British Journal of Community Nursing*, 10(7), pp.318–22.

McIntyre, R. (1996) *Nursing support for relatives of dying cancer patients in hospital: improving standards by research*, PhD thesis, Department of Nursing and Community Health, Glasgow Caledonian University.

Narayanasamy, A. (2004) 'The puzzle of spirituality for nursing: a guide to practical assessment'. *British Journal of Nursing*, 13(9), pp.1140–4.

Nursing and Midwifery Council (2006) *Clinical supervision advice sheet*. London: NMC.

Parkes, C.M. (2000) 'Bereavement as a psychosocial transition: process of adaptation to change', in Dickenson, D., Johnson, M. and Katz, J.S. *Death, dying and bereavement* (2nd Ed.). Buckingham: Open University/Sage Publications.

Parkes, C.M. and Weiss, R.S. (1983) *Recovery from bereavement*. New York: Basic Books.

Payne, S., Smith, P. and Dean, S. (1999) 'Identifying the concerns of informal carers in palliative care'. *Palliative Medicine*, 13(1), pp.37–44.

Pearce, C. and Lugton, J. (1999) 'Holistic assessment of patients' and relatives' needs', in Lugton, J. and Kindlen, M. (editors) *Palliative care: the nursing role*. Edinburgh: Churchill Livingstone, pp.61–87.

Picardie, R. (1998) *Before I say goodbye*. London: Penguin.

Prior, D. and Poulton, V. (1996) 'Palliative care nursing in a curative environment: an Australian perspective'. *International Journal of Palliative Nursing*, 2(2), pp.84–90.

Ramirez, A., Addington-Hall, J. and Richards, M. (1998) 'The carers', in Fallon, M. and O'Neill, B. (editors) *ABC of palliative care*. London: BMJ Books, pp.50–3.

Scottish Partnership for Palliative Care (1994) *Palliative cancer care guidelines*. Edinburgh: SPPC.

Sherwood, P.R., Given, B.A., Doorenbos, A.Z. and Given, C. (2004) 'Forgotten voices: lessons from bereaved caregivers of person with a brain tumour'. *International Journal of Palliative Nursing*, 10(2), pp.67–75.

Skilbeck, J., Mott, L., Smith, D., Page, H. and Clark, D. (1997) 'Nursing care for people dying from chronic obstructive airways disease'. *International Journal of Palliative Nursing*, 3(2), pp.100–6.

Sloan, G. (1998) 'Clinical supervision: characteristics of a good supervisor'. *Nursing Standard*, 12(40), 24 June, pp.42–6.

Smith, V. (1995) 'Support for the family in bereavement', in David, J. (editor) *Cancer care: prevention, treatment and palliation*. London: Chapman and Hall, pp.323–49.

Strang, P. (1997) 'Existential consequences of unrelieved cancer pain'. *Palliative Medicine*, 11(4), pp.299–305.

Wilkes, L., White, K. and O'Riordan, L. (2000) 'Empowerment through information: supporting rural families of oncology patients in palliative care'. *Australian Journal of Rural Health*, 8(1), pp.41–6.

World Health Organization (1990) *Cancer pain relief and palliative care*. Geneva: WHO, (Technical report no. 804).

World Health Organization (2002) *Definition of palliative care*, Geneva: WHO. **www.who.int/cancer/palliative/en** accessed 30/6/08.

Wright, H. and Giddens, M. (1994) *First principles for professional practice*. London: Chapman Hall.

Chapter 2

Essential Concepts

Elaine Stevens and Norrie Sutherland

INTRODUCTION

In Chapter 1 we set the scene for palliative care. We described what it was, explained who provided it, how and where. We stressed the importance of a holistic approach to palliative care. In this chapter we move on to look at several concepts that are essential in the practice of palliative care.

Palliative care is usually delivered by a team and, consequently, effective communication and effective teamwork are vital. For a patient to experience seamless care there must be no gaps in care, no pieces of information that get lost through poor communication. In Chapter 1 we mentioned the impact on care of the nurse's attitude and, in this chapter, we extend that concept to look at several models of nursing, with a view to enabling you to select and implement the model that will most enhance the palliative care you provide to patients. We review the variety of coping mechanisms that patients and families might use, so that you will better understand what they are doing and why, and so that you will be more able to support them. We consider a tool that you can use to analyse complex ethical dilemmas and, finally, we introduce the concept of reflective practice. It is important for all health care professionals to be ethical, reflective practitioners if we wish to improve patients' quality of life.

LEARNING OUTCOMES

When you have completed this chapter, you will be able to:
- explain the importance of effective teamwork and effective communication in palliative care;
- interpret the variety of reactions to loss and relate these to the use of coping mechanisms by patients and family members in the context of palliative care;
- compare and contrast a number of models of nursing and consider whether they are appropriate in palliative care;

- critically evaluate the ethical implications of your practice of palliative care;
- use a model of reflective practice to foster continuous improvement in your nursing practice.

Preparation

In Activity 2, we ask you to talk to some patients about the care they receive from the specialist palliative care team. Before you do this, discuss it with your manager and colleagues so that they are aware of what you are doing and why. If it is likely that patients will be disturbed beyond what would be normally required for clinical management, you should seek approval from your organisation's ethics committee before starting this activity.

In Activity 9, we ask you to obtain a copy of the following book: Seedhouse, D. (1998) *Ethics: the heart of health care* (2nd Ed.). Chichester: Wiley.

We suggest you start looking into how to get hold of a copy now, so that you have the book when you reach the activity.

The final activity, Activity 11, is a reflection upon a critical incident from practice. In it, we ask you to reflect upon an incident that had negative outcomes for a patient's quality of life. You may already have such an incident in mind, where you know things could be done to improve the outcomes for the patient, or other patients, in the future. We recommend that you bear this incident in mind throughout this chapter. The activity asks you to perform a literature search for the evidence on which your actions during the incident were based. It's probably a good idea to start your literature search now too, so that you are prepared for the activity when you reach the end of the chapter.

EFFECTIVE TEAMWORK

The WHO guidelines (2002) state that palliative care requires a team approach, which recognises that all health care workers have a role to play. Each person brings with them skills and knowledge that may be useful to the patient at some point, and the combined skills and knowledge of the team are greater than any individual could ever maintain. The patient and their family contribute a knowledge of the patient's past and current experiences, and their hopes for the future. Only patients can identify which needs are of the greatest importance to them and, without this information, it is not possible to design a care package which will best meet all of their needs.

Furthermore, the WHO guidelines (2002) indicate that in palliative care leadership of the team may vary depending on the patient's problems and needs. Again, this is very different from the curative model, where the consultant or GP is often the team leader. If leadership varies according to the patient's problems and needs, it therefore varies according to the knowledge and skills of the team members – rather than depending on seniority, or job title, for example. This flexibility means that every member of the team needs to understand how teams function, and how to run an effective team.

Activity 1: Your team

The aim of this activity is to enable you to identify all the members of your own team, and to identify what everyone does. Explain to everyone what you are doing before you start the activity. Explain that the aim is to improve the quality of care received by the patient. (People may fear that it is to check up on what they are doing.)

Note down the name and responsibilities of each member of your team, make brief notes on how you interact with them and on what you think they do in relation to patient care. The next time you see them, ask them what they do. (If you feel silly about doing this, explain that this activity requires a description in their own words.) Ask them what they think you do. (You may be surprised by their answers!)

Try to build up a picture of the tasks that your team performs. As well as asking your colleagues what they do, you could follow the care of a patient for five days or so. Note down what members of the team they see and what each member does for them. Is there anyone the patient didn't see but whom you think they ought to have seen?

Identify any areas of overlap, where tasks may be being duplicated, or gaps – tasks that you thought were being carried out (or believe should be carried out) that you have discovered are not being performed.

Feedback

Discuss any gaps in care or areas of overlap with your manager and colleagues to try to identify ways in which the team can be made more effective. Remember that you should all be focusing on providing the best possible quality of care for the patient. Compare your findings with those of the other members of your AL set.

In the next activity we ask you to interview patients. Discuss this with your manager and colleagues before approaching any patients. If you feel that the patient will be disturbed beyond what would be normally required for clinical management, you should seek approval from your organisation's ethics committee before starting the activity.

Activity 2: What does the patient want?

You now know who supports the patients and what they do for them. In this activity you are going to find out if this is what the patients want, and, if not, what they do want.

Ask a few of your patients if they would mind helping you with your work on this book by answering a few questions. If they are happy to help, ask them the following questions, but try to guide them to focus on tasks rather than personalities.

- What aspects of the care you receive are you most happy with?
- What aspects of the care you receive are you least happy with?
- Are there things that you would like team members to do for you that they don't currently do?

Feedback

Patients may describe personal characteristics of team members rather than the tasks that they perform. Make notes on the aspects of care (rather than personalities) that patients say they like or dislike. Discuss these aspects with your manager and colleagues, and agree how the patients' comments can be acted upon. Bear in mind, however, that patients may say what they think you want to hear.

A common request is simply for health care professionals to be able to spend more time with patients, talking to them and, perhaps more importantly, listening to them. Being empathic and caring towards patients is an important aspect of palliative care. We will look at the importance of the therapeutic relationship later in this chapter and in greater depth in Chapter 5. Unfortunately, nurses and other caregivers are often under so much pressure that they just don't have the time they would like to have with patients, and are so stressed that appearing caring seems almost impossible. These are often symptoms of a team that is not functioning effectively.

Researching the factors that affect the effectiveness of teams, Ajemian (1996) identified the following potential problem areas.

- **Role ambiguity.** Roles are poorly defined and team members are unable to focus on the purpose of their role within the care framework. Some people encroach into other people's areas, taking on too much work. Other people guard the boundaries of their role zealously, perhaps letting certain necessary tasks go undone because it is not their area. Other tasks may remain undone because everyone believes that someone else is doing them. This ambiguity has a negative impact on the quality of patient care.
- **Role conflict.** The ideas and inputs of each discipline are not considered equal. This may occur, for example, where there are differences in

educational background, professional qualifications, culture or social class. This may lead to the care being provided not covering all aspects of the patient's needs. It is particularly problematic if the patient's inputs are considered unimportant, or if the patient is unable to articulate their opinions.

- **Role excess.** One team member is given an excessive – unmanageable – workload. They will therefore be unable to meet all their commitments, thus delaying plans of care and compromising the quality of care provided. Furthermore, some people may actively choose to take on an excessive workload, perhaps because they feel unable to delegate.

- **Team decision making.** In hierarchical teams, the leader traditionally makes all the decisions, with little consultation with the other members. In palliative care teams, all members are equal so the decision-making process can become protracted, sometimes to such an extent that it impinges on the quality of care. When dealing with patients who may have only a little time left, it may be important to move quickly.

Activity 3: Problems related to professional roles

Look back to the work you did in Activity 1. Can you now identify any of the gaps or overlaps you noted as being due to role ambiguity, role conflict or role excess? Make brief notes under each heading, identifying what happened and why you think it happened.

Bearing in mind the definitions of these problems, what ways can you suggest in which problems within your team might be solved? Discuss these issues with your AL set.

Feedback

We would suggest that frank and open discussions in team meetings may help with these problems. Role ambiguity can be reduced if everyone agrees what each individual is responsible for, and it is ensured that no gaps are left. Role conflict can be reduced through negotiation and compromise, and through the determination of those who are having trouble being heard. If certain members of the team have difficulty making themselves heard, perhaps an assertiveness training session will help. Role excess can be managed if the overloaded person can delegate tasks to another person of their own discipline, or to another person in the multidisciplinary team. If they do not want to delegate, find out why not. Some individuals think that they know everything, and don't trust others' knowledge, skills or commitment. Negotiation and compromise should help improve the situation, although it may be necessary to set up a process through which work can be shared more evenly by all team members.

Activity 4: Decision making in a multidisciplinary team

Think about how decisions are made in your team.

Are appropriate members of the team – including the patient – involved in decision making? If not, why not, and what can be done to make sure that they are included?

Does the team have trouble reaching decisions? If so, why do you think that is?

Are any steps being taken to speed up the decision-making process? If so, what are they?

What steps do you think should be taken in a team with a flat hierarchy to make the decision-making process as efficient as possible?

Discuss these issues with your AL set and your colleagues.

Feedback

Many teams have trouble reaching decisions and sometimes this is because of the personalities within the team. However, if a team can agree a process for decision making, that's a good start. We would suggest a process that, for each decision, involves identifying:

- who has the information which will enable the decision to be made;
- who needs to be consulted before the decision is made;
- who needs to be informed after the decision has been made.

Team decision making can be accelerated by ensuring that everyone who should be involved is involved at the correct point in the process. This should ensure that the correct decision is reached in the minimum amount of time, therefore optimising the quality of care provided for the patient.

Activity 5: The importance of good teamworking

From your work on this book so far, and from your experience of caring for patients who are terminally ill or have life-threatening illnesses, why would you say good teamwork is important in palliative care?

Feedback

Good teamwork – 'seamless care' – is essential in palliative care because it directly affects the quality of care received by the patient. It ensures that everyone knows who does what and that no gaps are left. Equality and respect among members in the team ensures that all aspects of patient care are covered. Team members are not overworked and all tasks are completed as agreed. The team makes the right decisions as quickly as possible, thereby making care more efficient and improving the patient's quality of life.

Many teamworking problems are rooted in communication problems. We will look at communication next.

EFFECTIVE COMMUNICATION

Effective communication is a vital component of palliative care and forms the basis of good practice (Wilkinson *et al.*, 1999). Effective communication between the members of the team, including the patient and their family, can lead to:

- a trusting relationship between the patient and the nurse;
- the patient (and their family) receiving the information they need;
- the prevention of collusion;
- effective teamwork;
- a high standard of care for the patient and therefore an improved quality of life.

A trusting relationship is essential if the patient needs to discuss personal or distressing issues with you (Clayton *et al.*, 2005). Parle *et al.* (1996) found that patients who feel unable to discuss such issues, and who are left with unanswered problems, become anxious and depressed. However, Booth *et al.* (1996) found that nurses commonly use techniques which block communication and that this occurred more often when patients were disclosing their feelings. They found that:

> they [nurses] find it difficult to deal with their patient's concerns and feelings.
>
> Booth *et al.* (1996: 526)

In a study of nurses' empathy for cancer patients' distress, Reid-Ponte (1992) found, much to her surprise, that the more skilled a primary nurse was in 'perceiving, feeling and listening', the more distress patients experienced. She suggested that this was because a good listener may elicit more distress responses from patients. So, as your communication and empathy skills improve, don't be surprised if your patients seem more distressed. You are helping your patients by listening to their problems, and providing an opportunity to discuss them. Furthermore, you may be able to identify and refer on problems before they become too serious.

Patients, and their families, understandably want to know about the diagnosis, treatments and the progress of their disease (Faulkner, 1998b). Nichols (1993) found that the provision of accurate information promotes psychological wellbeing in patients.

Wilkinson (1995) found that not receiving enough information is a major source of distress for patients and families, but also that not all patients want to know everything about their illness. So when you are talking to patients you need to judge just how much they want to know. You need to avoid telling them more than they want to know if you are to prevent unnecessary distress. Questions like, 'Would you like me to tell you more?' allow patients to govern how much information you give them. 'What other concerns do you have?', and other similar questions, enables them to ask for further information if they want to.

If your own relationship with the patient and their family is open and honest, you can promote good communications between the patient and their family. This may prevent collusion, in which the patient or family withhold the full details of the illness or prognosis from each other (Buckman, 1998, 2000). This can lead to the breakdown of trust and damage the relationships between patients and their families. This inevitably causes increased anxiety in everyone involved. Effective communication between nurse and patient is essential in building a therapeutic relationship. Building such a relationship takes time, and trust is an important factor. (We will look at the therapeutic relationship briefly later in this chapter in the 'Nursing models' section, and in greater depth in Chapter 5 on 'Breathlessness'.)

As we mentioned earlier, in the section on 'Effective teamwork', it is important to promote effective communication within the team, to combat role ambiguity, role conflict and role excess, so as to ensure that all aspects of the patient's care are fully covered. It is also important to foster good communications with health care professionals whom you may not immediately consider to be a member of the team, such as nursing home matrons, who are in contact with the patient, or who may need to be in the future. Communication between all sectors involved ensures continuity of care for the patient. Furthermore, Nichols (1993) found that patients tend to be less anxious if they know that all the professionals involved in their care are in contact with each other. However, this doesn't mean telling everyone everything. Before sharing information about a patient, you should consider the ethical issues of who has right of access to the information, who the patient wants informed, and the issue of patient-held records. (We will consider ethics later on in this chapter.)

Activity 6: Ensuring effective communication

We have suggested that communication is important in palliative care because it can ensure:

- a trusting relationship between patients and their carers;
- the patient (and their family) receiving the information they need;
- the prevention of collusion;
- effective teamwork;
- a high standard of care for the patient and therefore an improved quality of life.

Identify a recent problem you encountered where it was clear that poor communication was a major contributory factor. Make notes on how this problem could be avoided in the future.

Feedback

You may have identified a situation in which something important to or for a patient in your care was not known, perhaps because the patient, their family or a colleague failed to pass on a piece of information. This may have seriously reduced the quality of care they experienced. Strategies for avoiding such failures in communication include making sure you ask questions about any factors that are important to the patient or may have an impact on the patient's quality of life, rather than waiting for others to tell you. Your attitude can make an important difference too. If patients and their families feel that you are open, honest, trustworthy, warm and caring, they are more likely to share information with you.

Often communication goes wrong and misunderstandings arise – after all, we are human. Reflecting on what happens when communication goes wrong can help you to learn – and help you to avoid making the same mistakes again. We look at a model of reflective practice at the end of this chapter.

If you want to learn more about communication skills, we would suggest the following materials as further reading: Faulkner (1998a), Buckman (1998, 2000) and Wilkinson (1995).

COPING WITH THE LOSSES ASSOCIATED WITH LIFE-THREATENING ILLNESS

A life-threatening illness is inevitably associated with loss. Weston *et al.* (1998: 4) suggest that 'to lose something or somebody is to be deprived of and separated from a presence, often taken for granted, around which or whom we have organised our lives'. This signifies a change and interruption to our lives, which give rise to reactions and feelings while our lives are being reorganised and we adjust to the loss (Weston *et al.*, 1998). Parkes (1998) refers to this as changes in our assumptive world. Many unique losses are incurred by individuals when they are threatened with a life-threatening illness – too many to list them all here. However, some examples are given in Table 2.1.

Area	Physical	Psychological	Social	Spiritual
Loss of:	Health. Body function, leading to disability.	Role. Self-worth. Self-esteem.	Friends. Hobbies. Place in society.	Religious faith. Hope. Life ambitions.

Table 2.1 Examples of losses associated with life-threatening illnesses

Folkman and Greer (2000) define 'coping' as the way in which individuals employ their thoughts and behaviours in order to manage a crisis that is causing distress, thus affecting the outcome of the situation. Ways of coping often include trying to manage the emotions from the crisis as well as problem-solving to deal with what is causing the crisis. For example, when a patient is told that they have an illness that is going to result in death, this creates a crisis for them and may include changes in financial security, physical ability/disability and so on. Emotions will be provoked and these will lead to practical changes that need to be addressed. The severity of the reaction to a loss is determined by the importance the person attaches to that which is being lost (Bowlby, 1969; 1973; 1980).

To give you a deeper understanding of the concept of coping with associated losses, and the way in which heightened anxiety may result from this process, we will consider three models of coping with loss:

- Kubler-Ross's five-stage model (1970);
- Parkes' four-stage model (1998);
- Buckman's three-stage model (1988, 1998).

Note that these mechanisms are not tools intended for your use. They are models that you can use to help you understand what a patient might be going through. A knowledge of the ways in which people cope with their losses will enable you to provide better support. People experience and express many emotions (e.g. fear, anger, guilt), and exhibit many different reactions (e.g. denial, acceptance), when dealing with loss and grief. These models will enable you to identify and validate these emotions and reactions, and thereby understand the patient more fully.

Kubler-Ross's five-stage model

Kubler-Ross (1970) suggested that in order to come to accept the losses incurred during a terminal illness, the individual had to work through five stages of grief.

1 Denial – 'it can't be happening to me'.
2 Anger – levelled at anyone whom the patient believes is not doing enough to help them.
3 Depression.
4 Bargaining – a temporary pretence that makes the patient feel that they still influence their life pattern through their behaviour.
5 Acceptance – a sense of peace and tranquillity that emerges when the patient accepts the loss that has been incurred.

However, Kubler-Ross (1970) indicated that to reach acceptance, the patient did not have to move through these stages in the above order, only that all stages had to be experienced to allow the patient to come to accept the loss. Recently this model has been out of favour, primarily because it has been abused. It has been used prescriptively to ensure people experiencing loss move through all the stages systematically so that they recover as quickly as possible from grief, but with little regard to the person as an individual, with their own personal experiences and emotional make-up. Furthermore, Buckman (1988, 1998) noted that the model omits to mention a number of emotions that people encountered when experiencing a life-threatening illness, namely fear, guilt, hope, despair and humour. Despite the criticisms of Kubler-Ross's (1970) model, knowledge of this model can be useful and can allow you to understand more fully some of the reactions patients may have to the losses incurred during their illness.

> The knowledge of these emotions and how they affect palliative care patients enhances the insight that health care professionals have, allowing them to address patients' needs more effectively.
>
> Co-ordinator, palliative day care

Parkes' four-stage model

Parkes (1998) conceived a model of the grief process, through his investigations of grief in palliative care. It describes how an individual comes to accept a loss, whether it has occurred through bereavement or during a life-threatening illness, by providing a model which separates the feelings generated by the person trying to cope with loss into four stages.

1 Numbness – disbelief in the situation.
2 Acute grief – including the urge to scream or cry, heart searching, anger, guilt, anxiety, restlessness, palpitations, nausea, insomnia and tiredness.
3 Depression and despair – characterised by the expressions of mourning.
4 Resolution – this occurs when the person has worked through the previous stages and is distinguished by their ability to recognise their loss without being distressed by it.

This model describes other emotions that may be experienced during different phases of the grief period, and recognises that anxiety is one of the emotions that individuals naturally experience when adjusting to the losses incurred during a terminal illness. Movement through the stages may take many years.

Buckman's three-stage model

Buckman (1998), having extensively investigated coping mechanisms within palliative care, offered a new three-stage model of the process of dying, which was based on two main propositions.

- Patients who are dying display a variety of responses and reactions which are individual to them and are not exhibited as a result of the diagnosis or being at a particular stage of the dying process.
- Proceeding through the dying process is identified, not by an alteration in the variety or kind of emotions, but in the patient's ability to resolve their feelings.

This three-stage model is illustrated in Table 2.2.

This model indicates that the following are all natural responses:

- the emotional experience of coping with loss (i.e. fear, despair and anxiety);
- the behavioural strategies that individuals may employ to help them cope with their losses (i.e. denial, bargaining, humour, anger);
- dealing with problems that they can resolve.

Individuals will employ coping strategies that they have used successfully in the past when threatened with loss or other stressors.

The use of denial is a legitimate coping mechanism for patients who are unable to face the enormity of their situation (Faulkner, 1998b). As long as it does not interfere with the patient's emotional wellbeing, it is better

Initial Stage (Facing the threat)	Chronic Stage (Being ill)	Final Stage (Acceptance)
A mixture of reactions which are characteristic of the individual and which may include any or all of: • fear; • anxiety; • shock; • disbelief; • anger; • denial; • guilt; • humour; • bargaining; • hope/despair.	Resolution of those elements which are resolvable. Diminution of intensity of all emotion (monochrome state). Depression is very common.	Defined by the patient's acceptance of death. Not an essential state provided that the patient is not distressed, is communicating normally, and is making decisions normally.

Table 2.2 Buckman's three-stage model (1988, 1998)

not to challenge this strategy. Faulkner found that as the disease process advances, this denial usually diminishes, as the patient is able to face the reality of their situation. Heightened anxiety may result from this process of adjustment. In some situations denial is not a helpful strategy. For example, if a single parent has no one to look after their child after their death, it is important to find a sensitive way around denial so that the patient can begin preparing the child for the parent's death.

The use of humour is 'an appropriate and effective coping mechanism for emotional and physical pain and loss' (Kanninen, 1998: 110). Although it may seem odd for patients who are facing death to appear cheerful, it is their own way of coping with their situation and helps reduce their feelings of anxiety. The use of humour may be a very potent agent in heightening a patient's feelings of wellbeing, reducing feelings of anxiety and increasing feelings of self-worth and motivation. However, nurses must use humour selectively and be sure that its use is appropriate, as not everyone will be able to find anything funny in their situation and some patients may therefore find the use of humour inappropriate and distressing.

Activity 7: Coping with loss

Think about the patients you have worked with recently. Did one of them perhaps display raw emotions that were not understood by the care team?

Review the incident and answer the following questions:

- Can you identify many of the emotions or reactions identified in the three coping models we have discussed?
- Do you now feel that you have a better understanding of why someone might feel about, or react to, a life-threatening illness in a certain way?
- What support do you feel you can offer?

Feedback

You probably identified many of the emotions and reactions we have listed, if not all of them.

The best support you can offer someone – patient or family – is to acknowledge and validate the way they feel from day to day. Each individual is likely to move through different stages in different orders and to spend different periods of time in each one. Remember that we stressed that the models are not tools for you to use. You are supporting the patient's own coping mechanisms, not making them jump through theoretical hoops.

The following extracts are taken from the article 'The angry person' (Faulkner *et al.*, 1995). This article emphasises the importance of acknowledging anger, with a view to defusing it, identifying its causes and managing those causes.

It is important to acknowledge the anger and, when appropriate, to acknowledge its legitimacy. This gives individuals permission to express their feelings.

Complaints can be a legitimate cause of anger. If the complaint is about the behaviour of a health professional, it is important to avoid the temptation to defend colleagues since this is only likely to spiral the anger upwards, e.g. 'Yes, go on and defend him – you lot all stick together!' It is still possible to show understanding without being defensive, e.g. 'I can see that you are angry that your appointment was delayed – and I guess I would be too.'

However, if the . . . professional has been involved in a legitimate error, it is important to apologise by saying, for example, 'Yes, I'm afraid we did get it wrong. We did think he would do better than he has done. I'm sorry.'

Faulkner *et al.* (1995: 83–4)

Other ways of supporting patients' coping mechanisms include building a good relationship with the patient, particularly the use of the therapeutic relationship, as discussed briefly later in this chapter and in detail in Chapter 5. In Walters' (1996) work he emphasises the importance of individuals being able to talk about their loss to someone who cares and who has an understanding of the meaning of that loss. It can be seen from this that the formation of a therapeutic relationship between the nurse and patient is of the utmost importance. Another relevant theme is that of effective teamwork (discussed earlier in this chapter). Good teamwork can ensure that patients are supported whenever they need it. Furthermore, as it can be extremely difficult and emotionally draining to support someone who is distressed, good teamwork will ensure that you are supported and helped to deal with your own stressors while helping patients who are in anguish. We discussed the importance of caring for carers – professional carers as well as lay carers – in Chapter 1.

NURSING MODELS

A nursing model is a framework or foundation on which you can reflect on elements of your care. The model that you probably know best is the medical model of care. The medical model of care focuses on the part of the human body that is not functioning as it should and relies on drugs, surgery or some other medical form of care to correct the problem. The focus is on the disease rather than on the patient and sometimes little attention is paid to how the patient's mood, social circumstances, relationships, intellect and spiritual needs may impinge on their illness. The medical model is a 'reductionist' model of care, so-called because it reduces the focus to physical/medical concerns only.

In this book we promote the concept of holistic care, where the patient is seen as more than a collection of cells and tissues, some of which may be diseased. Instead, we acknowledge the patient as a person of worth. A patient is not 'the appendix in bed 7', but 'Mr Andrews who has had an appendectomy'.

In this section we will consider four models of nursing:

- the activities of living model (Roper *et al.*, 1996);
- the supportive care model (Davies and Oberle, 1992);
- the psychotherapeutic model;
- the therapeutic model.

We will look at the first two in some depth and at the second two more briefly. More information on the therapeutic model, and recommended reading about it, is provided in Chapter 5 'Breathlessness'.

Activities of living model

This model is based on the following activities of living (Roper *et al.*, 1996):

- maintaining a safe environment – health, safety and hygiene issues;
- communicating – talking, writing and body language;
- breathing;
- eating and drinking;
- eliminating – urinary and faecal elimination;
- personal cleansing and dressing;
- controlling body temperature;
- mobilising – movement produced by the use of groups of muscles;
- working and playing;
- expressing sexuality – through physical appearance, strength, odour and clothes, through communication, in relationships and in choices relating to work and play, as well as through sexual intercourse;
- sleeping;
- dying.

The activities of living can be used very effectively within the framework of the nursing process, with the nurse and patient working together to discover which areas require intervention and support. Although every activity of living is important in the process of living, some are more vital to life than others. The activity of breathing is obviously of prime importance.

Problems with this model include the fact that Roper herself is strongly opposed to a non-scientific approach to nursing assessment and care. This militates against nurses using their intuition. Furthermore, the model primarily focuses on the individual, rather than on relationships and psychological support. It is most effective as a prompt, where nurses have excellent communication skills, such as an ability to ask questions that can provide a depth that is lacking in the model itself. However, not all nurses have such excellent communication skills, or are experienced enough to see what may be lacking in the model.

The supportive care model

This model is based on a research study which investigated the supportive role of the nurse in palliative care (Davies and Oberle, 1990). The authors discovered components of the role that could be applied in almost any field of care. They identified the following dimensions of care (see Figure 2.1):

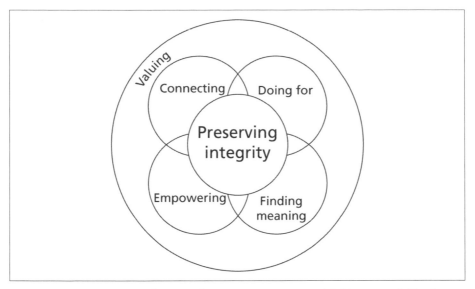

Figure 2.1 Dimensions of care in the supportive care model (Davies and Oberle, 1990: 89). Republished with permission of the Oncology Nursing Society, from Davies, B. and Oberle, K. (1990) 'Dimensions of the supportive role of the nurse in palliative care', *Oncology Nursing Forum*, 17(1), pp.87–94; permission conveyed through Copyright Clearance Center, Inc. **www.ons.org** (Site accessed 30/6/08)

- valuing – believing in patients' worth and in their strength and capabilities;
- connecting – forming a relationship with patients;
- empowering – helping patients to find or build strength or skills within themselves or nurses doing the same for themselves;
- doing for – providing physical care and technological interventions, but with the full involvement of the patient, so that it is empowering rather than disempowering;
- finding meaning – helping patients to make sense of what is happening to them in the context of the health care system;
- preserving integrity – nurses must maintain their own wholeness if they are to be able to provide support to others and they must enable patients to do the same.

The model involves family members and other informal carers and discusses such areas as developing trust and acknowledging death, as well as the importance for nurses of valuing themselves and acknowledging their own grief reactions. It also includes the 'tasks' of care such as managing pain and symptoms. Davies and Oberle (1990) state that the nurse as 'person' cannot be separated from the nurse as 'professional' and that belief in the worth of others is paramount if the nurse is to successfully deliver care in the palliative care setting.

Psychotherapeutic and therapeutic models

These are complex and ever-expanding areas, so we will only give you a brief introduction here. Psychotherapy is a term used to describe any method of psychological treatment that relies primarily on talking. Hall (1982) divides psychotherapy into two categories – directive and non-directive – and gives examples for each – rational-emotive therapy and person-centred counselling respectively.

The therapeutic use of self is defined by Travelbee (1971) as the ability to use one's personality consciously and in full awareness, in an attempt to establish relatedness and to structure nursing intervention. It requires:

- self-insight;
- self-understanding;
- an understanding of the dynamics of human behaviour;
- the ability to interpret one's own behaviour as well as the behaviour of others;
- the ability to intervene effectively in nursing situations.

In essence, therapeutic means 'being with' (rather than 'doing for'), while the psychotherapeutic model uses cognitive and behavioural strategies with the aim of leading to a beneficial outcome. We refer to the use of therapeutic and psychotherapeutic models in Chapters 4–7, and focus specifically on the therapeutic model in Chapter 5, 'Breathlessness'.

Activity 8: Nursing models

Think about the model of nursing that you use in your own practice. Even if you are not aware of using a nursing model, compare your nursing practice with the models described above. Identify which one most closely matches your own practice.

In the context of palliative care, we would recommend that you use the supportive care model, the psychotherapeutic model and/or the therapeutic model, depending upon the situation and the patient. (Although these models are valid in all forms of nursing practice.)

If you are currently using another model, consider how you can move towards the supportive care model or therapeutic model.

Feedback

You are probably aware of the medical model and may use the activities of living model, as this is one of the most commonly used models in the UK. To move towards the supportive care model, the psychotherapeutic model and/or therapeutic model, we recommend that you first perform a literature search to obtain more in-depth information about these models. You will also find it helpful to talk to nurses who use these models in practice. Find out if anyone in your team or AL set uses one of the models, or if they know anyone who does, and discuss with them the impact of the model on their practice.

Discuss your findings with your manager or your AL set facilitator, and agree ways in which you may be able to implement relevant aspects of these models into your practice. For example, in this pack we recommend the therapeutic model as the main approach for supporting patients experiencing breathlessness (see Chapter 5 for full details).

THE ETHICS OF PALLIATIVE CARE

Extraordinary advances in medical science and technology have made it possible to prolong life in the face of previously insurmountable barriers. The advances also present us with many perplexing questions: should every effort be made to save an individual, no matter what deterioration occurs in their quality of life? When survival can be prolonged almost indefinitely by mechanical means, who decides if the machinery should be switched off?

It is generally agreed that four important moral principles should guide medical decision making: respect for autonomy, justice and beneficence/non-maleficence (Beauchamp and Childress, 2001).

- **Autonomy** – Kendrick (1995) suggests that autonomy involves the self-governing person deciding on his/her course of action based on a plan chosen by him/herself, and that the autonomous person also considers and chooses plans and is able to act on the basis of those thoughts and considerations. Respecting others' autonomy acknowledges their right to their own choices, opinions, values, goals and freedom to act without interference. In medicine, respect for autonomy allows patients to make their own decisions in consonance with their values.
- **Justice** – this principle requires that all people be treated fairly. All similar cases should be treated similarly, the needs of all should be taken into consideration in allocating scarce resources and everyone should receive equal access to the benefits of medicine. Fair treatment also includes the concepts of privacy and confidentiality.
- **Beneficence/non-maleficence** – This is the concept of the duty to do good (beneficence), and the duty to do no harm (non-maleficence). Kendrick (1995) suggests the difficulty here lies in balancing the harm an action may do with the good that it may do. This introduces the concept of consequentialism, where one judges the rightness or

wrongness of an act only on the grounds of whether its consequences produce more benefits than disadvantages.

The National Council for Hospice and Specialist Palliative Care Services (NCHSPCS) has published guidelines on conducting research in palliative care (NCHSPCS, 1995) that also have these ethical principles as their major tenets.

The ethical grid

Figure 2.2 illustrates the ethical grid (Seedhouse and Lovett, 1992). Seedhouse (1998) suggests that when considering the ethics of a situation using the grid as a tool, it is possible to consider that the most significant principles are those at the centre of the grid. The outer boxes are of decreasing importance as you move (or spiral) to the outer limit of the grid. However, he acknowledges that this method may not be appropriate in all cases. Furthermore, each box is independent and detachable, although all the boxes have strong relationships with each other.

Seedhouse makes it clear that it is not claimed that the grid represents a new advance in ethical reasoning, rather he asserts that it makes some processes of moral reasoning more clear for those who are unfamiliar with the discipline. If you look at the grid you will see that it echoes the ethical principles above: autonomy, beneficence/non-maleficence and justice.

Activity 9: The ethical grid

Obtain a copy of the following book: Seedhouse, D. (1998) *Ethics: the heart of health care* (2nd Ed.). Chichester: Wiley.

Read Chapters 9 and 10, making notes on what you consider to be the most important points.

Identify an incident from practice that put you in a moral dilemma. Make notes of what happened, how you felt and what you did.

Use the moral grid to analyse the situation. Refer to the case studies in Chapter 10 if that helps – often the implementation of an abstract concept is easier to follow when presented as an incident from real life.

Start by considering the issue without reference to the grid. Make notes on what you feel would have been the best course of action and give reasons for your choice.

Then consider the issues using the grid as a tool. Consider the core issues first (probably, but not necessarily, the inner four boxes), followed by the other issues. Finally, make your

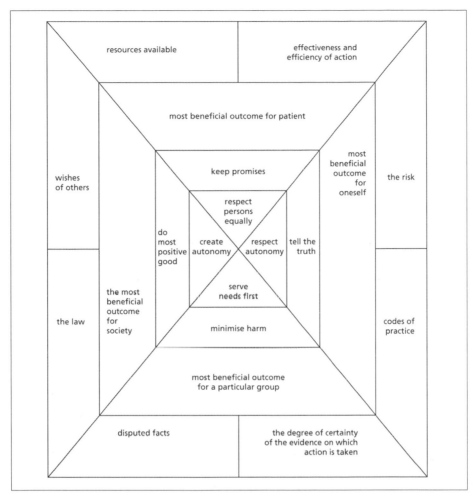

Figure 2.2 The ethical grid (Seedhouse and Lovett, 1992, cited in Seedhouse, 1998: 209, Figure 30). From *Ethics: the heart of health care* (2nd Ed.) by Seedhouse, D. (1998). © John Wiley & Sons Limited. Reproduced with permission. **eu.wiley.com/WileyCDA/ WileyTitle/productCd-0471975923.html** (Site accessed 30/6/08)

decision about what was the best (most moral or ethical) action you could have taken in the situation.

Compare the results of your deliberations without the grid and with the grid. Are they are different? Are there points that occurred to you while using the grid that didn't occur when you first thought about the problem? If so, what were they?

Feedback

Seedhouse makes it clear that the tool is not a substitute for your own moral reasoning. It is just something that you can use to help you think out issues more clearly and more comprehensively. So don't be surprised if you uncovered factors that you had not previously considered with respect to the practice incident when you used the grid.

> ... it is an aid both to understanding and to confidence ... it can throw light into unseen corners, and it can suggest new avenues of thought.
>
> Seedhouse (1998: 129 and 140)

If you wish to improve your abilities in moral reasoning, it is important to practise. Seedhouse suggests that you bring the ethical grid into play at every opportunity:

> For instance, when reading of moral issues in newspapers, or when watching television documentaries, or when reading literature, or when considering friends' problems in life, or when considering the way in which one deals with situations in one's own life.
>
> Seedhouse (1998: 142)

You can practise on hypothetical cases, or on incidents from your past, as in Activity 9. Seedhouse suggests that your ultimate goal should be to become proficient in moral reasoning so that you no longer need to refer to the grid.

Activity 10: Moral reasoning

Practise using the ethical grid as suggested by Seedhouse (when watching TV, reading, etc.). Apply it to ethical considerations within your own practice with patients who are receiving palliative care. Select an incident from the past or the present involving a moral dilemma. Discuss the incident with your AL set, using the ethical grid as a tool to comprehensively analyse the ethics of the situation.

You may also like to select topics that raise ethical issues, such as:

• Resuscitation. Is there a point at which you can say resuscitation should not be attempted for a particular patient? How do you decide when that point is reached? Who decides?
• Euthanasia/physician-assisted suicide. Should patients be allowed or enabled to end their own lives? On what grounds? Should their relatives be involved? Should health care professionals be involved?
• Resources. How should sometimes scarce palliative care resources be used? Who decides and how?
• Access. Do all patients have equal access to palliative care? If not, why not, and how can this inequality be redressed?

Feedback

In time and with practice you should become proficient at identifying the ethical implications of your actions (and of those of others). This is essential not only for health care professionals working in the area of palliative care, but for all health care professionals.

Resuscitation, euthanasia, resources and access are major, often interlinked, ethical issues in palliative care, and are too large to be covered here. There are many websites addressing these topics, and a few useful and interesting ones are listed below.

---

www.bma.org.uk
Provides a link to BMA guidance on ethical issues. (Full details of the book on withdrawing and withholding life-prolonging treatment is in 'Recommended sources of information'.) Site accessed 30/6/08.

www.patient.co.uk
Patient UK is a directory of UK health, disease and related websites. It is edited by two GPs. The entry for euthanasia, for example, provides links to Christian, ethical and moral aspects of health care. Site accessed 30/6/08.

www.donoharm.org.uk
The aim of 'First Do No Harm' is to bring together doctors who are opposed to the current campaign for euthanasia, and to exchange information. Site accessed 30/6/08.

www.rcn.org.uk
Provides guidance on ethical decision making for nurses in the United Kingdom. Site accessed 30/6/08.

A MODEL OF REFLECTIVE PRACTICE

Using reflective practice allows you to look back on an incident (reflection on action) in a structured way, investigating:

- what actually happened;
- what you thought and how you felt about the experience;
- the appropriateness of the actions you took during the incident, and the effectiveness of the care you provided, based on the evidence that underpins good practice;
- what you learned from the incident and how you can improve your future practice.

This model encourages you to evaluate current practice in relation to research and other literary evidence and, more importantly, to improve future practice.

Marks-Maran and Rose (1997) designed a simple model of reflective practice (Figure 2.3).

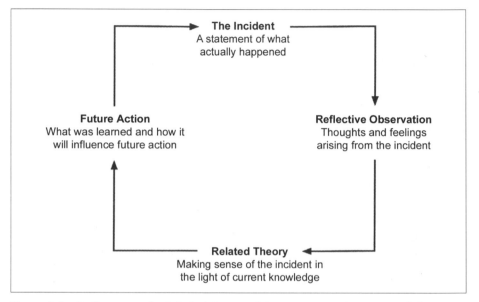

Figure 2.3   Reflective cycle (Marks-Maran and Rose, 1997:128). Reprinted from Marks-Maran, D. and Rose, P. (1997) *Reconstructing nursing: beyond art and science*, with permission from Elsevier. **www.elsevier.com** (Site accessed 30/6/08)

Activity 11: Reflective practice

Using the model of reflective practice we have given you (or another that you are already familiar with, if you prefer) reflect upon a recent incident which had negative outcomes for a patient's quality of life.

Start off by making brief notes on what actually happened, focusing on the actions that you took (or didn't take) and their consequences.

Then note down what you thought about the experience, and how it made you feel.

If you have not already done so, perform a literature search to identify the evidence surrounding the type of incident you have chosen. Comparing your actions with the evidence you have identified in the literature, consider their appropriateness and the effectiveness of the care you provided. Ask yourself questions like:

- What actions did I consider?
- Why did I choose to take some actions?
- Why did I decide against some actions?
- Who else was involved – other health care professionals? The patient's family and friends?
- What were their interests/involvement in the incident?

Compare your answers with the evidence you have found. Remember, however, that your overriding concern is the patient's quality of life. It is possible that the decisions you took, even though not recommended in the literature, may have been the best choice for that particular patient in that particular situation. Remember that your own experience is valuable evidence.

Now makes note on what you learned from the incident, either through simply reflecting upon it or from your review of evidence.

Reflect upon how you could improve the outcomes should a similar incident occur in the future. Make notes on the ways in which the steps you identify have been influenced by what you have learned in Chapter 1 and in this chapter:

- your new understanding of what is meant by palliative care and the importance of a positive attitude towards palliative care and patients receiving palliative care;
- your knowledge of palliative care professions, teams and settings;
- the value of effective teamwork and communication;
- the importance of holistic palliative care and caring for the carers;
- nursing models;
- coping strategies;
- ethics in palliative care.

Feedback

Don't be concerned if you found this activity more challenging than you were expecting. Becoming self-reflective and self-critical is quite difficult to begin with, and it takes time to change practice. We recommend that you consider keeping a reflective or learning diary (see the 'Introduction to this text book', page xxii, for full details). Keeping such a diary can be a part of making a real commitment to the process of becoming self-reflective and self-critical.

SUMMARY

In this chapter we looked at several concepts that are essential for you to grasp and to implement to become an effective, ethical, reflective practitioner. Having completed this chapter, you should be able to:

- explain the importance of effective teamwork and effective communication in palliative care;
- interpret the variety of reactions to loss and relate these to the use of coping mechanisms by patients and family members in the context of palliative care;
- compare and contrast a number of models of nursing and consider whether they are appropriate in palliative care;
- critically evaluate the ethical implications of your practice of palliative care;
- use a model of reflective practice to foster continuous improvement in your nursing practice.

RECOMMENDED SOURCES OF INFORMATION

Titles followed by O/P are out of print – but you may be able to find library copies.

On communication

Brewin, T. and Sparshott, M. (1996) *Relating to the relatives: breaking bad news, communication and support*. Oxford: Radcliffe Medical.

Faulkner, A. (1998) *Effective interaction with patients* (2nd Ed.). New York: Churchill Livingstone.

On teamworking

Belbin, R.M. (1993) *Team roles at work*. Oxford: Butterworth-Heinemann.

Blanchard, C. and Johnson, S. (2000) *The one minute manager builds high performance teams*. London: HarperCollins Business.

Johnson, S. (1998) *Who moved my cheese?* London: Random.

Morris, S., Willcocks, G. and Knasel, E. (1999) *How to lead a winning team*. London: Prentice Hall. O/P

Newstrom, J. and Scannell, E. (1998) *The big book of team building games*. London: McGraw-Hill.

Robbins, H. and Finley, M. (2000) *Why teams don't work*. London: Texere.

www.reviewing.co.uk/reviews/teambuilding.htm

Provides reviews and links to a number of recent books on teamwork and teambuilding. Site accessed 13/5/08.

On the therapeutic relationship

Sources for this topic can be found at the end of Chapter 5.

On ethics

The *Journal of Medical Ethics*

> *Journal of Medical Ethics* is a leading international journal that reflects the whole field of medical ethics. The journal seeks to promote ethical reflection and conduct in scientific research and medical practice. It features original articles on ethical aspects of health care, as well as case conferences, book reviews, editorials, correspondence, news and notes. To ensure international relevance *JME* has Editorial Board members from all around the world including the US, Europe, Australasia and Far East.
>
> Taken from the website, **jme.bmjjournals.com/info/about.dtl** Access to articles via the website is by paid subscription only. Site accessed 13/5/08.)

British Medical Association (2001) *Withholding and withdrawing life-prolonging medical treatment: guidance for decision making* (2nd Ed.). London: BMJ Books.

Randall, F. and Downie, R.S. (1999) *Palliative care ethics: a companion for all specialties* (2nd Ed.). Oxford: Oxford University Press.

Seedhouse, D. (1998) *Ethics: the heart of health care* (2nd Ed.). Chichester: Wiley.

REFERENCES

Ajemian, I. (1996) 'The interdisciplinary team', in Doyle, D., Hanks, G. and MacDonald, N. (editors) *Oxford textbook of palliative medicine.* Oxford: Oxford University Press, pp.17–28.

Beauchamp, T.L. and Childress, J.F. (2001) *The principles of biomedical ethics.* Oxford: Oxford University Press.

Booth, K., Maguire, P.M., Butterworth, T. and Hillier, V.F. (1996) 'Perceived professional support and the use of blocking behaviours by hospice nurses'. *Journal of Advanced Nursing,* 24(3) pp.522–7.

Bowlby, J. (1969) *Attachment and loss, volume 1: attachment.* London: Hogarth Press.

Bowlby, J. (1973) *Attachment and loss, volume 2: separation: anxiety and anger.* London: Hogarth Press.

Bowlby, J. (1980) *Attachment and loss, volume 3: loss: sadness and depression.* London: Hogarth Press.

Buckman, R. (1988) *I don't know what to say.* London: Macmillan.

Buckman, R. (1998) 'Communication in palliative care: a practical guide', in Doyle, D., Hanks, G. and MacDonald, N. (editors) *Oxford textbook of palliative medicine* (2nd Ed.). Oxford: Oxford University Press, pp.141–56.

Buckman, R. (2000) 'Communication in palliative care', in Dickenson, D., Johnson, M. and Katz, J.S. (editors) *Death, dying and bereavement* (2nd Ed.). Buckingham: Open University/Sage Publications.

Clayton, J.M., Butow, P.N. and Tettersall, M.H.N. (2005) 'When and how to initiate discussion about prognosis and end of life issues with terminally ill patients'. *Journal of Pain and Symptom Management*, 30(2), pp.132–44.

Davies, B. and Oberle, K. (1990) 'Dimensions of the supportive role of the nurse in palliative care'. *Oncology Nursing Forum*, Jan.–Feb., 17(1), pp.87–94.

Davies, B. and Oberle, K. (1992) 'Support and caring: exploring the concepts'. *Oncology Nursing Forum*, 19(5), pp.763–7.

Faulkner, A. (1998a) *Effective interaction with patients* (2nd Ed.). Edinburgh: Churchill Livingstone.

Faulkner, A. (1998b) 'Communication with patients, families and other professionals', in Fallon, M. and O'Neill, B. (editors) *ABC of palliative care*. London: BMJ Books, pp.47–9.

Faulkner, A., Maguire, P. and Regnard, C. (1995) 'The angry person', in Regnard, C. and Hockley, J. (editors) *Flow diagrams in advanced cancer and other diseases*. London: Edward Arnold, pp.81–5.

Folkman, S. and Greer, S. (2000) 'Promoting psychological well-being in the face of serious illness: when theory, research and practice inform each other'. *Psycho-Oncology*, 9(1), pp.11–19.

Hall, J. (1982) 'Psychology and nursing', in Hall, J. (editor) *Psychology for nurses and health visitors*. London: Macmillan, pp.7–17.

Kanninen, M. (1998) 'Humour in palliative care: a review of the literature'. *International Journal of Palliative Nursing*, 4(3), pp.110–14.

Kendrick, K. (1995) 'Ethical pathways in cancer and palliative care', in David, J.A. (editor) *Cancer prevention, treatment and palliation*. London: Chapman Hall, pp.224–44.

Kubler-Ross, E. (1970) *On death and dying*. London: Tavistock.

Marks-Maran, D. and Rose, P. (1997) *Reconstructing nursing: beyond art and science*. London: Baillière Tindall.

National Council for Hospice and Specialist Palliative Care Services (1995) *Guidelines on research in palliative care*. London: NCHSPCS.

Nichols, K.A. (1993) *Psychological care in physical illness* (2nd Ed.). London: Chapman and Hall.

Parkes, C.M. (1998) *Bereavement: studies of grief in adult life* (3rd Ed.). London: Penguin.

Parle, M., Jones, B. and Maguire, P. (1996) 'Maladaptive coping and affective disorders among cancer patients'. *Psychological Medicine*, 26(4), pp.735–44.

Reid-Ponte, P. (1992) 'Distress in cancer patients and primary nurses' empathy skills'. *Cancer Nursing*, 15(4), pp.283–92.

Roper, N., Logan, W.W., Tierney, A.J. (1996) *The elements of nursing* (4th Ed.). New York: Churchill Livingstone.

Seedhouse, D. (1998) *Ethics: the heart of health care* (2nd Ed.). Chichester: Wiley.

Seedhouse, D. and Lovett, L. (1992) *Practical medical ethics* Chichester: Wiley, cited in Thomas, A.J. (1997) 'Patient autonomy and cancer treatment decisions'. *International Journal of Palliative Nursing*, 3(6), pp.317–23.

Travelbee, J.P. (1971) *Interpersonal aspects of nursing* (2nd Ed.), Philadelphia: Davis, cited in Marriner-Tomey, A. (editor) (2002) *Nursing theorists and their work* (5th Ed.). St Louis: Mosby.

Walters, T. (1996) 'A new model of grief, bereavement and biography'. *Mortality*, 1(1), pp.7–25.

Weston, R., Martin, T. and Anderson, Y. (1998) *Loss and bereavement: managing change*. Oxford: Blackwell Science.

Wilkinson, S. (1995) 'Communication', in David, J. (editor) *Cancer care: prevention, treatment and palliation*. London: Chapman and Hall, pp.204–23.

Wilkinson, S., Bailey, K., Aldridge, J. and Roberts, A. (1999) 'A longitudinal evaluation of a communication skills programme'. *Palliative Medicine*, 13(4), pp.341–8.

World Health Organization (2002) *Definition of Palliative Care*. Geneva: WHO. **www.who.int/cancer/palliative/en** Site accessed 30/6/08.

Chapter 3

Generic Assessment in Palliative Care

Norrie Sutherland and Elaine Stevens

INTRODUCTION

> The need for holistic assessment [in palliative care] is indisputable,
> but the nurse must do more than simply hear the patient's story.
>
> Maher and Hemming (2005: 318)

The World Health Organization (WHO) (1987) defines assessment as
the initial part of the nursing process, consisting of systematically
collecting information from various sources. Assessment is a vital process,
because you need to know what the patient's needs are before you can
plan effective care. It ensures that treatments are prioritised correctly,
and reflects the patient's right to be in control. Assessment can be
particularly difficult in palliative care because patients may have many
complex problems.

The NHS and Community Care Act (Parliament, 1990) made the needs
assessment for the provision of services a legal requirement for health
boards and health authorities. The Act also requires that patients and
their carers contribute to these assessments.

LEARNING OUTCOMES

When you have completed this chapter, you will be able to:
- explain the need for holistic assessment and patient involvement;
- describe the assessment process, and identify factors that can help
  or hinder assessment;
- perform a general palliative care assessment (screening assessment)
  and identify what should be investigated further in a focused
  assessment.

Further steps in the assessment process are planning effective nursing care and critically evaluating the effectiveness of the nursing interventions. We assume that you are already proficient in planning care and we look at the evaluation of interventions in Chapter 8 'Quality improvement'.

Preparation

In Activity 12 we ask you to read the following article: Dunne, K., Coates, V. and Moran, A. (1997) 'Functional health patterns applied to palliative care: a case study'. *International Journal of Palliative Nursing*, 3(6), pp.324–9.

We suggest that you start looking for it now, so that you have it to hand when you reach the activity.

THE NEED FOR ASSESSMENT

> Health needs assessment is a newly developing approach to planning care. It is based on the rational premise that a comprehensive assessment of needs should precede the implementation of services, allowing these to be more sensitively tailored to local conditions and concerns. In palliative care where what might be called *emotional planning* has often predominated over more systematic approaches, the importance of careful assessment of needs is of major importance.
>
> Clark and Malson (1995: 55; original emphasis)

The aim of assessment is to identify the patient's needs as perceived by the patient, their family and friends and the professional team, so that the patient's care plan can be based on current, accurate information. It also enables you to:

- establish a rapport with the patient;
- give information (as well as receive it);
- give the patient a sense of being understood;
- give the patient hope;
- 'travel' with the patient;
- help the patient to tell their story ('patient narratives').

The meaning that an illness or symptom has for a patient can be enormously significant, and it is important that you explore this area with the patient when performing an assessment. Sadock and Sadock (2005) and Popay and Williams (1994) are among those who have studied the meanings of symptoms and the significance and consequences of those symptoms to patients and families. Lenz *et al.* (1995, 1997) also refer to the meaning of symptoms in their theory of unpleasant symptoms (discussed in Chapter 1). Kleinman's (1988) work on illness narratives, however, is still classed as seminal in the investigations for meaning of illness (Doyle *et al.*, 2004).

Symptoms as meaning

There is evidence to indicate that through examining the particular significances of a person's illness it is possible to break the vicious cycles that amplify distress. The interpretation of illness meanings can also contribute to the provision of more effective care. Through those interpretations the frustrating consequences of disability can be reduced. This key clinical task may even liberate sufferers and practitioners from the oppressive iron cage imposed by a too intensely morbid preoccupation with painful bodily processes and a too technically narrow and therefore dehumanising vision of treatment, respectively.

This alternative therapeutic approach originates in the reconceptualisation of medical care as (1) empathic witnessing of the existential experience of suffering and (2) practical coping with the major psychosocial crises that constitute the menacing chronicity of that experience. The work of the practitioner includes the sensitive solicitation of the patient's and the family's stories of the illness, the assembling of a mini-ethnography of the changing contexts of chronicity, informed negotiation with alternative lay perspectives on care, and what amounts to a brief medical psychotherapy for the multiple, ongoing threats and losses that make chronic illness so profoundly disruptive.

Kleinman (1988: 9–10)

Activity 1: The need for assessment

Read the following quotation and then discuss it with the members of your team.

> Palliative care of patients with cancer has greatly improved over the years. However, patients with serious illnesses (other than cancer) may be relatively disadvantaged in terms of accurate assessment of their needs and the quality of care they receive.
>
> Pearce and Lugton (1999: 63)

Is this true in your experience? If so, discuss with the members of your team what you can do to ensure that all palliative care patients in your clinical area receive appropriate assessment.

Feedback

Patients in your clinical area may be fortunate enough to be assessed thoroughly, regardless of their illness. However, if you are aware that there is an imbalance, everyone in your team should be involved in considering why this is so. Reasons may include a lack of time, pressure of work, a lack of skills or expertise, or a failure to understand the importance of assessment. Sometimes there is a failure to provide palliative care for patients who do not have cancer, or a failure to realise that the care provided for non-cancer patients (e.g. those with heart failure, COPD, advanced HIV disease or MS) is (or should be) palliative care. Discuss with your manager and colleagues whether it would be possible to organise a training session or workshop for the whole team to review skills and share expertise. You could also suggest the creation and implementation of a policy or standard to ensure that assessments are carried out routinely and thoroughly. We will look at setting standards in Chapter 8.

THE HOLISTIC APPROACH

Although Wilkinson *et al.* (1998) found that assessment tended to focus on the physical aspects of care, a holistic approach is important in assessing palliative care patients because of the wide-ranging and complex nature of the problems they may experience. Roper *et al.* (1996) identified the need for assessment of the following areas:

- physical;
- psychological;
- social;
- spiritual;
- the needs of the patient's family.

To this we will add the need for assessment of the patient's cultural background, and any problems associated with professional carers having little knowledge of a patient's culture. You will remember that these are the six areas that we considered as key to a holistic approach in Chapter 1.

Activity 2: The need for holistic assessment

Discuss the concept of addressing all areas of a patient's life (physical, psychological, social, spiritual, cultural and the needs of the family) in the assessment process with your colleagues or with members of your AL set.

Discuss the procedures that are currently followed, and the forms or tools that are used, with the team member who carries out assessments.

If you do not take a holistic approach to assessment, give your reasons.

Discuss with your colleagues or with members of your AL set how barriers to holistic assessment may be overcome.

Feedback

Reasons for omitting items from the assessment process may include thinking it's too time consuming, not having thought to ask about certain areas, feeling uncomfortable or ill-equipped to ask about certain areas, or believing that such a thorough assessment is only necessary for certain patients (e.g. those with cancer).

It should be possible to overcome most barriers to a holistic approach to assessment. Nurses who consider it too time consuming may need more practice and experience. A skilled practitioner may be able to assess all areas of a patient's life with surprising speed and accuracy, as they will be able to pick up subtle cues and make links between issues that a nurse inexperienced in assessment might miss. Nurses who forget to ask about certain areas may need to use a checklist to help them, and those who believe thorough assessment is not necessary for all patients may come round to the idea if you can present the arguments for its importance clearly enough.

Assessing physical needs

Here you are attempting to identify the patient's physical needs, usually by interviewing them and asking them what symptoms they are experiencing, how much the symptoms distress them, what they think is causing them, what makes the symptoms better or worse and so on. Patient involvement is vital here, because they are the only ones who can tell you how they feel. You are unlikely to be able to guess how they feel. For example, Schafheutle *et al.*'s (2004) research on pain assessment by nurses discovered that they greatly underestimated the pain that patients experienced after surgery. And while pain may be underestimated, other symptoms, such as fatigue, are often completely overlooked. (We will look at fatigue in Chapter 6.)

You can also observe the patient during the interview (how they move, for example) and later on you will carry out a short examination. Observation and examination will give you more information on the patient's physical state. For a fuller description of physical assessment, see Dunn (2000).

Activity 3: Physical assessment

You can gain a lot of information about a patient's physical state through interview, observation and examination. Having gathered the information, you need to analyse it rigorously and make appropriate decisions regarding suitable interventions.

Read through the notes of the last two or three assessments you performed, focusing on physical symptoms. Critically evaluate the inferences you made from those symptoms. With the benefit of hindsight, were there any symptoms that you failed to focus on clearly enough, or identify properly? Make a list of these items, together with the consequences for the patient (if known).

Feedback

As every patient is different, any items that you missed may differ from patient to patient. However, if there is a particular item that appears several times in your list, then you should probably pay careful attention to that item with every patient. As we have already mentioned, nurses often underestimate patients' pain. If you are aware that you do this, make a special effort with every patient not to discount how much pain they say they are experiencing. It may help to use formal tools for this and we will look at these later in this chapter and again in Chapter 7.

The management of physical needs can often improve all other areas of the patient's life, for example, lessening anxiety, improving their ability to get out and about to meet friends or to attend cultural festivals or religious meetings. Because of the often profound meanings that physical symptoms may have for patients, the assessment and management of these symptoms can make a huge difference, triggering a far greater improvement in patients' quality of life than you might expect.

Assessing psychological needs

In this part of the assessment you are looking for negative emotions or states that may be impairing the patient's ability to cope:

- depression;
- anxiety;
- emotional withdrawal;
- sadness;
- discontent;
- fear;
- anger.

Such emotions or states may be due to a number of factors, including the diagnosis of a terminal illness, how the patient and the family cope with the news, how the illness affects the patient and the relationships within the family, and so on.

Let's consider examples of areas in which patients may experience and exhibit psychological distress.

- Symptoms which impact upon patients' ability to express themselves sexually may be greatly distressing to the patients and to their partners.
- Patients who become aware of the waning of their intellectual powers may become anxious or depressed. They may have noticed an inability to concentrate, or to complete intellectual tasks that are a normal part of their everyday life, e.g. crosswords or reading.

However, these problems may be due to fatigue, treatment or medication, which may be managed or altered to improve the patient's quality of life. These examples show again how one area can impact on another and highlight the importance of a holistic approach to assessment.

There are special tools, notably the General Health Questionnaire (Goldberg, 1972), that are useful for assessing psychological wellbeing. If you feel you need guidance when assessing a patient's psychological state, you could use one of these tools, perhaps just as a guide to the sorts of questions you could ask. We look in more detail at tools for assessing anxiety and depression in Chapter 4 'Anxiety and depression'.

Activity 4: Assessing psychological needs

What factors do you find most challenging when performing psychological assessment? Make a few notes on this subject.

Feedback

You may be worried that patients will ask difficult questions, e.g. about whether they are dying and how long they have left to live. If you feel uncomfortable about being asked these questions, ask your manager if you can go on an advanced communications skills course. Advanced communication skills incorporate both communication skills and aspects of counselling skills, but do not constitute counselling training. Such a course will help to enhance the skills you have and help you to develop new ones. In our experience, courses that incorporate role-play and the production of audio tapes are the most useful for this purpose.

You may be concerned that you do not have the specialist skills to properly assess a patient's psychological state, or feel you need help, for example when dealing with patients who may be suicidally depressed. Discuss this with the mental health specialist on your team. You should be able to refer patients to the specialist when necessary, or it may be possible for you to receive training in this area.

Assessing social needs

Pearce and Lugton (1999) identify four areas of social need:

- altered relationships/social isolation;
- ill health/disability of another family member;
- loss of work/role;
- financial problems.

We defined these in full in Chapter 1. You might find it helpful to look back at that chapter if it is a while since you worked on it.

Social needs are extremely complex, and are interconnected with each other and with needs in other areas of the patient's life. When discussing these issues with patients, think carefully about how you will ask your questions. For example, 'Are you having financial problems?' may seem rude or threatening. It may be better to tell the patient that people in their situation sometimes have financial difficulties and that you have some information you could bring them if they would like. If you start out by discussing general issues, patients may slowly become more forthcoming and reveal their personal situation. If you start off by being extremely direct, they may not tell you anything at all.

Activity 5: Assessing social needs

Ask a patient whom you know well whether they would be prepared to talk to you in detail about their social needs. Explain what you need to know and why. Find out:

- which members of their family are most affected by the patient's illness (include friends or carers who are not members of the family, if they are close to the patient – the patient may consider them as family);
- how each person is affected (keep the notes you make on what you are told – you will need them for Activity 8);
- what the patient's normal routines and habits were before they became ill and how these have changed;
- if any financial difficulties have arisen because of their illness.

You might find it helpful to keep your notes on this activity in your reflective or learning diary.

Feedback

As you are talking to a patient you know well, you may be surprised by how much more you may be able to find out. You probably knew who among their family was most affected, but you may not have appreciated how badly they were affected, or how much other members of the family (or friends/carers) were affected.

The patient may have been a youth leader, a keen competitor or spectator at some sport, they may have been used to going to evening classes, or dancing, swimming or working out at the gym. They may miss talking to the people they met while walking their dog. They probably miss their friends and colleagues at work. Patients who can no longer make love with their partners, or share other expressions of intimacy, may feel that the relationship has changed, or that a part of it is now missing. They may be concerned that they won't see relatives or friends who live far away before they die.

Patients may be reluctant to discuss their financial difficulties with you, but you need to explain that it may be possible for you to arrange for them or their families to get help – if you know about the problem(s).

This activity may have given you useful information about a patient you know well. Having obtained all this information, it is important that you act upon it. Identify how you can help the patient with their social needs – many of them may be newly identified and may not have been addressed as yet.

Activity 6: Reflection on assessing social needs

Reflect upon your experiences in and following Activity 5. Make notes in your learning diary about:

- what happened – what did you do and say and why? How was your approach different from the usual way in which you approach a patient?
- what you thought and felt about the experience;
- what you learned from the activity;
- how you can improve your practice – is there anything you would do differently next time?
- any questions you would have liked to have asked, but didn't.

Feedback

You may find it helpful to discuss your experience and thoughts with a colleague, or with members of your AL set.

Assessing spiritual needs

In a study by Milligan (2004), it was suggested that nurses felt ill-equipped to deal with the spiritual needs of patients. This may be because spiritual needs are often difficult to assess. The patient may not be aware of what their spiritual needs are, or be able to tell you what they are. People often have difficulty with the very concept of spirituality. We looked at a definition of spirituality in Chapter 1. You may find it helpful to look back over your notes on the importance of a holistic approach if it is some time since you worked on Chapter 1.

Although Ross (1994) found that the nurses she surveyed had a tendency to view spiritual need in religious terms, the assessment of spiritual needs is more than that. It is about identifying the patient's beliefs and values. For example, vegetarian and vegan patients may not wish to take medicines that are contained in gelatine-based capsules.

Spiritual needs do, of course, include religious needs and this may be problematic if the nurse has little knowledge of the practices of the patient's religion. Once again, it is important to include the family in the assessment process, as they will be able to explain the requirements of the patient's faith. There may also be community leaders who can talk to you about the spiritual needs of patients from particular cultures. Spiritual and cultural needs are often intertwined. We will look at this in Activity 7. Stanworth (1997) is a particularly good source if you feel you need guidance when assessing a patient's spiritual needs.

Assessing cultural needs

If the staff and patients in your clinical area are from the same culture, then you probably have similar expectations about what the patient's experience will be. You will therefore, in many ways (and without considering the concept too hard), be able to anticipate and provide for your patients' cultural needs. However, if you and your patient are from different cultures, you may still assume that they will want what you would want in a similar situation. Unfortunately, your assumptions may well be wrong, or you may be completely unaware of some of their needs.

As with spiritual needs, the best sources of knowledge about the patient's cultural needs are the patient themselves and their family. Showing respect for a person's way of life means, among other things, never laughing at or about their culture or beliefs. Not only should you not do this yourself, you should discourage it in other members of your team. Even if the only reason for a cultural belief or behaviour is 'because it is always done like this', you should still respect the patient's need to act in that way. If you cannot successfully negotiate with a patient, seek support and advice from your manager and supervisor.

Activity 7: Cultural assessment

What cultures are present in the catchment area for your clinical area? Find out whether there are community leaders who would be willing to talk to you about the cultural and religious needs of people from their community. They may also be able to suggest a source of interpreters if there are people within their community who speak little or no English. You could create some information sheets to help nurses in dealing with patients from these cultures.

Feedback

Many towns in the UK are inhabited by people from a variety of cultures, including Indian, Pakistani, Chinese and Afro-Caribbean communities. Community leaders are often keen to help those who express an interest in widening the knowledge of their culture. They may also be able to help you with information about the spiritual needs of patients from their culture. As we mentioned earlier, spiritual and cultural needs are often intertwined together, as well as with the psychological, physical and social needs, and the needs of the family.

Assessing the needs of patients' families

Holistic assessment should involve the patient's family, including the children as well as the adult members. A patient's carers often experience physical, emotional, social and economic burdens as a result of the patient's illness. Too often professionals regard this as inevitable and do nothing, when they should be trying to help the carers with a view to improving the patient's quality of life. Given *et al.* (2001) say that carers need:

- information regarding the disease, including probable symptoms and expectations;
- assistance in structuring care activities, including co-ordination of care and financial implications;
- continued guidance to alleviate stressors, overall burden and associated depression.

Activity 8: Assessing the needs of patients' families

Re-read the notes you made in Activity 5 on the effects of the patient's illness on their family. Identify any ways in which you can help family members, and make notes on how you intend to implement those plans.

Feedback

You may be able to provide some help, but you may also need to turn to others, or tell patients and their families about the existence of other individuals and services who may be able to help them. For example, you may not be able to co-ordinate domiciliary support or provide specific financial advice, but you may know who can do so. Voluntary agencies and charities are often a valuable source of support and information for families.

INVOLVING PATIENTS

As we mentioned at the start of this chapter, the NHS and Community Care Act (Parliament, 1990) requires that patients and their carers have input into the assessment process. However, there are many other reasons why patients should be involved.

Activity 9: Involving patients

Why should patients and their families be involved in the assessment process? From your own experience, note down as many reasons as you can think of for involving patients and their families. Try to aim for five reasons.

Feedback

Reasons you have identified probably include:

- Only patients can tell you how they feel.
- It helps to establish a relationship with the patient.
- It builds trust.
- Families can help you with further details of the patient's physical, psychological, social, spiritual and cultural background, or perhaps act as interpreters.
- There may be differences in perceptions between patients and families, so you need to involve them all.
- You can't provide appropriate care if you don't know what the problems are.
- You need the patient's involvement and co-operation to make the interventions as successful as possible.
- You may discover myths/fears about illness and treatment that you can allay.
- You need the patient's feedback on the effects (positive and negative) of the interventions to decide whether to continue with those interventions.
- You may identify the family's needs too.

In support of the first point, Warden *et al.* (1998) found that graduate nurses held a neutral view of suffering and ineffectively managed hypothetical pain scenarios. This emphasises a point we made earlier in 'Assessing physical needs'. Nurses tend to underestimate patients' pain.

In relation to the fourth point, it is often better to assess a patient initially without a family member present, as Maguire *et al.* (1995) assert that people often deliberately withhold important information if they are first seen with a partner, relative or friend. If the patient doesn't speak English, you may need to find an interpreter from outside the family.

These points clearly show that patient involvement is essential to the assessment process and for the management of the patient's symptoms. Furthermore, understanding problems from the patient's perspective is vital to developing and implementing appropriate care. It is important to help the patient to tell their own story – how they feel and experience their illness and problems.

THE ASSESSMENT PROCESS

Pearce and Lugton (1999) identify the three stages of assessment as:

- a review of the database;
- a screening assessment;
- a focused assessment.

We will consider the third of these points only briefly, as focused assessment for specific needs will be explored in Chapters 4–7. We will then consider assessment as a continuous process and investigate factors that can help or hinder effective assessment.

A review of the database

This is defined as reading any existing documentation to find out who the patient is, why they are here, what the provisional diagnosis is and how they are progressing. We would also suggest that other professionals are a good source of information. Hospital nurses and district nurses often provide each other with a wealth of information when a patient is being transferred from hospital to the community or vice versa.

Activity 10: Sources of information

Make a list of the sources of information you seek out before interviewing the patient or their family.

Feedback

Information sources you have identified probably include:

- patient case notes;
- care plans;
- questionnaires that the patient has completed;
- test results;
- members of your team who have already come in contact with the patient;
- case conferences;
- admission/transfer letter;
- GP's referral letter;
- notes of phone calls from district nurse/hospital nurse/nursing home staff.

A screening assessment

This comprises a brief patient interview (if the patient is conscious and competent), observation of the patient and a short examination, if this is relevant. It is best to see the patient alone, as we have already mentioned. Similarly, family members may have things they wish to tell you, but feel unable to do so in the patient's presence. Consider the issues of confidentiality and collusion carefully in this sort of situation. It is essential to listen to what the patient and the family tell you, and to be aware that patients who have stopped verbalising their needs are not necessarily feeling better, they may just have given up asking because they feel that no one has done anything to help them.

When planning a screening assessment, consider the location of your interview. Can you go somewhere where the patient will be guaranteed privacy? Patients are more likely to talk openly and frankly if they are not concerned about being overheard.

Think about the beginning of the interview. How will you put patients at their ease? It helps to reassure a patient if you introduce yourself properly (if you have not already done so), and explain carefully what the purpose of the assessment is and what you intend to do. Agree a time limit on the interview with the patient, but let them know that they can take a break if they need to. Something as simple as offering the patient a cup of tea/coffee or glass of water can help them to relax.

Consider the patient's physical appearance, body language and mental and emotional state. If they are obviously anxious, tearful, frightened or bewildered, it is still more important to take time to reassure them.

Focus on your own body language and show that you are interested and supportive. If possible, don't sit on the other side of a desk from the patient – this physical barrier can translate into a communication barrier. Be discreet with paperwork, so that the patient does not become unnecessarily alarmed. Show you are listening by maintaining eye contact. Don't allow looking at the notes you are writing to become a barrier between yourself and the patient. See Faulkner (1998) for guidance in conducting a successful patient interview.

When performing an assessment it is helpful to have something like a list, questionnaire or form to help you structure the interview, and ensure that you perform a thorough and holistic assessment. As we mentioned earlier, in 'Assessing psychological needs', a useful example is the General Health Questionnaire (GHQ). The GHQ is a self-administered screening test designed to identify short-term changes in mental heath (Goldberg and Williams, 1988). When working through a list or a form to help you assess a patient, think about the types of questions you can use. Questions are a common feature of interviewing and of ordinary conversation, and so they are familiar ways of eliciting information, showing interest and allowing a session to flow.

Questions can be divided into 'open' and 'closed'. Open questions (such as 'Would you care to say more about that?') invite a further, possibly quite detailed, response. Closed questions (such as 'Did that hurt?') invite yes/no answers. Generally speaking, open questions are more effective in facilitating communication by broadening the topic, helping the patient to explore what they think and feel, and what decisions they want to make. Questions can be helpful, but there are some dangers associated with asking them, primarily because a question implies the need for an answer. In particular, the use of leading questions, such as 'That didn't hurt, did it?' encourages the patient to give a specific answer – which, in this example, is 'No'. Table 3.1 shows some examples of how questions may be useful or dangerous.

When asking patients about their experiences and feelings, it's helpful to reflect their answers back to them, as they will then feel that they are being listened to and understood. It also helps to make sure that you understood what they were trying to tell you.

Helpful use of questions	
Elaboration	Would you care to say more about that? Could you expand on what you've just said?
Being specific	When you say he upsets you, what happens? What exactly is it that you don't like about this?
Focusing/prioritising	How do you feel about that? Which of these difficulties would you like to focus on first?
Dangers	
Timing	Poor timing may interrupt patients when they are thinking, exploring something for themselves or expressing emotion.
'Why' questions	May invite intellectualisation and may be experienced judgementally.
Leading questions	Put the answer into the other person's mouth.
Closed questions	Limit the answer to yes, no or don't know.
Probes	May overstep the levels of trust existing in the relationship.

Table 3.1 Use of questions

Assessment tools for screening assessments

During her research into the support of patients with breast cancer by health visitors, one of the authors of this report (Lugton) found that a Domiciliary Assessment Form adapted from a form devised by Tait *et al.* (1982) helped to ensure that health visitors made a holistic assessment of patients' needs. Health visitors reported it to be a valuable tool. The form included general observations about the patient, her physical adjustment to breast disease, effects of the disease on key relationships, her interactions with the health care team since leaving hospital, social adjustment and psychological adjustment. The assessment of psychological adjustment included guidelines on the recognition of clinical depression and anxiety state. In the final section of the form, key problems were identified and the actions taken or pending were described.

Pearce and Lugton (1999: 67)

Before we go on to look in detail at some tools that may be used for screening assessments (in the next section, 'Assessment tools'), we will look briefly at the third and 'final' part of the assessment process, focused assessment, and at the importance of maintaining continuous assessment, where we suggest that assessment is a never-ending process.

A focused assessment

This is much more thorough and investigates a specific problem (or number of problems). We will consider focused assessments for anxiety and depression in Chapter 4, breathlessness in Chapter 5, fatigue in Chapter 6 and pain in Chapter 7.

Sateia and Silberfarb (1996) recommend that a brief review of sleeping patterns should be obtained from all patients requiring palliative care, as inadequate sleep can result in fatigue, depression and increased pain. Sleep can be a welcome respite from the stresses of experiencing a terminal illness and inadequate sleep can reduce a patient's quality of life. We revisit this concept in Chapter 4.

CONTINUOUS ASSESSMENT

Assessment is a continuous process (see Figure 3.1) and you need to decide how often you need to reassess a patient, based on your knowledge of the patient and the patient's state, and the solutions that have been implemented.

We have given you some suggestions about ways of identifying patients' needs by researching the database and performing a screening assessment in this chapter. We will explore focused assessment and possible solutions to needs for the management of anxiety and depression, breathlessness, fatigue and pain in Chapters 4, 5, 6 and 7 respectively. Tools for the evaluation and audit of nursing interventions are given in Chapter 8.

Activity 11: Different needs at different times

How does an assessment at the point of diagnosis differ from an assessment where the patient is admitted for palliative care? Discuss this with your colleagues and make a list of the reasons for any differences you identify.

Feedback

The initial assessment is often more difficult than following assessments. This may be because admission to palliative care is often preceded by a crisis. There may have been a sudden worsening of the patient's condition, or patients may have reached a point where they can no longer carry on at home, perhaps because of a loss of physical function/independence. Patients may be extremely breathless, anxious or experiencing great pain. They may believe or be aware that they are dying and will therefore require a great deal of reassurance. Furthermore, the family may be more heavily involved with an initial assessment, as they may have to speak on the patient's behalf. When performing assessments, you will often find it necessary to focus on different aspects of the patient's situation at different times.

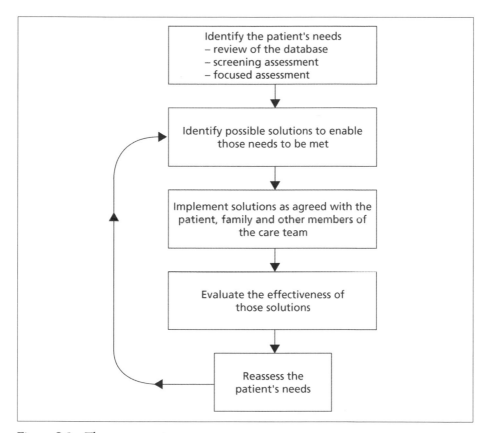

Figure 3.1   The assessment process

ASSESSMENT TOOLS

One theory of unpleasant symptoms (Lenz *et al.*, 1997 – see Chapter 1) suggests that we measure the intensity, timing and quality of the symptoms, and the distress associated with them. Symptoms are defined through several dimensions:

- **Intensity** refers to the severity, strength or amount of the symptom the patient experiences. It is usually measured by patients indicating the intensity of the symptom on a visual analogue or numeric rating scale representing the continuum of intensity (e.g. from 'No pain' to 'Worst pain I can imagine'). (We look at visual analogue/numeric rating scales for measuring breathlessness, fatigue and pain in Chapters 5, 6 and 7 respectively.)

- **Timing** includes the frequency of an intermittent symptom, the duration of a persistent symptom, or a combination of the two. It can also refer to the timing of a symptom's occurrence relative to specific activities such as the temporary experience of nausea associated with eating. Timing variables such as frequency and duration may be measured by self-report or observation.
- **Quality** is often reflected in the way in which the patient describes the symptom. Pain, for example, may be throbbing, pounding or flickering; breathlessness may be a feeling of suffocation or tightness in the chest. Quality can be ascertained by asking patients to describe their symptoms or by working through a checklist of words that can be used to describe the system.
- **Distress** refers to the degree to which the patient is bothered by the symptom. A symptom of a given severity may cause far more distress to some individuals than to others. Asking patients how much they are bothered by a symptom can give you an understanding of how they are interpreting the experience, and what meaning they assign to it. It is also the dimension that contributes most to the patient's quality of life. Distress can be measured either quantitatively (e.g. using visual analogue/numeric rating scales) or qualitatively (e.g. in-depth interviews).

The theory also suggests that measuring a single dimension of unpleasant symptoms is not too helpful, as the patient is often experiencing several symptoms that impact on each other, all of which affect and are affected by the patient's psychological, physical and social situation. In effect, the theory of unpleasant symptoms suggests that a holistic approach to assessment is necessary to 'capture' the patient's experience.

In this section we will look at two tools you can use to perform a holistic screening assessment, the functional health patterns (FHP) model and the Palliative Outcome Score (POS), but first we will look at some of the less complex tools. You need to be aware, however, that tools are only as good as their explanation, use and interpretation. When selecting a tool, you need to consider whether it is helpful and whether it is possible for the patient to complete (many are self-reporting tools). For example, patients with rheumatoid arthritis may not be able to use a pen to mark a scale and patients with fatigue may not be able to use tools which are long or complex.

Visual analogue scales (VAS)

Visual analogue scales are perhaps the simplest and commonest unidimensional tool. A scale usually consists of a line (horizontal or vertical) with statements at the extremes of the continuum of the symptom at either end, e.g. 'no pain' at one end and 'severe pain' at the other (Figure 3.2).

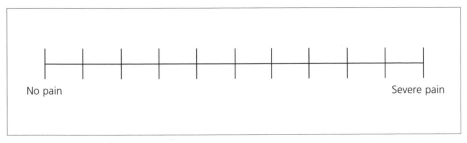

Figure 3.2 Visual analogue scale

Numeric rating scales (NRS)

These are a form of VAS (Figure 3.3). The patient rates the symptom on a scale from 1 to 10.

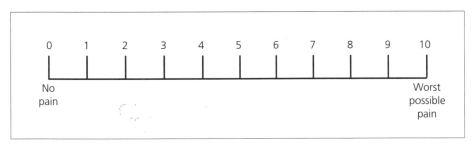

Figure 3.3 Numeric rating scale

Likert scales

The Likert technique presents a set of attitude statements. Subjects are asked to express agreement or disagreement of a five-point scale. Each degree of agreement is given a numerical value from one to five (see Figure 3.4). Thus a total numerical value can be calculated from all the responses.

Verbal rating scales (Figure 3.5)

The patient rates the symptom verbally, e.g. 'none', 'mild', 'moderate' or 'severe'.

It may be possible to use a variant of these tools to measure a symptom in the focused assessment, but it very much depends on the ways in which the patient is able to describe the symptom. For example, a patient

For each of the statements below, please indicate how much you agree or disagree by putting a tick in the appropriate box.

1. I frequently have pain.

Strongly agree	Agree	Undecided	Disagree	Strongly disagree

2. I have pain that is controlled by pain medications.

Strongly agree	Agree	Undecided	Disagree	Strongly disagree

Figure 3.4 Examples of Likert scales

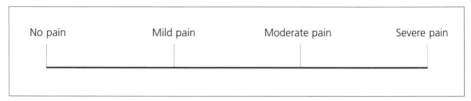

Figure 3.5 Verbal rating scale

may not be able to assign their pain a number. In this case you would have to use a different scale.

Often more complex tools include a number of these simpler tools to build up a picture of the patient's symptoms. They may also include prompts for structured or semi-structured interviews. We will now go on to look at two useful tools for performing holistic screening assessments.

A conceptual framework for needs assessment: the functional health patterns model

Gordon (1994) proposed a functional health patterns (FHP) model of assessment with a view to ensuring holistic assessment. The 11 aspects of this framework are as follows:

- health perception/health management pattern;
- nutritional/metabolic pattern;
- cognitive perceptual pattern;
- assessment of pain;
- self-perception pattern;
- role–relationship pattern;
- elimination pattern;

- activity/exercise pattern;
- sleep/rest pattern;
- coping/stress tolerance;
- value/belief pattern.

Activity 12: FHP applied to palliative care

Obtain a copy of the following article: Dunne, K., Coates, V. and Moran, A. (1997) 'Functional health patterns applied to palliative care: a case study'. *International Journal of Palliative Nursing*, 3(6), pp.324–9.

Read the article and make notes on any parts that you feel are particularly important or relevant to your situation.

Reflect upon the care of a patient whom you have recently assessed. Would your assessment have been:

- more thorough;
- more holistic;

if you had used the FHP model?

What do you like or dislike about the model?

Discuss your opinions on the FHP model with members of your AL set.

Feedback

Dunne *et al.* (1997) believed that the FHP model enabled them to understand the patient's needs well and to identify all problem areas. They felt that it enabled them to gather data from the patient's perspective rather than from the health care professional's perspective, an important aspect of patient-centred care.

Palliative care outcome scale (POS)

POS (Higginson, 1998) was developed in 1998 as a national tool to be used in the audit of palliative care. It was felt at the time that there was no generic tool which could assess the outcomes (including the quality of life and care of patients and families) of palliative care. Existing tools and measures were felt to be limited by:

- having been developed in only a small number of settings;
- having been designed for patients who were in earlier stages of illness, who were more able to complete complicated questionnaires;
- missing important components of palliative care, such as family needs.

POS took components that appeared to work well in earlier measures, e.g. the Support Team Assessment Schedule (STAS – Higginson, 1993), and includes aspects concerned with pain and symptom control, patient and family psychosocial needs and communication and information. (Source: **www2.edc.org/lastacts/archives/archivesJan00/POSDescription.asp** Site accessed 30/6/08.)

The POS homepage is: **www.kcl.ac.uk/schools/medicine/depts/palliative/qat/pos.html**

There are two versions of the questionnaire, one for patients:

www.kcl.ac.uk/content/1/c6/01/29/23/pt_q_v1.pdf Site accessed 30/6/08.

and one for staff:

www.kcl.ac.uk/content/1/c6/01/29/23/staff_q_v1.pdf Site accessed 30/6/08.

but the contents are similar. Using a 0–4 scale, the questionnaire asks the patient to review each of the following items over the last three days:

- pain;
- other symptoms, e.g. nausea, coughing or constipation;
- anxiety or worry about illness or treatment;
- family or friends' anxiety or worry;
- how much information the patient and family or friends have been given;
- whether the patient has been able to share how they are feeling with family or friends;
- whether the patient has felt that life was worthwhile;
- whether the patient has felt good about him- or herself as a person;
- how much time the patient feels has been wasted on appointments relating to their health care, e.g. waiting around for transport or repeating tests;
- whether any practical matters resulting from the patient's illness, either financial or personal, have been addressed;
- what the patient's main problems have been.

The Palliative Care Outcome Scale is copyright. However, you are free to use it, in full or as individual items, adapt it to your local circumstances or reproduce it without charge providing that you complete the registration form (**www.kcl.ac.uk/schools/medicine/depts/palliative/qat/pos-form.html** (Site accessed 13/5/08)) and agree to the following conditions:

- The Palliative Care Outcome Scale, Professor Irene Higginson and the POS Development Team will be acknowledged in any publication, reports or oral presentations.
- If POS is copied for others, you undertake to ensure they register to use the scale by contacting the POS Development Team.
- POS will not be sold, either in its original or adapted form.

Activity 13: Assessment tools and frameworks

When you perform a screening assessment, what tools or framework do you use (if any)?

Does the tool or framework ensure that your assessment is holistic?

If so, how?

If not, how could the tool or framework be improved to ensure more holistic assessments?

Feedback

You may be using a tool that is specifically designed for the palliative care context, such as POS, but you may be using a general tool such as the activities of daily living (Roper et al., 1996 – we introduced this in Chapter 2). In this case (or if you don't use any tool) you may decide that it would be helpful to include items from the FHP model or POS. Discuss any changes you decide are necessary with your colleagues. Implement the changes with your colleagues' agreement.

Activity 14: A screening assessment

The next time that you know you will have to perform an assessment, work through the following list first:

- perform a review of the database;
- review good practice for the patient interview, observation and examination;
- ensure that you have the appropriate holistic assessment tool/framework/form to hand.

Perform the assessment using the new or improved tool that you have chosen, based on your work in Activity 13.

Identify what needs require a focused assessment.

Feedback

Your assessment of the patient should be more thorough than those you carried out previously, as you have reviewed and revised your approach with a view to making it more holistic.

FACTORS THAT CAN HELP OR HINDER ASSESSMENT

For the assessment process to run effectively, it helps if nurses have a sound knowledge of:

- the illness from which the patient is suffering and its symptoms;
- the interventions used to manage that illness and their side-effects;
- emotions or states related to having an incurable illness;
- the limits of their own knowledge;
- who to go to for help;
- how to find evidence about interventions (evidence-based practice).

It helps too if the patient and family are co-operative and your team is working well. However, from your own experience you can probably identify many factors that can hinder the assessment process.

Activity 15: Hindrances to good assessment

Reflect upon the last two or three assessments you performed. If possible, include an assessment of a patient from a culture different from your own. For each assessment, make notes of the factors that made the process harder. Keep your notes, as you will need them again for Activity 16.

Feedback

Difficulties you might have encountered include:

- The patient's records are missing or illegible, or other team members won't hand them over.
- The patient and/or family or other team members won't talk to you candidly, or refuse to co-operate at all.
- Negative attitudes of other team members to patients from cultures or faiths different from their own.
- The patient's first language is different from your own, or the patient is inarticulate, and you have difficulty communicating with them.
- The patient has needs that they are embarrassed to express, e.g. sexual needs.

- The patient is too tired or too ill to take part in the assessment process, or is unconscious.
- The patient's family are tired, anxious or too stressed or short-tempered to be of much help.
- You do not have enough time to carry out a thorough assessment.
- Different team members using assessment tools in different ways, therefore invalidating some data.
- You can't read your own notes, or realise that you didn't record several important facts.
- You feel that you lack knowledge of suitable interventions.
- Other team members won't share their knowledge of suitable interventions with you.
- The patient requests interventions traditional to their culture that you feel you cannot be involved with.
- Budgetary constraints restrict the use of the interventions you have identified.
- The interventions you implemented managed one symptom, but caused an overall reduction of the patient's quality of life.

Having read the list above, you may wonder how you ever manage to perform a successful assessment! Many of these difficulties are communication problems, which can be solved in time, through reassurance, patience and perseverance. Unfortunately, time itself may be a scarce resource.

For assessment to be effective, nurses performing it need to have:

- good communication skills, in order to gain information about the patient and their situation and pass the information on;
- good analytical skills to enable them to interpret the data and to make appropriate decisions;
- the ability to produce clear documentation of the assessment, so that an adequate care plan can be formulated.

When you interview a patient, you need to have good questioning and listening skills. You need to be able to question the patient in such a way as to elicit as much information about how they are feeling as possible, bearing in mind that you may only have a short time in which to do so. You also need to listen actively to what the patient says – listen to the tone of voice in which they give their answer and observe their body language. If you don't share a language with the patient, you will need to find an interpreter. Above all, the patient needs to trust the interpreter and be prepared to tell them the full story. You may not find out everything you need to know if the patient is not prepared to be completely open with the interpreter. As we mentioned earlier, it is probably best if the interpreter is not a family member, but you may have no alternative. The notes you make during the interview need to be brief but accurate summaries of what you have learned from questioning, listening to and observing the patient.

Once you have collected information through interview, observation and examination, you need to be able to analyse it and make decisions about what to do about the patient's situation and how to do it. If you feel that you don't know enough about certain aspects of the situation, discuss them further with the patient, their family or other members of your team. If there are certain symptoms that you are still concerned about, do a literature search to find out what the current evidence-based approach is to managing those symptoms. You should then have enough information to enable you to make the best decision about appropriate interventions with regard to improving the patient's quality of life.

Finally, you should write up your notes from your first interview, observation and examination of the patient, notes on any further interviews or research and notes on how you made your decisions. These should be clear and concise, as other members of your team will need to read and understand them.

There's no point in assessing if we don't pass on the information.

Lecturer in palliative care

Pooling information with members of your team helps to prevent duplication. Multidisciplinary meetings and shared notes will assist with this process. Sharing information makes your team more effective and means that the patient is not unnecessarily stressed by being asked the same questions again and again. However, it is important to check back with the patient if you identify any areas that need clarification.

Knowing the patient

At the first interview you may not have met the patient before and this may be a little problematic. However, by the time you need to make decisions about reassessment, you may know the patient a little better – or even a lot better, depending on the situation. Benner *et al.* (1996: 22) define knowing the patient as knowing their:

- responses to therapeutic measures;
- routines and habits;
- coping resources;
- physical capacities and endurance;
- body topology and characteristics.

A good knowledge of all these areas, and a good relationship with the patient and their family, will help you to make decisions more quickly and with greater confidence.

The effects of personal prejudices

Prejudice is defined as a negative belief of a social group or individual that has no factual base or is unfounded (Crandall and Eshleman, 2003). Nurses' beliefs about patients' suffering are often based on their own culture, socioeconomic level and ethnic background, and prejudices may arise as a result of poor understanding of the culture of others. While this is a problem, it can be overcome if nurses work to understand other cultures and beliefs and make an effort to empathise with patients.

A far more serious hindrance to assessment is the involvement of people who consider that their own beliefs and practices are right and those of others are wrong. Such people may be tempted to discount or even mock the beliefs and practices of others, saying, for example, that traditional healing methods have no place in the modern world. However, doctors and nurses in South Africa work with traditional healers and witchdoctors, and we have already mentioned that you should have no problem incorporating traditional healing methods into the patient's treatment, as long as they will do no harm. Similarly, it should be possible to provide suitable food for all patients, no matter how many limitations there are on their diet, whether designated by culture or religion. Some health care professionals may find it frustrating to treat people with what they consider to be self-inflicted problems, such as smokers who develop lung cancer, or people who have fungating wounds that they have left untreated. However, everyone has a right to treatment and patients should be treated with respect regardless of the cause of the problem.

Activity 16: Personal prejudices

Read back through the notes you made in answer to Activity 15, where you reflected upon hindrances to assessment. Consider whether any of the difficulties you identified were related to your own personal prejudices. You may at the time have identified the cause of the problem as:

- the patient or family being too demanding for no good reason that you could see;
- the patient or family not clearly voicing their desires;
- requests you couldn't understand or couldn't see the point of;
- the patient or family acting in ways that seemed to you not to be in the patient's best interests.

Reflect once more upon the situation. Try to identify any ways in which your expectation that the patient would have the same sorts of requirements and expectations as you would have in the same situation might have affected how you behaved. Consider, for example, your reactions to their social class, culture (if different from your own), the relationships within the family, whether you felt the problem was self-inflicted, and so on.

If you now know the patient better, you might realise that there were requests you discounted, or needs you failed to identify, based solely on the patient's 'difference'.

Feedback

You might have realised that you failed to recognise the importance of a festival or of facing the right way while praying. You may not have realised that the patient would be distressed if you asked them to take medicines that contained gelatine or alcohol or if all the meals available contained things that they could not or would not eat.

If you consider your work practices to be anti-discriminatory, and yourself to be egalitarian, you will be dismayed if you discover that you have latent prejudices. Try to be alert to such responses when dealing with patients from different cultures, social classes or walks of life. Ask yourself what you are doing and why, and identify what you should be doing.

This 'thinking about what you are doing as you do it' is sometimes referred to as 'reflection-in-action'. This is one of three constructs of Schön's theory of reflection (Schön, 1983, 1987). The other two constructs are knowing-in-action (or professional 'know how') and reflection-on-action (when you reflect upon a past incident). Reflection-on-action was discussed in Chapter 2 and we gave you a reflective model to allow you to reflect on action.

Reflection-in-action occurs at a time when you can still make a difference to the particular practice situation, i.e. it's 'on-the-spot' reflection. You may be surprised by an event in practice – an unexpected outcome, either pleasant or unpleasant – and find that your practice is interrupted by an immediate reflective response, that is, you are thinking about what you are doing as you do it.

Reflection-in-action has a critical function. It questions the assumptions that underpin our knowing-in-action. It gives rise to on-the-spot experimentation because of our awareness and observation of new phenomena or things that occur in our practice.

You may need to leave the final activity of this chapter (below) for some time. It depends on the implementation of any changes that have been identified as necessary to improve the general assessment of patients receiving palliative care.

Activity 17: Assessment

After the first few times you have followed any new assessment procedures (or used new assessment tools), reflect upon any changes that have occurred in your care planning or in the effectiveness of the nursing interventions that you have used.

Make notes in your learning or reflective diary on your answers to the following questions:

- What changes have been made to procedures/tools/forms?
- How have these changes ensured that thorough and holistic assessments are routine for all patients?
- If assessments are not routine, thorough and holistic, how can you ensure they become so?
- What changes have occurred in your care planning – is it now holistic? If not, how can you make it so?
- When you evaluate the effectiveness of your nursing interventions, do you think that a holistic approach improves the patient's overall quality of life more than might otherwise have been the case?

Consider your approach to assessment and care planning. Reflect upon how you can become a more holistic practitioner.

Feedback

You may find it helpful to discuss these issues with your manager, colleagues and members of your AL set.

SUMMARY

In this chapter we have looked at the importance of assessing palliative care patients holistically and involving patients and their families in the assessment process. Having completed this chapter, you should be able to:

- explain the need for holistic assessment and patient involvement;
- describe the assessment process and identify factors that can help or hinder assessment;
- perform a general palliative care assessment (screening assessment) and identify what should be investigated further in a focused assessment.

RECOMMENDED SOURCES OF INFORMATION

Dunn, V.C. (2000) 'The holistic assessment of the patient in pain'. *Professional Nurse*, 15(12), pp.791–3.

Faulkner, A. (1998) *Effective interaction with patients* (2nd Ed.). New York: Churchill Livingstone.

Ingham, J.M. and Portenoy, R.K. (2005) 'The measurement of pain and other symptoms', in Doyle, D., Hanks, G., Cherney, N.I. and Calman, K. (editors) *The Oxford textbook of palliative medicine* (3rd Ed.). Oxford: Oxford University Press, pp.167–84.

Pearce, C. and Lugton, J. (1999) 'Holistic assessment of patients' and relatives' needs', in Lugton, J. and Kindlen, M. (editors) *Palliative care: the nursing role* (2nd Ed.). Edinburgh: Elsevier Churchill Livingstone, pp.61–87.

Robbins, M. (1998) *Evaluating palliative care: establishing the evidence base*. Oxford: Oxford University Press.

REFERENCES

Benner, P., Tanner, C.A. and Chesla, C.A. (1996) *Expertise in nursing practice: caring, clinical judgement and ethics*. New York: Springer.

Clark, D. and Malson, H. (1995) 'Mini review: key issues in palliative care needs assessment'. *Progress in Palliative Care*, 3(2), pp.53–5.

Crandall, C.S. and Eshleman, A. (2003) 'A justification–suppression model of the expression and experience of prejudice'. *Psychological Bulletin*, 129(3), pp.414–46.

Doyle, D., Hanks, G., Cherney, N.I. and Calman, K. (2004) *The Oxford textbook of palliative medicine* (3rd Ed.). Oxford: Oxford University Press.

Dunn, V.C. (2000) 'The holistic assessment of the patient in pain'. *Professional Nurse*, 15(12), pp.791–3.

Dunne, K., Coates, V. and Moran, A. (1997) 'Functional health patterns applied to palliative care: a case study'. *International Journal of Palliative Nursing*, 3(6), pp.324–9.

Faulkner, A. (1998) *Effective interaction with patients* (2nd Ed.). New York: Churchill Livingstone.

Given, B.A., Given, C.W. and Kozachik, S. (2001) 'Family support in advanced cancer'. *CA: A Cancer Journal for Clinicians*, 51(4), pp.213–31.

Goldberg, D.P. (1972) *The detection of psychiatric illness by questionnaire*. London: Oxford University Press.

Goldberg, D. and Williams, P. (1988) *A user's guide to the General Health Questionnaire*. Windsor: NFER-Nelson.

Gordon, M. (1994) *Nursing diagnosis: process and application* (3rd Ed.). St Louis: Mosby.

Higginson, I. (1993) 'Audit methods: a community schedule', in Higginson, I. (editor) *Clinical audit in palliative care*. Oxford: Radcliffe Medical, pp.34–47.

Higginson, I. (1998) For copies of POS, go to: **www.kcl.ac.uk/schools/ medicine/depts/palliative/qat/pos.html**

Kleinman, A. (1988) *The illness narratives*. New York: Basic Books.

Lenz, E.R., Suppe, F., Gift, A.G., Pugh, L.C. and Milligan, R.A. (1995) 'Collaborative development of middle-range nursing theories: toward a theory of unpleasant symptoms'. *Advances in Nursing Science*, 17(3), pp.1–13.

Lenz, E.R., Pugh, L.C., Milligan, R.A., Gift, A. and Suppe, F. (1997) 'The middle-range theory of unpleasant symptoms: an update'. *Advances in Nursing Science*, 19(3), pp.14–27.

Maguire, P., Faulkner, A. and Regnard, C. (1995) 'Eliciting the current problems', in Regnard, C. and Hockley, J. (editors) *Flow diagrams in advanced cancer and other diseases*. London: Edward Arnold, pp.1–4.

Maher, D. and Hemming, L. (2005) 'Understanding the patient and family: holistic assessment in palliative care'. *British Journal of Community Nursing*, 10(7), pp.318–22.

Milligan, S. (2004) 'Perceptions of spiritual care amongst nurses undertaking post registration education'. *International Journal of Palliative Nursing*, 10(4), pp.162–71.

Parliament (1990) *National Health Service and Community Care Act*. London: HMSO.

Pearce, C. and Lugton, J. (1999) 'Holistic assessment of patients' and relatives' needs', in Lugton, J. and Kindlen, M. (editors) *Palliative care: the nursing role*. Edinburgh: Churchill Livingstone, pp.61–87.

Popay, J. and Williams, G. (editors) (1994) *Researching the people's health*. London: Routledge.

Roper, N., Logan, W.W. and Tierney, A.J. (1996) *The elements of nursing* (4th Ed.). New York: Churchill Livingstone.

Ross, L.A. (1994) 'Spiritual aspects of nursing'. *Journal of Advanced Nursing*, 19(3), pp.439–47.

Sadock, B.J. and Sadock, V.A. (2005) *Kaplan and Sadock's comprehensive textbook of psychiatry* (8th Ed.). Philadelphia: Lippincot.

Sateia, M.J. and Silberfarb, P.M. (1996) 'Sleep disorders in patients with advanced cancer'. *Progress in Palliative Care*, 4(4), pp.120–5.

Schön, D.A. (1983) *The reflective practitioner: how professionals think in action*. New York: Basic Books.

Schön, D.A. (1987) *Educating the reflective practitioner*. San Francisco: Jossey-Bass.

Schafheutle, E.I., Cantrill, J.A. and Noyce P.R. (2004) 'The nature of informal pain questioning by nurses – barriers to post-operative pain management'. *Pharmacy World and Science*, 26(1), pp.12–17.

Stanworth, R. (1997) 'The imponderable: a search for meaning: spirituality, language and depth of reality'. *International Journal of Palliative Nursing*, 3(1), pp.19–22.

Tait, A., Maguire, P., Faulkner, A., Brooke, M., Wilkinson, S., Thomson, I. and Sellwood, R. (1982) 'Improving communication skills'. *Nursing Times*, 78(51), 22 December, pp.2181–4.

Warden, S., Carpenter, J.S. and Brockopp, D.Y. (1998) 'Nurses' beliefs about suffering and their management of pain'. *International Journal of Palliative Nursing*, 4(1), pp.21–5.

Wilkinson, S., Roberts, A. and Aldridge, J. (1998) 'Nurse-patient communication in palliative care: an evaluation of a communication skills programme'. *Palliative Medicine*, 12(1), pp.13–22.

World Health Organization (1987) *People's needs for nursing care: a European study: a study of nursing care needs and of the planning, implementation and evaluation of care provided by nurses in two selected groups of people in the European region.* Copenhagen: WHO Regional Office for Europe.

Chapter 4

Anxiety and Depression

Elaine Stevens

INTRODUCTION

Anxiety and depression in palliative care patients are seen as natural, inevitable reactions to living and coping with a terminal illness. However, recent research has indicated that, as these symptoms can severely affect the quality of life of patients with a life-limiting illness, a great deal can be gained from accurately diagnosing and treating them (McVey, 1998; Lloyd-Williams *et al.*, 2004).

The aim of this chapter, therefore, is to increase your knowledge of the assessment and management of anxiety and depression, and to enhance your nursing skills to ensure an optimum quality of life for your palliative care patients.

In this chapter we stress the importance of 'listening' and developing a relationship with the patient. Simply 'being there' for the patient can be therapeutic and yet it can be so very hard to do. Nurses may feel anxious when trying to help an anxious patient. They may feel hopeless, helpless or depressed when trying to help a depressed patient. It is important for you to acknowledge these feelings and work out how to deal with them. It is better not to simply distance yourself or to avoid patients whose demands you find difficult to meet, or to always rely on pharmacological strategies – both for yourself and for your patients. We suggest various support strategies (such as peer or clinical supervision) that may help nurses in such situations in 'Caring for the carers', in Chapter 1.

LEARNING OUTCOMES

When you have completed this chapter, you will be able to:
- give definitions of anxiety and depression;
- describe the manifestations, causes and predisposing factors of anxiety and depression in patients receiving palliative care;
- evaluate the different tools that can be used to assess anxiety and depression in your practice setting;

- compare and contrast the different approaches that can be taken to the management of anxiety and/or depression in your practice setting;
- critically evaluate how the management of anxiety and/or depression can impact on the quality of life of patients receiving palliative care.

Preparation

In the first few activities in Section 1: Anxiety, we are going to ask you to think about your own experiences of anxiety. It may therefore be a good idea to do the activities at a time and in a place where you feel safe, and where someone you trust will be around to support you if necessary. If this is not possible, try at least to find somewhere where you will not be interrupted.

You will need several photocopies of the checklist in Activity 2. It's a good idea to do that now, so that you are not caught unprepared for Activity 3.

Activities 7, 13, 16 and 23 involve talking to patients and their families. Before doing these activities, you should discuss what you intend to do with the members of each patient's health care team – including the patient. If they understand what you are doing and why, they are more likely to be willing and able to help you. Read through the activities before approaching the health care team. If it is likely that patients will be disturbed beyond what would be normally required for clinical management, you should seek approval from your organisation's ethics committee before starting these activities.

In Activity 15 we ask you to obtain copies of the following articles:

- McVey, P. (1998) 'Depression among the palliative care oncology population'. *International Journal of Palliative Nursing*, 4(2), pp.86–93.
- Billings, J.A. (1995) 'Depression'. *Journal of Palliative Care*, 11(1), pp.48–54.
- Lovejoy, N.C., Tabor, D., Matteis, M. and Lillis, P. (2000) 'Cancer-related depression, part 1: neurologic alterations and cognitive-behavioral therapy'. *Oncology Nursing Forum*, 27(4), pp.667–78.

Lloyd-Williams, M., Dennis, M. and Taylor, F. (2004) 'A prospective study to compare three depression screening tools in patients who are terminally ill? *General Hospital Psychiatry*, 26(5), pp.384–9.

We recommend that you start searching for them now so that you have them to hand when you reach the activity. They can be obtained from the National Library for Health and the NHS Scotland e-Library.

www.library.nhs.uk or **www.elib.scot.nhs.uk** Both sites accessed 13/5/08.

If you have problems sourcing the articles, please contact the RCN library **www.rcn.org.uk/development/library** Site accessed 13/5/08.

You might need access to a tape recorder for Activity 16.

SECTION 1: ANXIETY

Anxiety is defined as a 'universally experienced unpleasant emotion' (Twycross and Wilcock, 2001). Anxiety can be divided into two categories:

- acute anxiety – the feelings pass after a short time;
- chronic anxiety – the feelings persist for a long time.

Both types of anxiety have been shown to vary in intensity over time within individual patients and may have an adverse effect on their quality of life.

It is well recognised that anxiety is a natural response when people are given a diagnosis of cancer, when cancer recurs (Breitbart, 1995) or when disease is advanced (Lloyd-Williams *et al.*, 2004). Patients usually experience anxiety for a short period while they adjust to the situation and it may cause them little problem. Between a quarter and a half of all palliative care patients will suffer from some kind of psychological distress at some point in their illness (Greer and Moorey, 1997). A small but significant number of these individuals suffer from *heightened* anxiety, i.e. a subtle, ongoing feeling of being unsettled and fearful, which causes them to become unable to cope with their situation (Massie and Holland, 1992). We considered coping mechanisms in Chapter 2. It is *heightened anxiety* that requires expert assessment and management to ensure the patient has an optimum quality of life regardless of life expectancy. Heightened anxiety stemming from an inability to cope with stressors of any kind can increase to become acute or chronic, or have phases of both over a period of time.

> Having listened to many palliative care patients' stories when working within specialist palliative care for many years I have come to realise that many of them are anxious about their future, family, etc. when given a diagnosis of cancer. However, if the patients receive holistic care that meets their needs, as time progresses this anxiety diminishes. Those who remain overly anxious throughout their disease trajectory often have not had their needs met, and therefore have unresolved issues that need to be addressed.
>
> Co-ordinator, palliative day care

Activity 1: Reflecting upon anxiety

Think about the definitions of the various types of anxiety that we have given you:

- acute;
- chronic;
- heightened.

Consider a time when you have felt anxious. This may have been, for example, because you, or a member of your family, were ill, were experiencing job insecurity or change, or because of problems within a close relationship.

On a separate sheet of paper, make notes on your experience of anxiety:

- the cause(s);
- how you felt, or any changes in your behaviour;
- how you coped (or tried to cope) with your anxiety;
- anything you realise, with hindsight, might have helped, or that you intend to do should such a situation occur again.

You may find it helps to discuss these issues with someone you trust – perhaps a colleague, friend or member of your AL set.

Keep your notes with this book as you will need them for the next few activities.

Feedback

As you may be aware from the experiences you have just written about, anxiety can be an extremely debilitating state. Although the main incident that caused you anxiety may have been fairly catastrophic, you probably found that things that you would normally not even think about twice seemed to become extraordinarily difficult to deal with. In this state, and perhaps because of the ways your anxiety expressed itself – its manifestations – you probably found that you were less able to cope with difficult events in your life, big or small. You may have been able to employ your own coping strategies, or you may have had to seek help from professionals – either pharmacological or non-pharmacological help.

We will go on to consider the manifestations and causes of anxiety, and the assessment and management of anxiety in the following sections.

Manifestations of anxiety in palliative care patients

Patients' distress comes from the meanings they attach to their illness and the losses that are being incurred. This can result in a variety of symptoms being displayed in varying degrees. These include:

- being persistently tense and unable to relax;
- worrying a lot about many things;
- mood swings from which the patient cannot be diverted;
- poor concentration;
- interrupted or unrefreshing sleep;
- indecision;
- irritability;
- sweating attacks;
- tremors;
- nausea;
- panic attacks.

Severe anxiety results in feelings of hopelessness and helplessness and can lead to depression. We will consider depression in the second half of this chapter. Panic attacks can be very distressing and can cause sweating, dizziness, palpitations and hyperventilation. Conversely, hyperventilation may cause panic attacks, as may the fear of impending death, or strong feelings of fear or of loss of control. Panic attacks may come on suddenly for no apparent reason. They are very intense periods of anxiety and can last from five to 20 minutes. Strong feelings of fear about dying and losing control often result from these attacks.

Sleep disorders

Although the function of sleep remains largely a mystery, it can safely be said that an adequate amount of quality sleep is essential in order to feel alert, motivated and energised. Sleep is an important factor in promoting normal mood and cognitive function (Roth *et al.*, 1974; Johnson, 1969). It may play a role in musculoskeletal restoration/healing and immune function (Oswald, 1980; Moldofsky *et al.*, 1989) and can influence pain thresholds (Johnson, 1969). Finally, sleep may provide a respite from the pain, worry and hardship which can be associated with terminal illness. The inability to achieve adequate sleep may compromise the quality of life in the terminally ill, resulting in fatigue, drowsiness, depression and increased pain.

Sateia and Silberfarb (1996)

Activity 2: Manifestations of anxiety

Refer back to the notes you made in Activity 1.

Make several copies of this activity, as you will be using the checklist for Activity 3 too.

Using the checklist below, indicate which (if any) of the manifestations you felt you may have exhibited while you were experiencing anxiety. If you felt there were other signs you showed that are not on the list, add them on at the end.

- ☐ being persistently tense and unable to relax;
- ☐ worrying a lot about many things;
- ☐ mood swings from which you could not be diverted;
- ☐ poor concentration;
- ☐ interrupted or unrefreshing sleep;
- ☐ indecision;
- ☐ irritability;
- ☐ sweating attacks;
- ☐ tremors;
- ☐ nausea;
- ☐ panic attacks;
- ☐
- ☐
- ☐
- ☐
- ☐

Feedback

You may have experienced some or all of these symptoms, or had to add on others that are unique to you.

If you were ill at the time, you will have noticed one of the great drawbacks of anxiety. It will have made your experience of your illness even more unpleasant than it might have been in the first place, and may even have delayed your recovery. Palliative care patients will not recover from their illness or incapacity but, by managing their anxiety, they can at least experience a better quality of life.

Activity 3: Identifying anxiety

This activity asks you to consider the patients in your clinical area and, using the checklist of manifestations, identify whether any of them appear to be experiencing anxiety. It is not a real assessment tool, as it has not been validated as such. But you could, for example, refer to the checklist when conducting a semi-structured interview to ensure all areas are assessed. General assessment is discussed in Chapter 3 and validated assessment tools for anxiety are discussed later in this part of the chapter.

Using a copy of the checklist from Activity 2, identify each patient in your clinical area who is receiving palliative care and who is manifesting symptoms of anxiety.

- Indicate which symptoms they are exhibiting.
- Make a note of whether anxiety is documented in their care plan as being a problem for them.

Keep your checklists and notes, as we will be asking you to talk to these patients in Activity 7.

Feedback

We would hope that if, from your investigation, you considered a patient to be anxious, anxiety was marked as a problem on the care plan. If it was not, discuss with your team why it may not have been noted. First, of course, it may be a new symptom. On the other hand, there may be 'gaps' in the thoroughness of the assessment process or a lack of skills/experience in the team. (See Chapter 3 for details of the assessment process.)

It is important to realise, however, that the manifestations of symptoms of anxiety may not be quite so cut and dried. Anxiety may be masked by other symptoms and/or hidden from you by the patient.

Activity 4: Patient anxiety

Reflect upon a situation in which you nursed a patient who was particularly anxious. What symptoms did they display in the following areas:

- physical;
- psychological;
- social;
- cultural;
- spiritual.

Was the anxiety acute or chronic? Could the patient talk about their anxiety? What was the family's involvement? How did they cope?

What did you think and feel about the patient's anxiety?

Did you feel you could help the patient?

Feedback

You may find it helpful to discuss any issues you have about caring for anxious patients with your colleagues or members of your AL set.

Causes of patient anxiety

Heightened anxiety is a symptom of the underlying problems that patients are struggling to cope with during a terminal illness:

- physical problems;
- psychological problems;
- social problems;
- cultural problems;
- spiritual problems.

A patient's physical, psychological, social, cultural and spiritual problems are all interrelated and, furthermore, they may predispose the patient towards depression.

Case study

On admission to hospital Mrs Brown, 72, was extremely anxious and unable to make any rational decisions about her care. She had severe pain from metastatic breast cancer. On assessment it was noticed that the main pain was in her left hip. She was immediately prescribed painkillers to relieve the pain. Once pain-free, Mrs Brown's anxiety reduced and she was able to make informed decisions about her proposed care. An x-ray was ordered, which showed that she had a pathological fracture of her left femur, so an orthopaedic opinion was requested. It was decided that the best option was to operate and internally fixate the femur. Mrs Brown was to be transferred to the orthopaedic ward the next day.

Although Mrs Brown continued to take her painkillers, her pain returned and her anxiety levels rose once again. Even though her analgesia was significantly increased, the pain and anxiety did not get any better and she became extremely agitated. No one was sure of the cause of these symptoms and it was decided that she should be monitored overnight before any more medication was introduced. During a conversation with a nurse during the night, Mrs Brown admitted that she was very upset as she had been told she would only be in hospital for a short time, and she had left her home unattended and none of her neighbours knew she was away. As she had been burgled on a previous occasion when in hospital, she felt frightened about leaving her house empty. The nurse reassured her and enabled her to phone her neighbour to explain the situation. This reduced Mrs Brown's anxiety – and as the anxiety reduced so did the pain. By the time she was transferred to the orthopaedic ward, she was pain-free and although a little anxious about her operation, Mrs Brown was feeling content.

We will now go on to investigate each of the six areas.

Physical causes of anxiety

People suffering from severe illnesses, whether of malignant or non-malignant origin, are often anxious about the management of their illness (Folkman and Greer, 2000). Unrelieved or intractable symptoms such as severe pain, insomnia, nausea, weakness, breathlessness (dyspnoea), low blood sugar, brain impairment and concurrent psychiatric disorders have been shown to cause heightened anxiety in patients receiving palliative care (Twycross and Wilcock, 2001).

Physical symptoms caused by drugs can also induce feelings of anxiety. For example, morphine can cause hallucinations, corticosteroids can cause motor restlessness, and withdrawal from alcohol or benzodiazepines can cause restlessness and agitation. If these physical needs are unfulfilled, this can lead to feelings of low self-esteem, low self-worth and hopelessness (Maslow, 1987), which can compound the experience of heightened anxiety.

Psychological causes of anxiety

Psychological causes of anxiety include distress caused by changes of role that often occur in the palliative care patient. This is partly due to the losses resulting from these changes and to the feelings that are generated by the experience. We looked at coping with loss in Chapter 2.

Case study

Mr Green had high standing in the community and managed a company that meant he had responsibility for 100 staff. He was diagnosed as having motor neurone disease and he quickly became totally reliant on others for all his care needs. Mr Green lost his role within society, work and home within a short space of time. He therefore felt that he was no longer an active part of society, part of a team at work or a partner to his wife. This in turn led to feelings of hopelessness and of low self-worth and low self-esteem.

Feelings of self-worth and self-esteem have been shown to be an integral part of psychological wellbeing (Maslow, 1987).

Patients who are suffering from a life-limiting illness often display fear, which often leads to heightened anxiety. Buckman (1998) gives a summary of the common fears patients have about:

- **physical illness**, for example, physical symptoms (such as pain, nausea), disability (paralysis, loss of mobility);
- **psychological effects**, for example, not coping, 'breakdown', losing mind/dementia;
- **dying**, for example, existential fears, religious concerns;
- **treatment**, for example, side effects (baldness, pain), surgery (pain, mutilation), altered body image (surgery, colostomy, mastectomy);
- **family and friends**, for example, loss of sexual attraction or sexual function, being a burden, loss of family role;
- **finances, social status and job**, for example, loss of job (breadwinner), possible loss of medical insurance with job, expenses of treatment, being out of 'mainstream'.

Note how complex the situation becomes when you look closely at it. Although fear can be a cause of anxiety, there may be many and varied reasons for the fear. These reasons may often stem from any or all of the five key areas we are investigating.

Social causes of anxiety

Social causes of heightened anxiety are numerous. For example, the patient losing their job will put increasing financial pressure on the family. Patients may fear that the family cannot cope with the extra demands made on them during the illness or after their death. Housing issues also cause heightened anxiety. A disabled person may be a prisoner in their own home because they are unable to negotiate internal or external stairs.

Case study

Alan was 49. He was suffering from advanced motor neurone disease and was confined to a wheelchair. The toilet and the bedroom were upstairs in his house. He was unable to get downstairs or outside into his garden, which was his pride and joy. As the months went on, he saw his garden deteriorate and he became increasingly anxious and angry with his family, as they had neither the time nor the skills required to maintain the garden. A stair lift was eventually fitted and this gave Alan access not only to the garden but to the outside world. He began going to day hospice, where he showed off his gardening skills. His anxiety and anger started to dissipate. His wife remarked that she had the 'old' Alan back again and that a lot of the family tensions had resolved.

If the family cannot discuss the patient's diagnosis, treatments or prognosis, the patient may feel further isolated through being unable to discuss their anxieties and fears. Another source of anxiety is collusion, where the truth about the patient's illness and prognosis is withheld either from the patient or from a specific family member. This leads to mistrust and raised levels of anxiety in patients, families and professional carers.

Cultural causes of anxiety

Anxiety may stem from being in a hospital, hospice or other palliative care setting where the cultural norm is different from the patient's own, or from having carers from a different culture come into the patient's home. Difficulties may arise over the way in which things are done and who may carry out tasks for the patient (for example, same sex interaction only). There may be difficulties with language, particularly specialist medical language, and also body language. All of these areas may cause the patient anxiety over and above that related directly to their illness.

Spiritual causes of anxiety

Narayanasamy (2004) defines spirituality as:

> the essence of our being [which] gives meaning and purpose to our existence.
>
> Narayanasamy (2004: 1140)

It is acknowledged that when spiritual needs are not met then spiritual distress may ensue. Narayanasamy (2004) suggests that spiritual needs fall into the following areas:

- meaning and purpose;
- sources of strength and hope;
- love and relatedness;
- self-esteem;
- fear and anxiety;
- anger;
- relationships between beliefs and health.

Note that each patient will display his or her own unique mix of emotions when spiritually distressed, and heightened anxiety may be only one of a number of characteristics displayed.

Case study

Mr Smith was 70 and was suffering from end-stage cardiac failure. He was distressed that he had not seen his son for 30 years as he had been in prison and his father had disowned him. He had no idea where his son was, but wanted to see him before he died. The social worker took on the task of trying to trace the son and, after a few days, successfully contacted him through another family member. At this point Mr Smith became very anxious and then withdrawn. He then announced that he did not want any visitors, especially this son. This was unfortunate, as the son, after a lot of persuasion by the social worker, had decided to come and see his dad – although he was not keen to do so. The social worker went to speak to Mr Smith and after a period of silence he exploded with anger. He had not known where his son had been for many years and had been very worried about what had happened to him. However, when the social worker had investigated it was discovered that another close family member had never lost contact and had been keeping him updated about his father's deteriorating health. Mr Smith was very angry that he had not known about this relationship and that his health was being discussed behind his back. When the son arrived the social worker stayed in the room on Mr Smith's request and facilitated the reunion, which was very emotional for all concerned. Once Mr Smith had seen his son and talked to him about the missing years he was less anxious and felt that his last life wish had been fulfilled.

The needs of the family

We looked at caring for the carers and the importance of honest and open communication in Chapters 1 and 2 respectively. There we suggested that providing enough information to enable the family to take part in decisions about the patient's care can dispel the anxieties caused by doubt and fear. However, relatives often receive less information than patients although their anxiety is as great (Lugton, 1999).

There are also problems specific to those caring for patients suffering from heightened anxiety. For example, if the family is already struggling to cope, the emotional turmoil of the anxious patient may make the situation still more difficult to handle. The next activity is about supporting the patient's family. You may find it helpful to re-read bits of 'Caring for the carers' in Chapter 1.

Activity 5: Supporting the patient's family

Read the following case study, then answer the following questions. You may find it helpful to discuss this activity with the members of your AL set.

- What factors could be causing Ann's anxiety?
- How can you help Ann and what can be done to allow Alec's wishes to be fulfilled?

Case study: Alec and Ann

Alec and Ann have been married for 50 years and during this time have been inseparable. They have no family and their next of kin is a niece who lives in Canada. They receive some help from a neighbour, but in the main they support each other. For many years Alec has suffered from metastatic prostatic cancer. He is now nearing the end of his life. He was admitted to hospital as an emergency, as he had fallen at home. He desperately wishes to return home to die. Since he made these wishes known to the ward team, a discharge plan has been put into place so he can return home as soon as possible. However, since the issue of discharge has been raised with Ann she has become very anxious. She has been visiting less frequently and has been avoiding contact with the ward staff.

Feedback

Here are our brief suggestions – you and your colleagues may have come up with many other useful ideas.

- Ann's anxiety is probably based on fear of the unknown – not knowing how or when death may occur. She may be afraid that she will be unable to care for Alec. She may fear that she will lose emotional control as the end draws near. She may be afraid that Alec will fall again.
- It's important that you establish good communication with both Alec and Ann. Help them to identify any fears, and then set goals to enable them to overcome them. (We look at goal-setting later on in this chapter, in 'Behavioural interventions'.) Liaise with the community team about any problems and ensure that good discharge planning is taking place to cover all of Ann's and Alec's needs. The physiotherapist and occupational therapist should be involved so that appropriate assessment of Alec and his home can be arranged. If Ann is reluctant to have Alec at home, it may be necessary to compromise. She may be prepared to have him home for day visits at first and then perhaps an overnight stay. It may be possible to slowly build up the amount of time that Alec spends at home. If you intend to try this approach, you will need to explain to Alec that it may take time to resolve the issue.

Family members can have as many problems as the patient and they may therefore need a great deal of support. Furthermore, as we mentioned in 'Caring for the carers' (Chapter 1), patients and families sometimes have competing needs and therefore their goals are different. It takes careful negotiations to resolve the problems. Sometimes the patient and family members cannot resolve their differences and you need to help them reach a compromise by facilitating the negotiations.

Predisposing factors

There are a number of factors, identified by Barraclough (1998), which may increase the likelihood that certain patients will become anxious.

These predisposing factors are:

- organic mental disorders;
- poorly controlled physical symptoms;
- poor relationships and communication between staff and patient;
- past history of mood disorder or misuse of alcohol and drugs;
- personality traits hindering adjustment – such as rigidity, pessimism, extreme need for independence and control;
- concurrent life events;
- lack of support from family and friends.

By identifying the existence of any predisposing factors, you can identify those patients most at risk.

Activity 6: Causes of anxiety

Re-read the notes you made in Activity 1.

Make notes on a separate sheet of paper, or in your learning diary, to identify which of the causes of your anxiety were:

- physical;
- psychological;
- social;
- cultural;
- spiritual;
- related to the needs of your family.

You may not be sure which category a certain cause should go in and some causes may fit into several categories. Just ensure that the categorisation makes sense to you. Identify any predisposing factors you might have.

Feedback

As we said in the activity, you may not be sure which category a certain cause should go in and some causes may fit into several categories. This is because the categories are interrelated. In fact, it is unlikely that something that causes you anxiety would fall under only one category. If you had difficulty coping with your anxiety, you may now realise that it had knock-on effects in parts of your life that you had thought unaffected by it. Furthermore, you may not have considered the possibility of predisposing factors making you more prone to anxiety. Often people focus on the most apparent cause of anxiety, without considering the many complicating factors that are involved.

In the next activity you are going to talk to patients and their families about the causes of anxiety. If you have not already discussed this with the members of the health care team – including the patients – you should do this now, before attempting the activity. Make sure the patients understand what you intend to ask them about and that they are happy to help you. When interviewing the patients, don't delve too deeply. If a patient becomes slightly distressed, consider taking a break or moving onto a different subject. Ask them if they are prepared to go on. You do not want to reach a point where neither you nor the patient can cope with their distress, so be careful and sensitive in your questioning.

It's a good idea to limit the total number of people you interview to, say, five or even fewer if you feel that the activity will be too time-consuming.

Activity 7: Causes of anxiety in patients

Ask your manager and other members of your team for help in identifying several patients who are experiencing anxiety, and who may be prepared to talk to you about the anxiety they feel, its causes and manifestations, and how they are coping with it. Ask the patients you select if they would mind you talking to their families and check that this is also acceptable to the families. Alternatively, reflect on conversations of this type that you have had with patients in the past. If you are a lone worker and have not assessed patient anxiety before, it may be of use to have another team member for support when you do this for the first time.

Careful choice of patients is important, as you do not want to make anxious patients any more anxious than they already are. By asking them if they are prepared to be interviewed, you may make them more anxious. They may feel unable to say 'no'. They may have hidden their anxiety from their family (perhaps because they don't want to upset them) and wish to continue to do so, which will not be possible if you involve the family.

When you ask patients if they are prepared to talk to you, reassure them that they can withdraw or stop part way through if they want to.

You may find it helpful to tape record the conversation, but remember to obtain the permission of all participants. If you intend for others to listen to the tape, you must obtain written permission from the patient.

After the interview, make notes on the things they tell you.

Discuss with the patients in particular the six categories (physical, psychological, social, cultural and spiritual, and the needs of the patients' families) into which causes might be divided. Identify any predisposing factors in the patients' lives.

Ask the patients and their families how they are coping – some people, for example, use humour, some use anger or denial.

Ask patients and their families how they feel from day to day – you may find that they feel guilt, fear, disbelief or shock. Patients near the end of life may feel an acceptance of their fate.

Keep your notes, as they will be useful in later activities.

Feedback

You have probably encountered a wide range of causes and manifestations, and a variety of coping mechanisms. We looked at coping mechanisms in detail in Chapter 2.

The information you have gathered about the causes and manifestations of anxiety, and the strategies patients use to cope with anxiety, will give you a greater understanding of the anxious patient's experience of life. You will also be able to help and inform junior colleagues and unqualified staff who may misconstrue patients' behaviour or be puzzled or worried by it.

When supporting palliative care patients, it is useful to survey all areas in which the cause(s) of their anxiety might affect them. The care plan that you create can help you identify what is causing the patient the most distress. It may turn out that it is something that can be relatively easily rectified and you can improve the quality of the patient's life considerably by addressing this problem.

Unfortunately, it is likely that incurable or intractable problems are at least partly responsible for the patient's anxiety, in which case the most you can do is attempt to help them cope with the situation or identify ways in which the anxiety can best be managed. We looked at coping mechanisms in Chapter 2, and we will look at the management of anxiety at the end of this section of the chapter.

You may have been surprised to discover, when talking to the patients' families, that they too may have exhibited many of the symptoms of anxiety. You may have suspected that this is one of the causes of the patient's anxiety, although they may not have said as much. You may like to discuss this with them without the presence of their family. They are more likely to agree if this is the case. This is just one of the reasons why it is important to take a holistic view of the patient and for supporting the family as well as the patient. By relieving the distress felt by the patient's family, you can reduce the pressures felt by the patient, and this will improve their quality of life. We considered how to care for the carers in Chapter 1.

Assessment of anxiety in palliative care patients

A rigorous initial assessment should be undertaken to assess patients' actual and potential problems and needs (see Chapter 3). A holistic approach to the general assessment ensures that patients know you are interested in the needs of their families and the patients' psychological, social, cultural and spiritual concerns as well as their physical symptoms. They are more likely to tell you about their concerns in these areas in the future (Maguire *et al.*, 1996), thereby reducing the anxiety they experience (Parle *et al.*, 1996).

Once anxiety has been identified as being a problem for a patient, a more in-depth assessment into the causes of the patient's anxiety should be undertaken. You can do this by conducting an in-depth interview covering aspects such as the causes of the anxiety with the patient. You may find it useful to attend a communication skills course. This should enhance your ability to listen actively, ask questions appropriately and reflect and paraphrase patients' responses. Faulkner (1998) suggests the following guidelines for interviews:

- use a private room;
- ensure you will not be interrupted;
- allow the patient time to discuss problems;
- set an agenda;
- use different types of questions to allow the patient to impart the whole story, i.e. open questions allow explanation whereas closed questions only allow a 'yes' or 'no' answer, clarifying questions allow you to ensure you have understood what the patient has said;
- don't use questions which ask more than one question at a time as this can confuse the patient and can put them off the track they were on;
- don't use premature reassurance as this may stop the patient from exploring all their problems.

Taking notes is a good way of ensuring that none of the concerns the patient mentions are accidentally left out of the care package (Heaven and Maguire, 1997). You should, however, ask the patient's permission before taking any notes.

If patients and/or relatives are very distressed it may be a good idea to let the rest of the care team know where you are going to conduct the interview. If anything untoward happens, for example a very angry person begins using physical violence, they can come to your aid.

It is useful to interview the patient's family separately (with the patient's permission), as they often have different opinions about and perceptions of the patient's symptoms (Robbins, 1998). Both patients and their families may have issues that they are more likely to discuss with you if the others are not present.

Another way of making an objective measurement of anxiety is to use a valid and reliable assessment tool, such as:

- the Hospital Anxiety and Depression Scale (HADS) (Zigmond and Snaith, 1983);
- the General Health Questionnaire (Goldberg, 1972) – there are several versions of the General Health Questionnaire in a variety of lengths: GHQ12 (12 questions), GHQ20, GHQ28 and GHQ30 are all useful for assessing psychological wellbeing;
- the Mental Adjustment to Cancer Scale (MAC) (Watson *et al.*, 1988);
- the European Organisation for Research and Treatment of Cancer Quality of Life Questionnaire (EORTC QLQ-C30) (EORTC Quality of Life Study Group, 1995).

Several studies have suggested ways of using these tools (Urch *et al.*, 1998; Herrmann, 1997). Furthermore Robbins (1998) suggests that the results may be dependent on staff perceptions of patients' problems. The use of these tools is therefore not as unproblematic as could be hoped.

The next activity asks you to find out about the four tools we have just listed, with a view to finding a suitable tool for assessing anxiety in your workplace. In Activity 19 in Section 2: Depression, we will be asking you to perform a similar activity about tools for assessing depression.

Activity 8: Assessment tools

Perform a literature search to find out about the following tools:

- the Hospital Anxiety and Depression Scale (HADS) (Zigmond and Snaith, 1983);
- the General Health Questionnaire (Goldberg, 1972);
- the Mental Adjustment to Cancer Scale (MAC) (Watson *et al.*, 1988);
- the European Organisation for Research and Treatment of Cancer Quality of Life Questionnaire (EORTC QLQ-C30) (EORTC Quality of Life Study Group, 1995).

For example, McDowell and Newell (1996) provide a comprehensive summary of the uses of many assessment tools. Find out who within the health care team is responsible for assessing patients receiving palliative care, specifically those experiencing anxiety. Discuss with them the tools that they use. If tools for assessing anxiety are not used regularly, find out why. For each tool used, create a list of pros and cons regarding its use.

From your literature search and discussion with an experienced assessor, identify the tool that seems to be most useful in your situation. HADS, for example, is quick and easy for patients to complete, which is useful when working with patients receiving palliative care, but it is very much focused on the psychological aspects of a patient's life, rather than taking a holistic approach. Obtain a copy of the tool you have selected. A simple tool may be accompanied by instructions on how to calculate the patient's score, but more complex tools may be accompanied by an entire training package. Be aware that you may have to get permission from the authors or their publishers to use the tool you have chosen. Write a brief report on the tool you have chosen, explaining your reasons for choosing it. Also identify the other tools that you considered and give your reasons for not selecting them.

Discuss the possible implementation of the tool with your manager and colleagues from the multidisciplinary team. If necessary, do a further literature search to answer any questions they may have.

Once you have agreed on a tool, find out what training is necessary for you to be able to perform the assessment competently, and undertake the training.

Feedback

There may be a specialist on your team who is responsible for the psychological assessment of patients and there should also be a referral protocol – usually to a psychologist or another qualified specialist. The specialist should be able to discuss the pros and cons of various assessment tools with you and ways of introducing the tools into practice if they are not currently used regularly. The most suitable tool may vary from setting to setting and you and the specialist are probably the best people to identify which is most useful in your clinical area.

Before trying to use a new assessment tool in your clinical practice, make sure you have investigated its uses thoroughly and that you know exactly how to use it, when, why and with whom.

If you (or your manager) decide that an existing validated tool is to be used, all the professionals who will use it should have the rationale behind its use explained to them and be trained to use it properly. This ensures that everyone understands why it is being used and that it is used consistently. Without this education and training, there may be misinterpretations in the use of the tool and results of the assessments may be invalid.

It is important to continue to assess the patient's condition in a holistic manner and at regular intervals (Regnard and Tempest, 1998). Furthermore, you should re-evaluate the situation after each intervention (Lugton, 1999). This allows the health care team to evaluate the efficacy of the interventions and also to note whether the patient's condition, family circumstances, or any other external circumstances have changed, as this may result in a change in the plan of care.

The next activity depends upon your having done the training that will enable you to use the assessment tool you have selected. Note that before using a tool in practice, you must be properly trained in its use.

Activity 9: The assessment of anxiety

Use the tool you selected in Activity 8 the next few times you wish to assess a patient experiencing anxiety. Once you are familiar with the tool, draw up a list of pros and cons, drawing on the work you did in Activity 8, and on your experience of using the tool in practice. Identify any ways in which you can make the tool more suitable to your situation.

Feedback

Discuss any problems you encounter with the psychological assessment specialist on your team and discuss any changes that you think are necessary. Once you and the specialist are confident that the tool is suitable, discuss its implementation throughout your clinical area with your manager. Remember that all the people who will use the tool must have the appropriate training.

Management of anxiety in palliative care patients

Having assessed the patient and concluded that they are suffering from anxiety, the next step is to negotiate a plan of care with the patient and the care team. Note that accurate assessment of the underlying causes of a patient's problems leads to more effective treatment (Twycross and Wilcock, 2001), which should result in a better quality of life for the patient. Furthermore, as we mentioned in Chapter 2, effective teamwork is a vital component of effective palliative care.

Good communication skills are essential for the health care professional. They will enable you to explain fully to the patient the nature of the problem, the variety of interventions that may be employed to help relieve their suffering, their possible outcomes and side effects. The clear presentation of accurate information allows the patient to make informed decisions about the treatments they may be offered (Lugton, 1999). This encourages patient autonomy and increased feelings of control and self-esteem (Maslow, 1987) and may therefore reduce anxiety.

We will now investigate in greater depth some of the interventions that may be used to manage heightened anxiety in the patient receiving palliative care. This will help you to gain insight into the different treatment options that may be available to you. We will consider the nurse's role, non-pharmacological and pharmacological interventions.

The nurse's role

The nurse's role in the management of anxiety in patients is divided into two major parts: communication and helping the patient with coping strategies. Through clear and open communication you can establish yourself as someone to whom the patient can relate frankly and without fear. Although your role is about creating an environment that can ease anxiety, the way in which you present yourself and relate to patients receiving palliative care may be just as important. You may find it helpful to reflect upon the models of nursing that we presented in Chapter 1, as they identify helpful ways of 'being with' patients.

The nurse's role also includes the assessment and education of patients with respect to coping strategies, which we looked at in Chapter 2. Find out what coping strategies the patient has used and whether they are still proving effective. If they are not, the patient may find some of the interventions below helpful. Through the use of these interventions, patients may reach a state in which they are able to use their own coping strategies once again. However, this may depend on the meanings held for patients by their physical illness and the proximity of death, particularly if they are in the terminal stage of their illness.

Non-pharmacological interventions

While the patient is coming to terms with the realities of their situation, discuss their concerns and fears with them in an empathetic manner (Breitbart *et al.*, 1998). To help them to openly express their fears and concerns, patients may need the professional to help them to appraise their situation and to listen to their expressions of emotion (Lugton, 1999). This type of support enables the patient to cope with their situation and may in turn alleviate a number of the underlying causes of their anxiety. We will consider the following non-pharmacological interventions:

- behavioural interventions;
- cognitive interventions;
- complementary therapies;
- attendance at a day hospice.

We will also look at non-pharmacological interventions for panic attacks and at some simple leisure activities you can introduce to reduce patients' boredom and anxiety.

Behavioural interventions

Behavioural techniques aim to change the patient's behaviour, persuading them not to attempt tasks that are unattainable and therefore generate anxiety and encouraging them to undertake activities that have previously brought pleasure and generated feelings of personal control, and which have not been affected by the illness. Encouraging positive thinking increases feelings of self-worth and personal control, and reduces feelings of helplessness. This breaks the cycle of pessimistic thoughts that leads to reduced activity.

Goal setting is a useful intervention in palliative care, as it can be used to rehabilitate patients within the context of their disease. Patients set goals in agreement with the professionals caring for them (Tigges, 1998). The sense of achievement a patient feels on meeting a goal fosters hope and increases self-esteem (Hockley and Mowatt, 1996). Unfortunately, patients sometimes envisage meeting goals that are well outside their limits. It can be challenging to support a patient when they have to accept this and adapt to new, lesser goals. However, you can help to achieve this through sensitive management – allowing the patient to feel fulfilled and to have pride and self-esteem in what they can do (Tigges, 1998).

Relatives have an important part to play in helping a patient to set and reach goals, although they may be as anxious as the patient (Greer and Moorey, 1997). Goal setting, through giving both the patient and the family increased insight into the patient's capabilities, may therefore improve the quality of life of both parties.

Goal setting is also useful in the promotion of hope in patients with depression, as it directs their thoughts beyond their present state to the future (Stevens, 1996). For example, you could start by encouraging the patient to set him- or herself a small goal for tomorrow such as, for example, instead of staying in bed all day, get up and sit in a chair for an hour. Once the patient has accomplished this goal, you can discuss how the patient wants to move forward. The next goal, for example, could be to get dressed tomorrow. Once the patient has accomplished their second goal, you can discuss the next goal. For example, now they are up and dressed, you could suggest that they might want to try going out with their family at the weekend. The idea is to extend the timeframe while keeping it within easy reach of the patient's thoughts. The next goal could be to go to the hairdresser's/barber's. If the patient cannot achieve a goal, you need to discuss why the patient thinks this is. The patient may need to make the task easier, or extend the timeframe. However, if the patient's health is deteriorating, as is often the case with patients receiving palliative care, you need to be aware that a goal set on Monday and achieved on Tuesday may be unachievable by Saturday, and make allowances for this when discussing goal setting with the patient.

Patients may also find breathing exercises helpful – we look at these in depth in Chapter 5, 'Breathlessness'.

Cognitive interventions

The focus of cognitive interventions is to allow patients to investigate the negative, sometimes unrealistic, thoughts that they may experience. By doing this, they may be able to change the way they think about their illness, thus producing a more positive view of the future and restoring their feelings of personal control. For example, in one programme the patient keeps a diary, noting down every automatic negative thought they have. The therapist helps the patient to identify the roots of these thoughts and to challenge them, allowing the patient to consider whether their interpretation of these thoughts is realistic. For example, if a patient believes that they are a burden to their family, getting them to ask the family about it and receiving positive feedback challenges the assumption and relieves the negativity of it.

This type of programme is usually undertaken by trained therapists. However, the underlying principles of the therapy could be applied within any health care setting, providing the professionals have the necessary skills to explore the patient's personal concern, to address the issues that arise and to support the patient through the programme. For further information on cognitive interventions, see Adams *et al.* (2006) and Dein (2005).

Greer and Moorey (1997) have developed a programme of adjuvant psychological therapy (APT) for cancer patients to help them to cope with their cancer-related emotional stress, anxiety and depression. It is not suitable for those suffering from schizophrenia, manic-depressive illness, organic confusional states or dementia.

In the cognitive approach of APT, the patient and therapist explore the patient's major problems and how they can cope with them. The sessions aim to:

- induce the patient's 'fighting spirit' by highlighting the patient's individual coping strengths;
- promote autonomy by encouraging them to talk to their oncologist about treatments and participate in decisions about their treatments;
- illustrate the actions that they can take to increase personal control in their lives.

The patient is also encouraged to express their feelings in a supported environment where those feelings can be explored and evaluated. The feeling of wellbeing generated by the expression of these feelings may help some patients, but many require more specific behavioural and cognitive coping strategies.

Complementary therapies

There are many complementary therapies on offer to palliative care patients, including:

- aromatherapy;
- reflexology;
- massage;
- homeopathy;
- acupuncture;
- relaxation.

The aim of these therapies is to help the patient to relax and to relieve stress, which in turn help to relieve symptoms and lead to feelings of positive wellbeing (Bottrill and Kirkwood, 1999).

In my experience this is very evident in the patients who have received these therapies. The feeling of relaxation and wellbeing really increases their quality of life.

Co-ordinator, palliative day care

There are a number of studies examining the use of complementary therapies in the promotion of quality of life in palliative care patients (Milligan *et al.*, 2002; Hodgson, 2000; Corner *et al.*, 1995; Wilkinson, 1995). It is suggested that before embarking on the use of a complementary therapy within a health care setting, guidelines should be drawn up by the care team to ensure that safe practice is being undertaken and that the patient's quality of life is not diminished. For example, certain questions should be asked: Is the therapist experienced in working with cancer patients? It is known that some essential oils are not suitable for cancer patients undergoing chemotherapy (Bottrill and Kirkwood, 1999).) Is the therapist qualified? Does the therapist have insurance should anything go wrong? Current best practice on the implementation of complementary therapies for palliative care patients can be found in the *National guidelines for the use of complementary therapies in supportive and palliative care*. You can find them on The Prince of Wales Integrated Health website at **www.fih.org.uk** (accessed 30/6/08). Once on the site, put 'palliative' into the search box and the guidelines will be available to read or download.

Attendance at a day hospice

This has been shown to help improve a patient's psychological wellbeing through the implementation of an individualised rehabilitation programme. This may involve the use of therapeutic activities such as art therapy or music therapy, and the use of goal-setting techniques (Stevens, 1996). There may also be complementary therapies on offer. Also, the members of the day hospice team are experts in the holistic management of palliative care patients and have time and energy to spend in caring for and supporting patients while they try to adjust to their situation. Further information on palliative day care can be found at: **www.apdcl.org.uk**

Management of panic attacks

If a patient is aware of the feelings that start these attacks off, they may be able to control them by trying to relax or distract themselves from those feelings (Regnard and Tempest, 1998). The patient's state needs regular assessment and the help of a proficient companion who is able to stay throughout an episode (Fallon and O'Neill, 1998). The patient may require specialist help to resolve these panic attacks, i.e. a psychiatrist or psychologist, to unravel their problems and to provide counselling and support (Regnard and Tempest, 1998). We also look at panic attacks in Chapter 5, 'Breathlessness'.

Simple leisure activities

Simple craft activities that do not require much manual dexterity and where it is easy to achieve a quick outcome are useful for relaxation and distraction. Ask patients what sorts of things they would like to do. For example, patients may enjoy making cards for special occasions for family members using craft materials. This is simple and can be done in bed if required. It may cost a little to get the materials in the first place, but they can be used time and again. Patients may enjoy reading short stories or daily newspapers that do not require a lot of concentration to read. Jigsaw puzzles can allow the patient and family members to become involved in a joint venture. Smaller jigsaws (250–500 pieces) are more appealing, as they can be achieved in a fairly short time (depending on the patient's concentration span). If you want to supply crosswords, it's best to supply single crosswords on a page rather than a lot in one book. Crosswords can capture a patient's interest and, again, they can be done in bed or with family members or staff members. The production of relaxation tapes can be a useful exercise and helpful to patients. Simple games like dominoes and cards may be popular.

Activity 10: Investigating non-pharmacological interventions

1. Explore non-pharmacological interventions that could be employed to help alleviate the cause(s) of anxiety. You could investigate local complementary therapists with a view to offering the service to patients, or discuss purposeful activities with the occupational therapist. Is there a local psychologist who could help with the more distressed patients? Is there access to psychological therapies? Focus on your own workplace to see if there are any interventions that could be employed.

2. Along with other members of the multidisciplinary team, devise a simple activity that could be undertaken by patients in your area to take the focus of their attention away from the things that are making them anxious.

3. Compile a resource list of services that could be used to help a community-based palliative care patient suffering from anxiety who lives in your area.

Feedback

1. You may find that there are few services available to help the care team with the anxious patient. Resource implications may be raised – e.g. it may be good to have a complementary therapist, but who pays them? There may be no clinical psychologist. Discuss these issues with your team and with your AL set. Contact the organisations listed in parts 2 and 3 below, and other organisations in a similar situation to your own, and find out what advice or help they can offer. Can you obtain charitable funding?

2. Once you have found out what the patient is interested in, you might find that the family will supply crosswords, jigsaws, etc. But remember that an activity undertaken without patient involvement may cause further anxiety. The occupational therapy department may be able to supply useful items. You may find local voluntary agencies that will supply craft items, such as the Women's Royal Voluntary Service (WRVS).

3. Services that can help the palliative care patient include: self-help groups, community groups that provide lunch clubs, etc., for example Crossroads, local day hospice, the Red Cross, Macmillan Nurse Service, information services such as BACUP, Breast Cancer Care, the Chest, Heart and Stroke Association, Macmillan Cancer Support (which also provides money for individuals to help with financial problems), and the local specialist palliative care team.

Pharmacological interventions

In conjunction with non-pharmacological approaches to the management of anxiety, some patients require medication to relieve the suffering caused by their anxiety. The choice of drug should be based on the desire to keep unwanted side effects to a minimum, as this may adversely affect the patient's quality of life (Lloyd-Williams *et al.*, 1999). Patients should be advised of any side effects they may experience, as this reduces anxiety (McVey, 1998) and increases patients' co-operation/compliance. Some patients may be afraid they will become addicted to the drugs that are prescribed for their anxiety. When discussing side effects, encourage the patient to ask questions, express any concerns they might have and allay their fears where you can. If patients ask questions you cannot answer, check the manufacturer's literature and report back when you can. If you encourage patients to ask questions, you must be prepared to put some effort into finding answers to their questions.

Benzodiazepines

The main drugs and common doses used to treat depression in palliative care are listed in Table 4.1, together with the symptoms they are designed to alleviate. Individual prescribers will have their own ideas as to what is the correct dose. Prescribers could refer to the palliative care section of 'The British National Formulary' for further guidance, if they need it. All these drugs have the same side effects to a greater or lesser degree – drowsiness, flaccid muscles and postural hypotension.

Antipsychotics

Antipsychotics are classed as typical or atypical and can be used in the following situations:

Symptom	Drug	Dose
Sleeplessness	Temazepam	10–20 mg at night
Anxiety, tenseness of the muscles	Diazepam	2–5 mg three times a day, reducing over several days to a maintenance dose of 2–5mg at night
Panic attacks.	Lorazepam	0.5–1mg, sublingually
	Midazolam	5–10 mg, intravenously or subcutaneously

Table 4.1 Symptoms of anxiety and benzodiazepines that can be used to treat them

- when benzodiazepines do not control symptoms sufficiently;
- where an organic cause is suspected;
- where the patient has psychotic symptoms such as delusions or hallucinations (these may sometimes be induced by opioids).

Typical antipsychotics include haloperidol, methotrimeprazine, trifluoperazine and chlorpromazine. Atypical ones include risperidone and olanzapine. The adverse effects of these drugs include sedation, anticholinergic symptoms and hypotension in varying degrees. The atypical antipsychotics tend to have fewer side effects and are more favoured in palliative care where patients are frail with advanced disease.

Tricyclic antidepressants, opioids and beta-blockers

Tricyclic antidepressants (TCAs) such as amitriptyline and nortriptyline can be used if the patient is depressed as well as anxious. TCAs are useful in treating panic disorders. Their usefulness is often limited due to their anti-cholinergic and sedative side effects.

If anxiety is caused by breathlessness or cardiopulmonary processes, carefully titrated doses of opioids can be of use. They are especially useful in the treatment of respiratory distress in the terminal phase.

Beta-blockers (e.g. propanalol) are useful where there are somatic signs, i.e. tremors, sweating, diarrhoea.

Sources: *British National Formulary 51*, 2006; Twycross and Wilcock, 2001; Fallon and O'Neill, 1998; Regnard and Tempest, 1998.

It is important that once the patient's anxiety is being treated, regular, ongoing assessment of the outcomes of this treatment are recorded and discussed with the care team and the patient. Any changes to the plan of action should be fully discussed with the patient, their family and the multidisciplinary care team before a new avenue of treatment is explored and initiated. Remember that there are some patients who require more expert support, i.e. a psychiatrist or psychologist, to help investigate and treat their anxiety. The members of the care team should be able to recognise when they do not have the knowledge and skills to adequately care for and support a patient with difficult symptoms. They should be confident enough to refer such patients to other specialists who have the necessary knowledge and skills (Regnard and Tempest, 1998).

Activity 11: Investigating pharmacological interventions

Investigate which drugs could be prescribed to reduce anxiety in the palliative care patient. You could do this by performing a review of the case notes of previous patients to look at the prescribing patterns. Alternatively, you could interview the prescribers in your workplace – or you could do both. Compare the patterns or preferences you have identified with our suggestions.

Investigate protocols for the drug management of anxiety elsewhere, for example local hospices, hospital palliative care teams, Macmillan Nurse services, other wards in your hospital, other general practitioner (GP) surgeries. If your area does not already have a protocol, identify a suitable protocol for drug management of anxiety and discuss its introduction with the other members of your care team, particularly your manager and the doctors and pharmacists. Agree a strategy for its implementation.

Identify the side effects of these drugs, and make notes on how the side effects might impact on the patient's quality of life. You could produce an information leaflet for patients on the side effects – this may reduce the anxiety of having to take medication. It is important that you discuss this with your pharmacist.

Feedback

You may find that little prescribing of drugs is undertaken. You will need to think about how you can persuade prescribers that drugs may be required to treat these patients. You may find that no protocol exists for the drug management of anxiety, even though within specialist palliative care the use of protocols for the drug management of palliative care problems enhances the care given and the patient's quality of life.

Remember that patients may become more anxious if they are not involved in decisions about their care. Involving them in discussions of possible drug treatment and identifying possible side effects provides information and may therefore reduce their anxiety.

Activity 12: Reflecting on the management of anxiety

Using the reflective cycle provided in Chapter 2 (Marks-Maran and Rose, 1997), reflect on the care offered to an anxious patient in your clinical area. On a separate sheet of paper, make notes on your answers to the following questions:

- Was anxiety documented in the care plan as a problem?
- What interventions were planned to help this patient?
- What more could have been done to help this patient?

Keep your notes – they may be useful if a future patient presents with similar symptoms.

Feedback

We would hope that if you considered the patient to be anxious, anxiety was marked as a problem on the care plan. However, the general assessment that was carried out may not have identified anxiety as a symptom.

The interventions you have listed may include several of those we have described above, as well as others dealing with symptoms other than anxiety.

You may have felt that further interventions – pharmacological and non-pharmacological – should have been offered to help manage the patient's anxiety, especially if anxiety was not listed on the care plan.

Activity 13: Assessment, care planning and evaluation

Select a palliative care patient from your own workplace who, in your opinion, is anxious (possibly select one from your work in earlier activities), and who has anxiety documented in their care plan as a problem. As you perform the following tasks, make notes about them and keep your notes with this book.

- Agree a plan of care with the patient and their family to help alleviate the patient's anxiety and agree a timeframe within which the plan will be carried out.
- At the end of the agreed time, discuss the outcomes of the care package with the patient and their family. Record the impact that this care has had on the patient's quality of life.
- If the patient has achieved their goals, find out why they think the plan worked so well.
- If the goals have not been achieved, again find out why: were they too ambitious, or have other problems prevented the patient from achieving their goals?
- In both cases, identify whether new goals need to be set. What is the next plan of action to take the patient further (if this is what they want)? Have the patient's

priorities changed during the time the plan was being worked on? For example, the patient's condition may have deteriorated to such an extent that it is better to put the plan on hold or abandon it.

Feedback

As you can see, this is a continuous cyclic process. It is essential for effective care planning for all patients, not just those with palliative care needs.

Activity 14: Reflection on assessment, care planning and evaluation

Now that you have reflected on past practice and have undertaken a period of new practice, compare the notes you have kept about the care the patient received in Activity 13 to the reflective work completed for Activity 12. Ask yourself the following questions.

- What were the main differences in the two courses of action?
- Did any differences in the care provided have different effects on the patient's anxiety?
- How was the quality of the patient's life altered as a result of the care provided in both situations?

Feedback

Having developed your practice, you should be able to see improved quality of life in the patients. However, it may take some time for a whole team to change the way in which it works. It's important not to give up or become despondent. Try to get support from your manager or the medical consultant. If there has been little change in the way in which these patients have been cared for, there may be little change in their circumstances. Use the information collected from these activities to provide a report for your manager on the positive outcomes that can be achieved when managing anxiety in the patient receiving palliative care.

SECTION 2: DEPRESSION

The presence of intolerable distress that compromises the usual function of the patient requires evaluation, diagnosis and management.

Massie and Holland (1992)

Grief and depression are normal reactions to any diagnosis of a terminal illness and, although depression is one of the most common psychiatric complications of the cancer patient (Smitz and Woods, 2006), it is seldom diagnosed or managed correctly (Holtom and Barraclough, 2000).

Depression can be defined as 'a morbid sadness, dejection or melancholy' (Weller, 2000: 116–17). Although McVey (1998) has indicated that as there is no accurate definition of depression, the term can refer to a symptom, a syndrome, an emotional state or a disease. Casey (1998) suggests that the overriding feelings of depression in patients receiving palliative care are sadness and gloom, while Lovejoy *et al.* (2000: 668) suggest that depression is 'a complex, progressive neurologic-cognitive response to loss or deprivation'.

Studies suggest that between 4.5 and 77 per cent of all patients receiving palliative care suffer from depressive symptoms (Casey, 1998). This wide variation is thought to be related to the absence of reliable diagnostic criteria and the use of a variety of different assessment instruments. Twycross and Wilcock (2001) suggest that 5–10 per cent of palliative care patients suffer a major depressive illness. The numbers suffering from depression may be higher in patients with high levels of disability, far-advanced disease or poorly controlled symptoms (Breitbart *et al.*, 1998), especially pain (Massie and Holland, 1992). It has also been discovered that patients with certain types of cancer suffer from a higher prevalence of depression, e.g. pancreatic cancer (Sheibani-Rad and Velanovich, 2006). Depression can also be combined with anxiety and dementia (Payne, 1998).

It is important for the multidisciplinary team to be able to identify patients who are likely to suffer from depression, as the treatment can be highly successful and lead to a much-improved quality of life (McVey, 1998). Billings (1995) indicates that early treatment of depressive symptoms may also prevent a mood disorder becoming more severe. Untreated depression in palliative care patients can lead to other symptoms being intensified, poor compliance with treatments and longer hospital stays (Lovejoy *et al.*, 2000).

Activity 15: Why intervene?

In the introduction above, we give several reasons for helping patients to manage their depression:

- improving their quality of life;
- preventing mood disorders becoming more severe;
- preventing the intensification of other symptoms;
- improving compliance;
- making hospital stays no longer than necessary.

Talk to the other members of your team about how they feel about the treatment of depression in palliative care patients. Find out whether they think that depression in palliative care should be managed. Ask for the reasons that underpin their answers.

One reason for people thinking that depression need not be treated could be simply not having thought about the issue, especially if they are new to the team and unaware of the concept of palliative care. So it could be a good idea to create an information book about the importance of treating depression in palliative care patients.

Start your information book by tracking down the articles that we have referenced:

- McVey (1998);
- Billings (1995);
- Lovejoy et al. (2000);
- Lloyd-Williams et al. (2004)

Write brief notes on the contents of the articles and include them in your book. To increase the evidence base for your assertion that depression in palliative care patients should be treated, do a literature search to find other relevant articles. Again, include copies of the articles that you identify, or make notes on the relevant points.

Then create a section of anecdotal evidence, based on the responses you received from your colleagues. They may also have further references that you could research.

If you know any palliative care patients who are no longer depressed, ask them if they would mind contributing. Ask their family and friends too. Explain what you are doing and why, and make sure that they don't mind being quoted in your information book. They may, for example, be prepared to contribute, but wish to remain anonymous.

Feedback

Most of your colleagues will probably have given good reasons for agreeing that depression should be treated. After all, the basic tenet of palliative care is to improve the quality of the patient's life. Perhaps some of your colleagues said that they felt depression was an inevitable reaction to a diagnosis of terminal illness and that therefore there was no point in treating it. If so, reading the testimonials of patients whose quality of life has improved through the treatment of depression will hopefully convince them that it is worth treating, even if they are unconvinced by the research evidence that you present.

You could also include details of local and national support groups, and details of the services that are available from which patients can seek further help, such as local psychologists or psychiatrists.

Symptoms of depression

[The] most reliable indicators of depression are persistent dysphoria, feelings of helplessness, hopelessness and worthlessness, guilt, loss of self esteem, and wishes to die.

Billings (1995: 50)

It is often difficult to distinguish between feelings of sadness and true depression. Some of the symptoms of sadness and of depression are given in Table 4.2, below.

Sadness and depression	Features suggesting depression
Depressed mood	Low mood which differs from previous
Anxiety	experiences
Decreased sleep	Loss of all emotion
Decreased concentration	Not distractible from low mood but the severity
Loss of interest	varies throughout the day
Tearfulness	Sweating, panic attacks, tremor
Tiredness	Hopelessness, especially when thinking about
Anorexia	family and friends
Suicidal ideas	Strong feelings of guilt
	Intractable pain
	Suicide attempts
	Requests for euthanasia

(Adapted from Twycross and Wilcock, 2001)

Table 4.2 Symptoms of sadness and depression

Note, however, that a patient is not just a combination of symptoms. It is useful to be aware of lists of identifying symptoms such as the one given above – this may be the quickest way to identify depression, but it is most important to build up a therapeutic relationship with the patient. They may then feel safe enough to divulge their concerns to you. This may be the best way to find out how the patient feels and to identify problems such as depression. The development of trust takes time, however, and it is important that if depression is suspected, management strategies should be implemented as soon as possible. Furthermore, nurses may find depressed patients difficult to deal with and may feel hopeless, helpless or depressed themselves, and perhaps even begin to avoid the patient. If you find yourself in this situation, remember that help is available, as we outlined in 'Caring for the carers', in Chapter 1.

Activity 16: Symptoms of depression

The aim of this activity is to give you a deeper understanding of the experience of depression. You can do it in two ways, depending on your situation. If you cannot find a suitable patient with whom to discuss depression, or do not feel confident about discussing a patient's depression with them, consider a patient whom you have nursed who was depressed while you were nursing them. Use the reflective cycle we introduced in Chapter 2 to review your interactions with them. Focus on the symptoms and possible causes of their depression.

Otherwise, identify a patient who has been successfully treated for depression. It would be useful if you know them fairly well, as you will already have some knowledge of their situation. Ask them if they would be prepared to talk to you about their depression. You will be asking them:

- how they felt – emotional and physical feelings;
- what they thought the causes of the depression might be.

(Note: It is often difficult to engage in conversation with depressed patients and, unless you are properly trained in this area, it may not be helpful for them to talk to you about how they feel. In this case, reflect on a previous patient, as suggested above.)

Create a checklist based on Table 4.2 above. (If you wish to develop your information book from Activity 15, you could include a copy of your checklist.)

Make notes on your conversation with the patient or, if it is acceptable to them, tape record the conversation. As the conversation progresses, indicate on your checklist which of the symptoms the patient mentions.

Afterwards, listen to the tape, or read through your notes again. Identify any symptoms that they mentioned that aren't on your checklist.

From the tape or your notes, make a list of the causes the patient suggested for their depression. You will need this list for Activities 17 and 18.

Feedback

It is one thing to think about the differences between sadness and depression, and quite another to experience depression. You will know this if you or anyone close to you has been depressed. Other symptoms a patient might mention include loss of appetite, weight loss, fatigue, insomnia and agitation. They may list other symptoms that they experienced at the time that might not actually have been related to the depression but to an illness or any treatments for an illness. We will investigate this issue later on in the section on assessment.

Causes of depression in the palliative care patient

As we mentioned earlier, depression can be one reaction to a diagnosis of terminal illness and, therefore, the diagnosis itself can be considered a cause of depression. Other causes of depression in the palliative care patient can include persistent feelings of loss of control, leading to feelings of hopelessness and helplessness and depression (Greer and Moorey, 1997).

The associated pathophysiology of depression is thought to relate to biological disturbances of neurotransmitters, which reduce the secretion of norepinephrine and serotonin, thus reducing the activity of the central nervous system. The limbic system, which regulates emotion, and the diencephalon, which regulates sleep, appetite, energy and psychomotor function, are also affected by the reduction of these substances (McVey, 1998).

Chronic anxiety can lead to depression. When a patient experiences anxiety, the limbic system is under continual stimulation by the panic centre (locus ceruleus). This leads to reduced neurotransmitter levels, as they cannot be made quickly enough to meet demand (McVey, 1998). A more in-depth account of the related pathophysiology is given in Lovejoy *et al.* (2000).

It has also been recognised that a number of drugs that the palliative care patient may be prescribed may contribute to depression (McVey, 1998), including:

- anti-hypertensives;
- benzodiazepines;
- corticosteroids;
- antipsychotics;
- cytotoxics.

Furthermore, some medical conditions such as hypothyroidism, can cause depression.

Psychological distress varies from individual to individual. Massie and Holland (1992) suggest that this is dependent on three variable factors:

- medical – site, stage, treatment and clinical course of disease and the presence of pain;
- psychological – prior adjustment, coping ability, emotional maturity, the disruption of life goals, the ability to modify plans;
- social – availability of emotional support offered by family, friends and co-workers.

We would also suggest that you consider the situation holistically and investigate the patient's cultural and spiritual state, and how well the families' needs are being met, as well as the three areas identified by Massie and Holland above.

Activity 17: Causes of depression

You will need your notes from Activity 16 for this activity.

Read through your notes on the causes of the patient's depression, then quickly re-read the causes we have suggested. You might also like to identify the physical, psychological, social, cultural and spiritual causes of the patient's depression, as you did in Section 1 of this chapter for anxiety, and review the needs of the patient's family.

Feedback

On the causes of depression, your theory should be validated by the patient's experience. However, you may find you have quite a long list of causes that we haven't mentioned. This may be down to a difference in terminology. Where a patient has identified an event or situation as a cause, we may refer to it as a predisposing factor, i.e. something that makes someone more likely to develop depression. You will remember that we have already looked at predisposing factors for anxiety. We will go on to look at predisposing factors for depression next.

Predisposing factors

A number of risk factors have been shown to increase the likelihood of depression. Patients are more susceptible to depression if they:

- have a previous history of depression themselves or in other family members;
- are unable to express their emotions;
- have had mutilating surgery or highly visible/major surgery;
- are aware that the threat of death is apparent;
- are living in an environment where collusion is apparent;
- lack the support of a close relationship in which to share the effects of the illness;
- have a history of recent bereavements;
- have lost their independence;
- have a history of alcohol or substance abuse;
- suffer
  - spiritual difficulties;
  - persistent pain;

– hypercalcaemia (a life-threatening metabolic disorder commonly associated with cancer);
– concurrent life stresses;
– concurrent medical conditions.

Knowledge of a patient's possible predisposition to depression is useful. You can be alert for the signs and symptoms, and ensure that the patient receives early treatment.

Activity 18: Predisposing factors

You will need your notes from Activity 16 for this activity and a photocopy of the checklist in this activity.

Read through your notes on the causes of the patient's depression. From your notes, and any background knowledge you might have of the patient, go through the checklist of predisposing factors below, indicating which ones were present for this patient.

- ☐ a previous history of depression themselves or in other family members.
- ☐ unable to express their emotions.
- ☐ have had mutilating surgery or highly visible/major surgery.
- ☐ aware that the threat of death is apparent.
- ☐ living in an environment where collusion is apparent.
- ☐ lack the support of a close relationship in which to share the effects of the illness.
- ☐ a history of recent bereavements.
- ☐ have lost their independence.
- ☐ a history of alcohol or substance abuse.
- ☐ spiritual difficulties.
- ☐ persistent pain.
- ☐ hypercalcaemia.
- ☐ concurrent life stresses.
- ☐ concurrent medical conditions.

Feedback

It may be possible to identify whether a patient is likely to develop depression by investigating their predisposing factors – your completed checklist may be an example of this. If you wish to develop your information book from Activity 15, you could include a copy of the checklist.

It is important that you use this checklist only as a point of reference. If you want to use it with a patient, don't use it as a series of questions as the patient may find it upsetting or threatening to be asked directly about some aspects. Use your knowledge of the patient to decide what questions to ask and how to phrase them.

Assessing depression in palliative care

If a general assessment (see Chapter 3) suggests that a patient may be suffering from depression, you should carry out a more in-depth assessment of their condition. The main aim of this second assessment is to identify whether the patient is displaying signs of sadness or the symptoms of true depression. (The symptoms of sadness and of depression were given in Table 4.2, and you did some work based on the information in the table in Activity 16.) When doing this assessment, you should bear in mind, however, that patients may not divulge the extent of their depression, for fear of being stigmatised for having mental health problems (Sadock and Sadock, 2005).

One of the most effective ways to identify depression is to conduct a semi-structured interview with the patient. Unfortunately, this is often not possible because of a lack of time and properly trained professionals. This type of interview may allow the patient to divulge all their concerns and problems. The nurse creates a checklist (similar to the one in Activity 18, but extended to cover symptoms, causes, any existing treatments, etc.) as a prompt to ensure that the assessment is carried out thoroughly and that a holistic approach is taken. The Palliative Care Outcome Scale (POS), which uses a scoring system to measure the severity of symptoms, is often used as a general assessment tool during a semi-structured interview in palliative care (Higginson, 1998). We look at POS in Chapter 3.

We will look at assessment tools in more depth after considering the importance of assessing the patient's:

- psychological/emotional distress;
- medical condition;
- suicidal tendencies (if any).

In assessing these areas, you need to make use of your communication skills and skills in non-verbal assessment (i.e. reading the patient's body language). You also need to consider the role of the patient's family in their situation.

Psychological/emotional distress

Many of the somatic (physical) symptoms of cancer are also indicative of depression, e.g. anorexia, insomnia, fatigue and weight loss. This makes diagnosing depression in cancer patients difficult (Lloyd-Williams et al., 1999). It has therefore been suggested that rather than focusing on the somatic symptoms, assessment should be based on the patient's emotional state. Feelings of helplessness, hopelessness, worthlessness and inappropriate guilt should be assessed, together with the effect these are having on the patient's quality of life (Billings, 1995).

Twycross and Wilcock (2001) recommend that the following criteria be considered when assessing the palliative care patient for depression.

- Low mood, which the patient recognises as qualitatively and quantitatively different from normal variations in mood and from periods of previous unhappiness.
- Depression of mood which persists for at least two weeks and occupies over 50 per cent of each day.
- The patient is not able to banish the depression or be distracted from it.
- The patient has four other symptoms of depression from the 11-item list below that cannot be attributed to their physical disease:
  – sleep disturbance – repeated waking or early morning waking;
  – loss of weight;
  – loss of appetite;
  – impaired concentration;
  – problems in decision making;
  – feelings of hopelessness;
  – feelings of irritability;
  – feelings of guilt and unworthiness;
  – inability to enjoy life;
  – loss of interest;
  – increasing difficulty with daily chores.

Massie and Holland (1992) also suggest an in-depth assessment of:

- any previous psychological problems experienced by the patient or other family members;
- concurrent life stresses;
- substance abuse;
- social support mechanisms.

Nurses are ideally placed to carry out this assessment because they spend a great deal of time caring for patients and their families. You can ask (with appropriate sensitivity) about how a patient coped with any previous crisis in their life and whether this situation is more or less severe. You can ask whether they have taken prescribed medicine, or over-the-counter medicines, and it can help to elicit whether there has been substance abuse. You should ask about this topic sensitively, as patients may take offence or become defensive. Questions like this may help: 'Sometimes people in a similar situation have started drinking more than normal, or smoking cannabis, to try to get some relief. Does this relate to your own experience, or have you thought about it?'

It is important to find out the meaning that their illness has for patients, as psychological distress is dependent upon the way in which people cope with the losses associated with their illness (Bowlby, 1980). This is an essential part of the nurse's role. We considered coping strategies in Chapter 2.

Holtom and Barraclough (2000) suggest that the regular use of the Hospital Anxiety and Depression Scale (HADS, which we looked at in Section 1: Anxiety and will consider again later in this section) may help identify those patients who require a referral to psychiatry to aid the management of their depression.

Medical condition

You also need to assess the patient's medical condition, as a concurrent condition (such as hypothyroidism) may be causing or contributing to the patient's depression.

Suicidal tendencies

Suicidal ideas need to be carefully assessed to determine whether they are suicidal thoughts or passive death wishes, e.g., 'I wish I could go to sleep and not wake up' (Casey, 1998). Breitbart (1989) suggests risk factors associated with a high risk of suicide in cancer patients include:

- poor prognosis and advanced illness;
- depression and hopelessness;
- uncontrolled pain;
- delirium;
- prior psychiatric history;
- history of previous suicide attempts or family history of suicide;
- history of recent death of friends or spouse;
- history of alcohol abuse;
- few social supports.

These findings have also been reported more recently in a paper by Akechi *et al.* (2002).

Suicide and suicidal behaviour in the palliative care patient remains a rare occurrence (Casey, 1998). However, Billings (1995) suggests that if suicidal ideas appear serious or are expressed frequently then you should refer the patient for a psychiatric opinion. It is important that information about the expression of suicidal ideas by a patient are recorded and disseminated within the team, so that a full picture of the patient's state of mind is obtained and appropriate action taken.

Assessment tools

There are a number of valid, reliable tools that can be used to assess depression in palliative care, including:

- the Beck Depression Inventory (Beck *et al.*, 1961);
- HADS (Zigmond and Snaith, 1983);
- the General Health Questionnaire (Goldberg, 1978);
- the Edinburgh Postnatal Depression Scale (EPDS) (Lloyd-Williams *et al.*, 2002).

More information about these can be found in McDowell and Newell (1996), Robbins (1998) and Herrmann (1997). Payne (1998) performed a review of studies looking at the use of such tools in palliative care. Breitbart *et al.* (1995) suggest that the educated use of validated tools should be used to further research into depression in this group of patients.

Activity 19: Tools for assessing depression

Perform a literature search to find out about the following tools:

- the Beck Depression Inventory (Beck *et al.*, 1961);
- HADS (Zigmond and Snaith, 1983);
- the General Health Questionnaire (Goldberg, 1978);
- the Edinburgh Postnatal Depression Scale (EPDS) (Lloyd-Williams *et al.*, 2002).

For example, McDowell and Newell (1996) provide a comprehensive summary of the uses of many assessment tools, and there is more information in Robbins (1998) and Herrmann (1997).

Find out who within the health care team is responsible for assessing patients receiving palliative care, specifically those experiencing depression. Discuss with them the tools that they use. If tools for assessing depression are not used regularly, find out why. For each tool used, create a list of pros and cons regarding its use.

From your literature search and discussion with an experienced assessor, identify the tool that seems to be most useful in your situation. HADS, for example, is quick and easy for patients to complete, which is useful when working with patients receiving palliative care, but there are some doubts over the validity of the depression subscale in dying patients (Farrer, 1999). Furthermore, it is very much focused on the psychological aspects of a patient's life, rather than taking a holistic approach.

Obtain a copy of the tool you have selected. A simple tool may be accompanied by instructions on how to calculate the patient's score, but more complex tools may be accompanied by an entire training package. Be aware that you may have to get permission from the authors or their publishers to use the tool you have chosen.

Write a brief report on the tool you have chosen, explaining your reasons for choosing it. Also identify the other tools that you considered, and give your reasons for not selecting them.

Discuss the possible implementation of the tool with your manager and colleagues. If necessary, do a further literature search to answer any questions they may have.

Once you have agreed on a tool, find out what training is necessary for you to be able to perform the assessment competently and undertake the training.

Feedback

The psychological assessment specialist on your team should be able to discuss the pros and cons of various assessment tools with you, and any ways of introducing the tools into practice if they are not currently used regularly. The most suitable tool may vary from setting to setting, and you and the specialist are probably the best people to identify which is most useful in your clinical area.

Before trying to use a new assessment tool in your clinical practice, make sure you have investigated its uses thoroughly and that you know exactly how to use it, when, why and with whom.

If an existing validated tool is to be used in your clinical area, all the professionals who will use it should have the rationale behind its use explained to them and be trained to use it properly. This ensures that everyone understands why it is being used and that it is used consistently. Without this education and training, there may be misinterpretations in the use of the tool and results of the assessments may be invalid. Studies have shown that there can be substantial differences in the way these tools are used by professionals (McVey, 1998).

Professionals are not the only ones who may have difficulties using these tools. For example, patients, due to disabilities (McVey, 1998) or severe illness (Urch et al., 1998), may be unable to complete a self-reporting questionnaire (McVey, 1998).

Activity 20: The assessment of depression

Use the tool you selected in Activity 19 the next few times you wish to assess a patient experiencing depression. Once you are familiar with the tool, draw up a list of pros and cons, drawing on the work you did in Activity 19 and on your experience of using the tool in practice. Identify any ways in which you can make the tool more suitable to your situation.

Feedback

Discuss any problems you encounter with the psychological assessment specialist and discuss any changes that you think are necessary. Once you and the specialist are confident that the tool is suitable, discuss its implementation throughout your clinical area with your manager. Remember that all the people who will use the tool must have the appropriate training.

A medical method of assessing depression has been suggested by Lovejoy *et al.* (2000). They suggest that serum serotonin levels may indicate depression and that, therefore, the taking of routine blood samples may be a way of assessing the patient's condition and the ongoing efficacy of treatments. However, this type of invasive procedure may be an intrusion if patients are very ill and you should consider the ethical issues surrounding it very carefully. For example, if the patient won't live long enough for an anti-depressant to work, it would be unethical to carry out this procedure. (We considered ethics in Chapter 2.)

Management of depression in palliative care

Many health care professionals believe that depression is an inevitable reaction to a terminal illness and therefore it need not be treated. However, it is known that treating depression in this patient group has a high success rate (Billings, 1995), and can much improve their quality of life. Also, as we mentioned earlier, untreated depression can lead to other symptoms being intensified, poor compliance with treatments and longer hospital stays (Lovejoy *et al.*, 2000).

The use of enhanced communication skills (to elicit patients' views and the meanings their illness have for them) and effective team working are required for the effective management of depression (Craven, 2000). These topics are discussed in Chapter 2.

Encouraging the patient to undertake their own care can reduce feelings of helplessness and hopelessness, as can setting realistic goals to help encourage physical activity (McVey, 1998). (See Section 1 of this chapter for the principles of goal setting.)

Interventions that can be used to reduce depression fall into two main categories: psychotherapy and drug intervention (Massie and Holland, 1992). In the patient receiving palliative care, interventions can also include treating the underlying symptoms of the disease process and reintegrating the patient into society. However, before investigating psychotherapy and drug intervention, we will consider the importance of promoting hope.

The promotion of hope

In a study of patients with chronic heart failure, Rideout and Montemuro (1986) discovered that patients who are more hopeful maintain their involvement in life regardless of the physical limitations imposed by heart failure. They concluded that nursing interventions should contribute to the enhancement of hope for the future and active participation with others, and could therefore include:

- helping the patient to set realistic goals;
- encouraging the active involvement of the patient in decision making related to their current health status;
- directing the patient's thoughts beyond their present state to the future.

You can assess how likely a patient is to remain hopeful while receiving palliative care when exploring how they relate to the world during your investigation of their psychological and spiritual state. Assessing hope requires an individualised assessment which aims to understand the patient's motivations to allow hope to be well balanced within their capabilities (Rees and Joslyn, 1998).

You can direct patients' thoughts from beyond their present state to the future by introducing goal setting. We looked at goal setting in Section 1 of this chapter, in 'Behavioural interventions', in the section on the non-pharmacological management of anxiety.

What is hope?

Hope has been described as:

> an inner power that facilitates the transcendence of the present situation and movement toward new awareness and enrichment of being.

> Herth (1990: 1256)

This is a sentiment echoed by Urquhart (1999), who describes hope as:

> being an inner power or strength that can enrich lives and enable individuals to look beyond their pain, suffering and turmoil.
>
> Urquhart (1999: 35)

Considering these definitions, you can understand why Herth (2000) suggests that patients with serious illness tend to focus on the realistic aims in life rather than looking forward in the long term. It is a continuous struggle for these people to maintain hope.

Lynch (1965) suggests that 'hope is . . . characterised by the belief that there is a way out and that with help the individual can manage changes in his being'. As their disease progresses, patients can hope for the relief of their symptoms. Even near the end of life it may be possible to hold on to the hope that there can still be rewarding times ahead. Hope motivates a person to live through their illness from diagnosis until death itself. At the very end, there can still be hope for a peaceful death.

One drawback of the hope of prolonging life, however, is that patients may accept treatments that have very little hope of success, which may reduce the quality of their life, or shorten the time they have left.

Loss of hope and hopelessness

Threats to hope include abandonment, isolation, uncontrollable pain and the devaluation of the patient's personhood (Herth, 1990). A patient who has difficulty talking about the future may have lost feelings of hope (Peck, 1997). However, we would suggest that there is a vast difference between loss of hope and hopelessness.

Loss of hope is usually seen in patients who are aware of their fate and who can acknowledge that they will not be able to fulfil their life goals. The use of an individualised rehabilitation programme that focuses on the setting of new, realistic goals can help this type of person to realise that there is still hope of achieving some aims and goals. Penson (2000) suggests that a patient has a good quality of life 'when the patient's hopes are matched or fulfilled by his/her experiences of reality'.

More severe than loss of hope, hopelessness is characterised by severe psychological distress. Hopelessness may be caused by the patient's inability to acknowledge what the future holds for the hopes and dreams of themselves and their loved ones. It may be due to the patient realising that they have irrevocably relinquished their defined role and responsibilities, or that they will soon have to do so (Flaming, 1995). It may be the result of severe or untreated anxiety and may lead to depression. Patients experiencing hopelessness often become very withdrawn and become unable to discuss their situation. They may also display anger and despair at their situation.

Dealing with hopelessness is stressful for the care team and everyone involved in the care of the patient will need support. The patient's family will also require a great deal of support. As we suggested in Chapter 1, providing information about what is happening to the patient can help to relieve the family's anxieties. However, giving the patient too much information or inappropriate information can reduce hope and lead to hopelessness and despair (Penson, 2000). The patient who is suffering from hopelessness requires constant, empathetic professional care. Care team members should use advanced communication skills to try to encourage the patient to discuss their problems and to allow the patient to vent the feelings that may arise. If the care team is unable to help the patient resolve these feelings of hopelessness, then specialist psychological/psychiatric help may be needed.

However, there may not be a way to relieve the feelings of hopelessness in some patients. In this situation, the care team will need to be briefed at regular intervals to enable them to cope with the stresses that this distressing situation brings.

Case study

Mary had spent her life following the country fairs around the UK with her large family, which lived on the money made at the fairs. Unknown to her family, Mary had found a lump in her breast. It was only when her daughter noticed the odour from a fungating breast lesion, three years later, that medical aid was sought. By this time the tumour was very advanced and no curative treatment was offered.

Later that year, following a fall from her caravan step, Mary was admitted to the local hospital. She was found to have a pathological fracture of her femur and widespread bony secondaries. Mary declined all treatment for the fracture and bony secondaries, which were now causing her a lot of pain. She felt that as she was so ill, and as there was no hope of her returning to travelling with her family, there was no point in prolonging her life.

She was transferred to the local hospice for symptom control and continuing care. On admission to the hospice Mary was very quiet and offered no complaints. She told the admitting doctor that her life was over, as she would never be able to go back to her caravan and travel with her family, even though the doctor explained that if she received the treatment she had been offered, she might indeed get back home.

Over the next few weeks Mary became more and more despondent. She insisted that there was no hope for her and she just wanted to die, and that her family would be better off without her being a burden to them. Her bone pain was severe at times and, as she refused most of her medication, she slept very little. As time went on, Mary's despair became deeper. She stopped eating and refused even basic care to attend to her personal hygiene. Any attempts to talk to Mary, especially about her family who had now moved on to another area, met with anger and abuse. She threw crockery at the nurses when they attempted to persuade her to eat. She would not talk to the medical team or the hospice counsellor, or, after referral, to the psychiatrist. As her condition deteriorated, Mary's anger and bad language escalated. She refused to eat or drink, or accept any kind of care or medication.

Mary's family was contacted and her daughter came to visit. Mary cried solidly through her daughter's visit, but did not speak to her. Her daughter was very upset and decided she could not cope with seeing her mother like this as she had always been so strong. She asked to be contacted when her mother died. After her daughter's visit, Mary spoke to no one and took nothing orally. She lay and looked at the walls. Slowly her condition deteriorated and she died peacefully a week after her daughter had visited. Her daughter visited, saw her mother's body and was glad the situation was over for her and that she was now at peace.

The hospice counsellor held a debriefing session for the care team involved with Mary, as many of them felt that they had failed to help her, as they had been unable to connect with her and help her in her hopelessness. It took four debriefing sessions for all the care team members to come to accept that Mary had chosen her own path and that everything possible had been done to help her.

Activity 21: The patient's choice

Have you had an experience similar to the one described above? If so, use the reflective cycle we introduced in Chapter 2 to reflect upon the situation. Make notes on your answers to the following questions:

- What actually happened?
- What did you think and feel about the experience?
- How appropriate were the actions you took during the incident?
- How effective was the care you provided?
- On what evidence do you base your answers to the last two questions?
- What did you learn from the incident?
- How can you improve your future practice?

Feedback

It can be very hard to accept the situation when a patient doesn't seem to want your help. Although palliative care is about optimising the patient's quality of life, it is also about respecting the patient's autonomy. Patients must be allowed to make their own choices – no matter how vehemently you may disagree with them. You may find it helpful to discuss this issue with members of your AL set.

Promoting hope

Nurses are sometimes pessimistic about setting goals for patients or discussing the patient's future, because they do not want to give false hope. However, there are lots of ways of promoting hope. The list of suggestions below is based upon the work of Gardner (1991), Herth (1990), Herth (1996) and Urquhart (1999). You may notice that some of these suggestions are similar to the cognitive strategies that can be employed to relieve anxiety. Nurses can promote hope through their own positive attitudes and actions, and by:

- inducing a positive attitude in the patient;
- promoting the patient's sense of control;
- assisting the patient's development of effective coping strategies;
- improving communication between the patients and their partners and families;
- encouraging patients to openly express negative feelings, particularly anger;
- encouraging interpersonal connectedness – trying to ensure the presence of one or more meaningful shared relationships in the patient's life;
- encouraging lightheartedness (where appropriate) – encouraging the patient to allow feelings of delight, joy or playfulness, whether communicated verbally or non-verbally;
- agreeing attainable aims with the patient – giving purpose to the patient's efforts;
- encouraging patients to recall uplifting memories – positive moments and times;
- affirming the patient's worth – accepting, honouring and acknowledging the patient's individuality;
- emphasising the patient's potential, not their limitations;
- encouraging small successes;
- developing a sense of the possible;
- providing guidance and support when personal goals need to be refocused;

- supporting and encouraging personal attributes that are associated with hope, such as perseverance, endurance, courage, patience and toughness, determination and serenity;
- acknowledging that illness is only one part of a person;
- not communicating in a negative manner;
- not giving false hope;
- allowing the patient to realise that putting your affairs in order is not giving up;
- helping patients to assess what their hopes are;
- helping to make sense of what is going on;
- providing support during periods of change.

If in your assessment you realise that the patient has active spiritual beliefs and practices, and would appreciate the fostering of the spiritual aspect of hope, you should identify their religious needs and needs for spiritual comfort. You can then help patients to meet these needs, for example by allowing them time for quiet reflection, meditation, prayer or to read the holy book of their faith.

Case study

Mr Jones had always wanted to go on a boat trip but had never quite got round to it. He loved anything to do with boats and spent a lot of time at the local harbour watching them on his days off. He was due to retire soon and a boat trip was high on his list of things to do. Unfortunately, when admitted to hospital with severe weakness in his legs, he was diagnosed with spinal cord compression. The condition was found to be due to secondary bone cancer, which had spread from an undiagnosed primary prostate cancer. Following treatment he was admitted to the hospice where he was confined to bed. After some rehabilitation he was able to transfer from bed to chair, and was mobile in a wheelchair. He began attending the day hospice from the ward on a daily basis. His determination to overcome his disability was obvious but unfortunately over-optimistic. It became clear that the wish to go on a boat trip was still high on his agenda, although he believed that it could never happen as he would not be able to get off and on a boat in a wheelchair. This lost hope made him feel very useless and worthless.

However, the day hospice team decided to find a way around the problem. After discussion with Mr Jones and his care team, a trip on a barge on the local canal was arranged. This was possible as the barge was modified to take disabled groups including those in wheelchairs. The trip was free as the barge was run by a charity. As the barge held 12 people, it meant that some of the day hospice patients also had an outing that they thought would be too difficult or even impossible. The trip was a great success – Mr Jones was in his element and the trip was discussed within the day hospice for many weeks. Mr Jones told everyone about his trip and showed them the photographs that had been taken. His feelings of wellbeing from the trip lasted for many weeks, and talk of the trip still made Mr Jones smile even as his condition deteriorated, and even when he was very ill. His family was delighted that his psychological state had improved. After Mr Jones's death, his family had memories and photographs of his most recent happiest day, on which he achieved his goal of going on a boat trip.

Activity 22: Promoting hope

Compare your current practice with the list of suggestions we have just given you. Discuss with the other members of your team practical ways in which you can introduce the promotion of hope into practice in your clinical area.

Feedback

Hope means different things to different people – it is extremely subjective. Your strategies for promoting hope need to be general and yet you need to be able to 'customise' them for each patient. If, on comparing current practice with our list, there are practices you think should change, discuss these issues with your colleagues. Agree ways of implementing the amendments to practice.

Psychotherapy

Psychotherapy aims to help the patient change their negative thoughts into positive ones and teaches them how to challenge irrational thoughts and regain control of their lives through the use of cognitive and behavioural therapies (Greer and Moorey, 1997). Provision of emotional support and information can help the patient to cope and to alleviate the crisis they are facing (McVey, 1998).

Cognitive behavioural therapy as described by Lovejoy *et al.* (2000) may help reduce depression, by helping patients to investigate their current situation using positive and realistic ideas, thus reducing the negative perceptions that may be reducing the quality of their lives. Techniques such as cognitive distraction, imagery, music therapy, psycho-education, relaxation therapy and activity scheduling may resolve different depths of depression.

- Cognitive distraction involves 'superimposition of pleasurable reveries into conscious attention, forcing the mind to shift away from the negative thoughts that drive the depression' (Breitbart and Passik,

1993), e.g. focusing on pleasant memories rather than allowing the mind to dwell on problems.

- Musical interventions can range from simply playing music to patients to more formal music therapy. Pleasing musical pieces can relieve depression for many patients, even when they are confused or in the terminal stages of illness (Lovejoy et al., 2000). Formal music therapy uses the skills of a music therapist to relieve anxiety stress and distress. (Uses of music therapy can be found in Rykov and Salmon's (1998) bibliography for music therapy in palliative care.) It is thought that music therapy helps the depressed patient by stimulating the limbic system through the senses and increasing the production of neurotransmitters. This in turn reduces anxieties and helps the patient to relax (O'Callaghan, 1996). The use of music may be an inexpensive way of relieving feelings of depression in dying patients.

> Music, when played to very ill patients, does seem to lift their spirits.
>
> Co-ordinator, palliative day care

- Psycho-education helps patients to adjust to an unknown or altered future by providing information (Lovejoy et al., 2000), i.e. educating patients about what might happen.
- Relaxation therapy, which can include breathing techniques, massage, aromatherapy, imagery, tai chi, meditation, etc., again changes the focus of the patient's attention. Relaxation therapy can relieve muscle tension, autonomic arousal and mental distress (Breitbart and Passik, 1993).
- Activity scheduling encourages patients to become involved in pleasurable and constructive activities, which elevate their mood and restore their sense of control and produce positive comments from others on their achievements (Lovejoy et al., 2000).

However, cognitive behavioural therapy may take 12 weeks or longer to be effective and it would therefore not be useful in the terminal phase of a patient's illness (Lovejoy et al., 2000).

Constant observation and reassurance are necessary for suicidal patients and it is suggested that patients want to talk about their suicidal intentions and allowing them to do so actually reduces the likelihood of them attempting suicide. Billings (1995) suggests that if suicidal ideas appear serious or are expressed frequently then referral for a psychiatric opinion is necessary.

It is important to include the family when managing the patient with depression, as the family may be finding it difficult to talk to or interact with their loved one (Payne, 1998). Such involvement can help the family to understand what is happening and may give them ideas of how to help and support the patient through this difficult time. We looked at the care of the family in Chapter 1.

The next activity asks you to try a simple non-pharmacological intervention with a patient who is depressed but is not receiving any treatment for it. Discuss which patient might be suitable with the members of your team, and then consult the patient to make sure that they are prepared to try the intervention you suggest.

Activity 23: Non-pharmacological management of depression

Identify a patient who is depressed but is not yet receiving any treatment for it. Ask them if they would be prepared to try a relaxation or music tape (local libraries should have examples of these) or other form of relaxation therapy. You could also contact the occupational therapist for ideas, or the local hospice/Macmillan Nurse team.

After a few days, ask the patient how they feel. Ask the patient's family if they believe the relaxation has had a beneficial effect. Remember, however, that these strategies can sometimes take weeks or months to take effect. This is the major drawback in implementing them to help palliative care patients.

If there appear to have been improvements to the patient's quality of life, provide feedback on this to the team.

If there has been no improvement, or the patient's depression has deepened, do not simply give up on them. Find out what other interventions (including pharmacological ones, if necessary) might help them. If you start trying to help them and then give up, you will probably make matters worse. Your abandonment of them will lower their self-esteem, which is likely to have a direct effect on their depression.

Feedback

If there is a change in the patient's feelings of depression (for better or worse), it may or may not be as a result of the intervention. A deepening of depression may be due to the natural progression of the disease. An improvement may be due to the intervention – or it may be due to the fact that you are talking to the patient, are taking an interest in their problem and are trying to help.

If your strategy is not working, reflect upon the situation and try to identify why it is not working and how you might be able to improve it. It may take a few patients and lot more experience before you can observe changes, but at least you are actively trying to increase patients' quality of life, which is always worthwhile.

Drug intervention

Casey (1998) suggests that the opportunity to talk to professionals who provide support may not reduce the patient's symptoms alone and that antidepressants may also be required. Billings (1995) suggests that for moderate and severe depression medication will be necessary to alleviate the symptoms. Unfortunately, these drugs are often introduced so late in the patient's life that they do not have time to receive the full effect of the treatment (Lloyd-Williams *et al.*, 1999).

The choice of drug should be based on the desire to keep unwanted side effects to a minimum, as this may adversely affect the patient's quality of life (Lloyd-Williams *et al.*, 1999). Patients should be advised of any side effects they may experience at the beginning of a new treatment regime as this reduces anxiety (McVey, 1998).

The following list of drugs that can be used to manage depression is adapted from Twycross and Wilcock (2001), McVey (1998), Lloyd-Williams *et al.* (1999), Anderson *et al.* (2000) and the *British National Formulary* No 51 (2006). Good practice guidelines suggest that clinicians:

> match [the] choice of antidepressant drug to individual patient requirements as far as possible, taking into account [the] likely short- and long-term effects.
>
> Anderson *et al.* (2000: 9)

Tricyclic antidepressants (TCAs) and related antidepressant drugs

TCAs with sedative properties include amitriptyline, doxepin, dothiepin and trazadone. Those that are less sedating include imipramine, lofepramine and nortriptyline. Side effects of TCAs may include anticholinergic (dry mucous membranes, i.e. dry mouth and eyes, constipation, etc.), sedative and hypotensive (lower the blood pressure) effects. These drugs stop the uptake of serotonin and norepinephrine, thus improving central nervous system activity. They are often used in lower doses in palliative care patients and the elderly as they are more prone to the side effects. They can be used with patients who also have agitation and insomnia. There is little evidence to suggest they are less effective than newer, more expensive antidepressants.

Selective serotonin re-uptake inhibitors (SSRIs) and serotonin and noradrenaline re-uptake inhibitors (SNRIs)

SSRIs include fluoxetine, citalopram, paroxetine and sertraline. Their side effects include a sedative effect and they can cause gastro-intestinal upsets and reduce the appetite. They are, however, less sedating than the TCAs that are often the drugs of choice in this patient group. SNRIs include venlafaxine. Venlafaxine is reported to have a quicker onset in elevating mood and lacks the sedative effect of other antidepressants.

Other antidepressants

Mirtazapine is another drug which increases serotonin output and can be used with the depressed patient who is anxious/agitated. It may sedate at lower doses but this effect decreases as dosage is increased, and it may also produce feelings of wellbeing at higher doses. It is less sedative than traditional antidepressants.

Psycho-stimulants

These include methylphenidate and pemoline. These drugs produce feelings of wellbeing and reduce fatigue and increase appetite when given in small doses. They have few side effects, mainly sedation, but they can cause nightmares, insomnia and psychosis. As these drugs have a rapid effect, they are useful when time is short. They should be used under the supervision of a palliative care specialist.

Other drugs

Benzodiazepines – can be used in patients who have mixed symptoms of anxiety and depression.

Monoamine oxidase inhibitors (MAOIs) and lithium are usually used only in exceptional circumstances or for patients who have been treated successfully for depression with these drugs in the past. Problems with using these include the need to follow a special diet that may affect the already poor appetite of the palliative care patient.

Finally, when managing depression in palliative care, it is important for the members of a multidisciplinary team to acknowledge their limitations and refer the patient for a psychiatric opinion when the prescribed treatments do not appear to be effective (McVey, 1998).

Activity 24: Pharmacological management of depression

Identify a patient who is about to start on antidepressants. Make a note of the presenting symptoms and note down the drug(s) the patient is about to start taking. Review your notes on pharmacological and non-pharmacological treatments and identify why this particular treatment has been selected:

- What are the benefits?
- Are there any harmful side effects and, if so, are they counterbalanced by the benefits?

If you think there might be more suitable treatments (pharmacological or otherwise), discuss them with the team.

Obtain permission to re-interview the patient (and their family, if possible) after the period of time in which it takes the drugs to work. Your pharmacist or medical team should be able to advise you of the appropriate time. This could be at an outpatient clinic or with the district nurse/Macmillan Nurse – you will need to negotiate this with your manager. Note any differences in the quality of the patient's life

Feedback

Provide feedback to the team on the differences (improvements or otherwise) that the interventions have made to the patient's quality of life. If you believe alternative treatment strategies would have been more successful, perform a literature search to find out whether there is existing evidence on which to base your suggestions. Discuss the issue with members of your AL set. Reflect upon the various stages you have worked through. Discuss your findings with your colleagues.

SUMMARY

In this chapter we have looked at the causes and symptoms of anxiety and depression, and at how those symptoms can be assessed and managed. Having completed this chapter, you should be able to:

- give definitions of anxiety and depression;
- describe the manifestations, causes and predisposing factors of anxiety and depression in patients receiving palliative care;
- evaluate the different tools that can be used to assess anxiety and depression in your practice setting;
- compare and contrast the different approaches that can be taken to the management of anxiety and/or depression in your practice setting;
- critically evaluate how the management of anxiety and/or depression can impact on the quality of life of patients receiving palliative care.

RECOMMENDED SOURCES OF INFORMATION

Titles followed by O/P are out of print – but you may be able to find library copies.

Anderson, I.M., Nutt, D.J. and Deakin, J.F.W. (2000) 'Evidence based guidelines for treating depressive disorders with antidepressants: a review of the 1993 British Association of Pharmacology Guidelines'. *Journal of Psychopharmacology*, 14(1), pp.3–20.

Billings, J.A. (1995) 'Depression'. *Journal of Palliative Care*, 11(1), pp.48–54.

Bowlby, J. (1980) *Attachment and loss, volume 3: loss: sadness and depression*. London: Pimlico.

Buckley, J. and Herth, K. (2004) 'Fostering hope in the terminally ill'. *Nursing Standard*, 19(10), pp.33–41.

Buckman, R. (1988) *I don't know what to say*. London: Macmillan. O/P

Doyle, D., Hanks, G. and MacDonald, N. (2005) *Oxford textbook of palliative medicine* (3rd Ed.). Oxford: Oxford University Press.

Fallon, M. and O'Neill, B. (2006) *ABC of palliative care* (2nd Ed.). Malden: Blackwell Publishing.

Fisher, R.A. and McDaid, P. (1996) *Palliative day care*. London: Arnold.

Folkman, S. and Greer, S. (2000) 'Promoting psychological well-being in the face of serious illness: when theory, research and practice inform each other'. *Psycho-Oncology*, 9(1), pp.11–19.

Lovejoy, N.C., Tabor, D., Matteis, M. and Lillis, P. (2000) 'Cancer-related depression, part 1: neurologic alterations and cognitive-behavioral therapy'. *Oncology Nursing Forum*, 27(4), pp.667–78.

Lugton, J. and Kindlen, M. (2005) *Palliative care: the nursing role* (2nd Ed.). Edinburgh: Elsevier Churchill Livingstone.

McVey, P. (1998) 'Depression among the palliative care oncology population'. *International Journal of Palliative Nursing*, 4(2), pp.86–93.

Maslow A.H. (1987) *Motivation and personality* (3rd Ed.). New York: Harper & Row.

Nichols, K. (2003) *Psychological care for ill and injured people: a clinical guide*. Maidenhead: Open University Press.

Parkes, C.M. (1996) *Bereavement: studies of grief in adult life* (3rd Ed.). London: Routledge.

Payne, S. (1998) 'Depression in palliative care patients: a literature review'. *International Journal of Palliative Nursing*, 4(4), pp.184–91.

Regnard, C.F.B. and Tempest, S. (1998) *A guide to symptom relief in advanced disease* (4th Ed.). Hale: Hochland and Hochland.

Robbins, M. (1998) *Evaluating palliative care*. Oxford: Oxford University Press.

Twycross, R. and Wilcock, A. (2001) *Symptom management in advanced cancer* (3rd Ed.). Abingdon: Radcliffe Medical.

World Health Organization (1990) *Cancer pain relief and palliative care*. Geneva: WHO, (Technical Report no. 804).

REFERENCES

Adams, N., Poole, H. and Richardson, C. (2006) 'Psychological approaches to chronic pain management Part 1'. *Journal of Clinical Nursing*, 15(3), pp.290–300.

Akechi, T., Nakano, T., Akizuki, N., Nakanishi, T., Yoshikawa, E., Okamura, H. and Uchitomi, Y. (2002) 'Clinical factors associated with suicidality in cancer patients'. *Japanese Journal of Clinical Oncology*, 32(12), pp.506–11.

Anderson, I.M., Nutt, D.J. and Deakin, J.F.W. (2000) 'Evidence based guidelines for treating depressive disorders with antidepressants: a review of the 1993 British Association of Pharmacology Guidelines'. *Journal of Psychopharmacology*, 14(1), pp.3–20.

Barraclough, J. (1998) 'Depression, anxiety and confusion', in Fallon, M. and O'Neill, B. (editors) *ABC of palliative care*. London: BMJ Books, pp.27–30.

Beck, A.T., Ward, C.H., Mendelson, M., Mock, L. and Erbaugh, J. (1961) 'An inventory for measuring depression'. *Archives of General Psychiatry*, 4(6), pp.561–71.

Billings, J.A. (1995) 'Depression'. *Journal of Palliative Care*, 11(1), pp.48–54.

Bottrill, B. and Kirkwood, I. (1999) 'Complementary therapies', in Lugton, J. and Kindlen, M. (editors) *Palliative care: the nursing role*. Edinburgh: Churchill Livingstone, pp.163–91.

Bowlby, J. (1980) *Attachment and loss, volume 3: loss: sadness and depression*. London: Hogarth Press.

Breitbart, W. (1989) 'Psychiatric management of cancer pain'. *Cancer*, 63(11: supplement), pp.2336–42.

Breitbart, W. (1995) 'Identifying patients at risk for, and treatment of major psychiatric complications of cancer'. *Supportive Cancer Care*, 3(1), pp.45–60.

Breitbart, W. and Passik, S.D. (1993) 'Psychiatric approaches to cancer pain management', in Breitbart, W. and Holland, J.C. (editors) *Psychiatric aspects of symptom management in cancer patients*. Washington: American Psychiatric Press, pp.49–86.

Breitbart, W., Bruera, E., Chochinov, H. and Lynch, M. (1995) 'Neuropsychiatric syndromes and psychological symptoms in patients with advanced cancer'. *Journal of Pain and Symptom Management*, 10(2), pp.131–41.

Breitbart, W., Chochinov, H. and Passik, S. (1998) 'Psychiatric aspects of palliative care', in Doyle, D., Hanks, G. and MacDonald, N. (editors) *Oxford textbook of palliative medicine* (2nd Ed.). Oxford: Oxford University Press, pp.933–54.

British National Formulary (2006) BNF No 51, BMJ Publishing. **www.bnf.org** Site accessed 30/6/08.

Buckman, R. (1998) 'Communication in palliative care: a practical guide', in Doyle, D., Hanks, G. and MacDonald, N. (editors) *Oxford textbook of palliative medicine* (2nd Ed.). Oxford: Oxford University Press, pp.141–56.

Casey, P. (1998) 'Diagnosing and treating depression in the terminally ill'. *European Journal of Palliative Care*, 5(5), pp.152–5.

Corner, J., Cawley, N. and Hildebrand, S. (1995) 'An evaluation of the use of massage and essential oils on the well-being of cancer patients'. *International Journal of Palliative Nursing*, 1(2), pp.67–73.

Craven, O. (2000) 'Palliative care provision and its impact on psychological morbidity in cancer patients'. *International Journal of Palliative Nursing*, 6(10), pp.501–7.

Dein, S. (2005) 'Cognitive behavioural therapy in the palliative setting'. *European Journal of Palliative Care*, 12(4), pp.174–6.

EORTC Quality of Life Study Group (1995) EORTC QLQ-C30 (version 3) available from **www.groups.eortc.be/qol/questionnaires_qlqc30.htm** Site accessed 13/5/08.

Fallon, M. and O'Neill, B. (1998) *ABC of palliative care*. London: BMJ Books.

Farrer, K. (1999) 'Research and audit: demonstrating quality', in Lugton, J. and Kindlen, M. (editors) *Palliative care: the nursing role*. Edinburgh: Churchill Livingstone, pp.271–96.

Faulkner, A. (1998) *Effective interaction with patients* (2nd Ed.). New York: Churchill Livingstone.

Flaming, D. (1995) 'Patient suffering: a taxonomy from the nurse's perspective'. *Journal of Advanced Nursing*, 22(6), pp.1120–7.

Folkman, S. and Greer, S. (2000) 'Promoting psychological well-being in the face of serious illness: when theory, research and practice inform each other'. *Psycho-Oncology*, 9(1), pp.11–19.

Gardner, R. (1991) 'Rekindling hope'. *Nursing Times*, 87(15), 10 April, pp.50–2.

Goldberg, D.P. (1972) *The detection of psychiatric illness by questionnaire*. London: Oxford University Press.

Goldberg, D. (1978) *Manual of the General Health Questionnaire*. Windsor: NFER.

Greer, S. and Moorey, S. (1997) 'Adjuvant psychological therapy for cancer patients'. *Palliative Medicine*, 11(3), pp.240–4.

Heaven, C.M. and Maguire, P. (1997) 'Disclosure of concerns by hospice patients and their identification by nurses'. *Palliative Medicine*, 11(4), pp.283–90.

Herrmann, C. (1997) 'International experiences with the Hospital Anxiety and Depression Scale: a review of validation data and clinical results'. *Journal of Psychosomatic Research*, 42(1), pp.17–41.

Herth, K. (1990) 'Fostering hope in terminally ill people'. *Journal of Advanced Nursing*, 15(11), pp.1250–9.

Herth, K. (1996) 'Hope from the perspective of homeless families'. *Journal of Advanced Nursing*, 24(4), pp.743–53.

Herth, K. (2000) 'Enhancing hope in people with a first recurrence of cancer'. *Journal of Advanced Nursing*, 32(6), pp.1431–41.

Higginson, I. (1998) For copies of POS, go to : **www.kcl.ac.uk/schools/medicine/depts/palliative/qat/pos.html**

Hockley, J. and Mowatt, M. (1996) 'Part 1: philosophy: chapter 2: rehabilitation', in Fisher, R.A. and McDaid, P. (editors) *Palliative day care*. London: Edward Arnold, pp.13–21.

Hodgson, H. (2000) 'Does reflexology impact on cancer patients' quality of life?' *Nursing Standard*, 14(31), 19 April, pp.33–8.

Holtom, N. and Barraclough, J. (2000) 'Is the Hospital Anxiety and Depression Scale (HADS) useful in assessing depression in palliative care?' *Palliative Medicine*, 14(3), pp.219–20.

Johnson, L.C. (1969) 'Psychological and physiological changes following total sleep deprivation', in Kales, A. (editor) *Sleep: physiology and pathology*. Philadelphia: Lippincott, pp.206–20.

Lloyd-Williams, M., Friedman, T. and Rudd, N. (1999) 'A survey of antidepressant prescribing in the terminally ill'. *Palliative Medicine*, 13(3), pp.243–8.

Lloyd-Williams, M., Friedman, T. and Rudd, N. (2002) 'Criterion validation of the Edinburgh Postnatal Depression Scale as a screening tool for repression in patients with advanced metastatic cancer'. *Journal of Pain and Symptom Management*, 20, pp.259–65.

Lloyd-Williams, M., Dennis, M. and Taylor, F. (2004) 'A prospective study to compare three depression screening tools in patients who are terminally ill'. *General Hospital Psychiatry*, 26(5), pp.384–9.

Lovejoy, N.C., Tabor, D., Matteis, M. and Lillis, P. (2000) 'Cancer-related depression, part 1: neurologic alterations and cognitive-behavioral therapy'. *Oncology Nursing Forum*, 27(4), pp.667–78.

Lugton, J. (1999) 'Support processes in palliative care', in Lugton, J. and Kindlen, M. (editors) *Palliative care: the nursing role*. Edinburgh: Churchill Livingstone, pp.89–113.

Lynch, W.F. (1965) *Images of hope*. Baltimore: Helicon. Cited in Rideout, E. and Montemuro, M. (1986) 'Hope, morale and adaptation in patients with chronic heart failure'. *Journal of Advanced Nursing*, 11(4), pp.429–38.

Maguire, P., Faulkner, A., Booth, K., Elliott, C. and Hillier, V. (1996) 'Helping cancer patients disclose their concerns'. *European Journal of Cancer*, 32A(1), pp.78–81.

Marks-Maran, D. and Rose, P. (1997) *Reconstructing nursing: beyond art and science*. London: Baillière Tindall.

Maslow, A.H. (1987) *Motivation and personality* (3rd Ed.). New York: Harper Row.

Massie, M.J. and Holland, J.C. (1992) 'The cancer patient with pain: psychiatric complications and their management'. *Journal of Pain and Symptom Management*, 7(2), pp.99–109.

McDowell, I. and Newell, C. (1996) *Measuring health. a guide to rating scales and questionnaires* (2nd Ed.). New York: Oxford University Press.

McVey, P. (1998) 'Depression among the palliative care oncology population'. *International Journal of Palliative Nursing*, 4(2), pp.86–93.

Milligan, M., Fanning, M., Hunter, S., Tadjali, M. and Stevens, E. (2002) 'Reflexology audit: patient satisfaction, impact on quality of life and availability in Scottish hospices'. *International Journal of Palliative Nursing*, 8(10), pp.489–96.

Moldofsky, H., Lue, F.A., Davidson, J.R. and Gorczynski, R. (1989) 'Effects of sleep deprivation on human immune functions'. *FASEB Journal*, 3(8), pp.1972–7.

Narayanasamy, A. (2004) 'The puzzle of spirituality for nursing: a guide to practical assessment'. *British Journal of Nursing*, 13(19), pp.1140–4.

O'Callaghan, C.C. (1996) 'Pain, music creativity and music therapy in palliative care'. *American Journal of Hospice and Palliative Care*, 13(2) pp.43–49. Cited in McVey, P. (1998) 'Depression among the palliative care oncology population'. *International Journal of Palliative Nursing*, 4(2), pp.86–93.

Oswald, I. (1980) 'Sleep as restorative process: human clues'. *Progress in Brain Research*, 53, pp.279–80.

Parle, M., Jones, B. and Maguire, P. (1996) 'Maladaptive coping and affective disorders among cancer patients'. *Psychological Medicine*, 26(4), pp.735–44.

Payne, S. (1998) 'Depression in palliative care patients: a literature review'. *International Journal of Palliative Nursing*, 4(4), pp.184–91.

Peck, S.M. (1997) *The road less travelled and beyond*. London: Rider.

Penson, J. (2000) 'A hope is not a promise: fostering hope within palliative care'. *International Journal of Palliative Nursing*, 6(2), pp.94–8.

Rees, C. and Joslyn, S. (1998) 'The importance of hope'. *Nursing Standard*, 12(41), 1 July, pp.34–5.

Regnard, C.F.B. and Tempest, S. (1998) *A guide to symptom relief in advanced disease*. Hale: Hochland and Hochland.

Rideout, E. and Montemuro, M. (1986) 'Hope, morale and adaptation in patients with chronic heart failure'. *Journal of Advanced Nursing*, 11(4), pp.429–38.

Robbins, M. (1998) *Evaluating palliative care*. Oxford: Oxford University Press.

Roth, T., Kramer, M., Leston, W. and Lutz, T. (1974) 'The effects of sleep deprivation on mood'. *Sleep Research*, 3, p.154.

Rykov, M. and Salmon, D. (1998) 'Bibliography for music therapy in palliative care, 1963–1997'. *American Journal of Hospice and Palliative Care*, 15(3), pp.174–80.

Sadock, B.J. and Sadock, V.A. (2005) *Kaplan and Sadock's comprehensive textbook of psychiatry* (8th Ed.). Philadelphia: Lippincott.

Sateia, M.J. and Silberfarb, P.M. (1996) 'Sleep disorders in patients with advanced cancer'. *Progress in Palliative Care*, 4(4), pp.120–5.

Sheibani-Rad, S. and Velanovich, V. (2006) 'Effects of depression on the survival of pancreatic adenocarcinoma'. *Pancreas*, 31(1), pp.58–61.

Smitz, L.L. and Woods, A.B. (2006) 'Prevalence, severity and correlates of depressive symptoms on admission to inpatient hospice'. *Journal of Hospice and Palliative Nursing*, 8(2), pp.86–91.

Stevens, E.M. (1996) 'Promoting self-worth in the terminally ill'. *European Journal of Palliative Care*, 3(2), pp.60–4.

Tigges, K.N. (1998) 'Rehabilitation in palliative care: occupational therapy', in Doyle, D., Hanks, G. and MacDonald, N. (editors) *Oxford textbook of palliative medicine* (2nd Ed.). Oxford: Oxford University Press, pp.829–37.

Twycross, R. and Wilcock, A. (2001) *Symptom management in advanced cancer* (3rd Ed.). Oxford: Radcliffe Medical.

Urch, C.E., Chamberlain, J. and Field, G. (1998) 'The drawback of the Hospital Anxiety and Depression Scale in the assessment of depression in hospice inpatients'. *Palliative Medicine*, 12(5), pp.395–6.

Urquhart, P. (1999) 'Issues of suffering in palliative care'. *International Journal of Palliative Nursing*, 5, pp.35–9.

Watson, M., Greer, S., Young, J., Inayat, Q., Burgess, C. and Robertson, B. (1988) 'Development of a questionnaire measure of adjustment to cancer: the MAC scale'. *Psychological Medicine*, 18(1), pp.203–9.

Weller, B. (2000) *Baillière's nurses' dictionary* (23rd Ed.). Edinburgh: Baillière Tindall.

Wilkinson, S. (1995) 'Aromatherapy and massage in palliative care'. *International Journal of Palliative Nursing*, 1(1), pp.21–30.

Zigmond, A.S. and Snaith, R.P. (1983) 'The Hospital Anxiety and Depression scale'. *Acta Psychiatrica Scandinavica*, 67(6), pp.361–70.

Chapter 5

Breathlessness

Mary Bredin

INTRODUCTION

Breathlessness is a complex symptom to manage. Patients face a variety of problems that may include a limited ability in carrying out activities of daily living and a feeling of distress. The distress associated with breathlessness makes working with patients who are breathless very challenging, both professionally and personally. Compounding the problem is the fact that there are no straightforward solutions to managing breathlessness, since the evidence base for much medical treatment is fairly sparse.

In this chapter we suggest the use of an integrated approach for managing breathlessness, where the emotional aspects of the symptom are considered as important as the physical ones. You will be introduced to a variety of strategies that have been used by nurses to complement medical treatments and help patients cope with breathlessness. These strategies, originally reported to be of benefit to patients with breathlessness as a result of chronic lung disease, have since been refined and further developed to be used with patients with lung cancer. They may also be used within a palliative care setting, regardless of the patient's diagnosis, since they are about working with both the physical and emotional limitations breathlessness imposes rather than the underlying disease.

It can take time and confidence to learn new therapeutic strategies both for the practitioner and the patient. It would be good if you approach your learning as ongoing and experiential. Imagine that you are going to be looking into a toolbox where you can dip in and pick out a variety of tools. Some you will feel confident in using and others you will need to practise. The more you work with this book, share it and reflect upon it, the more confident you will become and the more help you will be to the patients you care for.

LEARNING OUTCOMES

When you have completed this chapter, you will be able to:
- explain the nature and causes of breathlessness;
- describe the impact of breathlessness on quality of life for patients and their families;
- clarify the importance of making a careful assessment of the patient's breathlessness;
- summarise the current medical treatments for breathlessness, the evidence base for them and the benefits and limitations of medical treatments alone, with special emphasis on the emotional and functional impact of breathlessness;
- describe current nursing strategies for managing breathlessness, emphasising the value of the integrative model for managing breathlessness and explaining the importance of the therapeutic relationship;
- describe how the successful management of breathlessness can improve the quality of life of patients receiving palliative care.

Preparation

For Activity 3 you will need a copy of the following CD-ROM: *A breath of fresh air: an interactive guide to managing breathlessness in patients with lung cancer.* This is a CD-ROM on the management of breathlessness in advanced lung cancer originally produced in 2001 by the Interactive Education Unit at The Institute of Cancer Research in London. A new and updated version of the CD-ROM was launched in 2007. For more details see: **www.icr.ac.uk/ieu/projects/Breathlessness Project/ConceptBens.htm.** (Site accessed 13/5/08.) The CD-ROM is available free of charge to health care professionals from the dedicated orderline: 0800 9177263 or by e-mailing **ieu@icr.ac. uk**. We recommend that you obtain a copy of the CD-ROM as we refer to it throughout this chapter. You can use either edition of the CD-ROM for the activities.

In Activity 4, we ask you to explore the patient's experience of breathlessness. It is worth mentioning this now to any patients who you feel might be prepared to help you with this activity by discussing their experience with you.

WHAT IS BREATHLESSNESS?

. . . you don't think you'll get it back again – like a suffocation, frightened the life out of me . . . breath is more important than water . . . .

Quote from a patient: O'Driscoll *et al.* (1999: 39)

Breathlessness, also known as 'dyspnoea', comes from the Greek *dys* meaning bad or difficult and *pneo* meaning breathing. Breathlessness on exertion – for example when running for a bus – is normal. Here, however, we are talking about breathlessness that is caused by an underlying disease pathology, which may be experienced by the patient as severe and disabling both physically and emotionally.

Breathlessness is not just a symptom of disordered breathing, it is a problem where there is a complex interplay between physical, psychological, emotional and functional factors (O'Driscoll *et al.*, 1999). It is also a highly subjective experience, as a patient may *appear* to be breathing relatively easily but they may complain of *feeling* severely short of breath (Carrieri *et al.*, 1984). It is different from tachypnoea (increased respiratory rate) or increased ventilation rate, since these are both objective measures of respiration.

In a study looking into the experience of breathlessness in patients with lung cancer, patients described breathing as the 'very essence of life' and they strongly associated the loss of that ability with death (O'Driscoll *et al.*, 1999). This is why breathlessness as a symptom of disease can seem so frightening and overwhelming to patients, as the quote above so powerfully suggests.

According to Twycross and Lack (1990a), 30 per cent of all terminally ill cancer patients, and 60 per cent of lung cancer patients, experience breathlessness. Breathlessness is also a major problem for patients with chronic obstructive pulmonary disease (COPD). Many of the symptoms experienced by patients with COPD are similar to those experienced by patients with lung cancer, but the symptoms develop at a far greater speed in patients with cancer, giving them little time to develop coping strategies.

Activity 1: Reflecting on breathlessness

The purpose of this activity is to help you think about your work with patients who are breathless. Carry out this exercise with a colleague. Discuss your responses with them, and make brief notes of your discussion. You may find it helpful to use the model of reflective practice given in Chapter 2, or use one that you are already familiar with.

Your task is to reflect upon the care you gave to a patient experiencing problems with breathlessness. If you have not cared for someone with breathlessness, find a colleague who has – ask if they would be prepared to discuss their experience with you.

Use the following questions as a guide:

- How/where did you first meet the patient?
- What were their main problems?
- What medical treatment did they receive for their breathlessness?
- What nursing interventions did they receive and why?
- How did they respond to these interventions?
- How did you feel when you were looking after this person?
- What interventions in your opinion may have helped/not helped them cope with their breathlessness?
- What else would have helped you to care for this person, e.g. resources, information, environment, etc.?

Feedback

We want you to start this chapter by reflecting upon the knowledge and expertise you already have when caring for patients with breathlessness. This will help you to then consider what skills you might want to develop further in your work.

CAUSES OF BREATHLESSNESS

Breathlessness may be due to a number of causes, including:

- cancer (particularly lung cancer and associated problems – see Table 5.1);
- chronic obstructive airways disease (COAD – now more commonly known as chronic obstructive pulmonary disease, COPD);
- pneumothorax;
- asthma;
- heart failure;
- pulmonary fibrosis;
- acidosis;
- congestive cardiac failure;
- mitral/aortic valve disease;
- motor neurone disease;
- bacterial, viral and fungal infection (Twycross and Lack, 1990b; Cowcher and Hanks, 1990; Corner *et al.*, 1997).

Although patients with conditions such as lung cancer, COPD and congestive heart failure are most likely to experience breathlessness, in the National Hospice Study patients without underlying pulmonary disease accounted for 25 per cent of those experiencing breathlessness (Reuben and Mor, 1986; Mosenthal and Lee, 2002).

The causes of breathlessness in cancer are also varied and complex (Moore *et al.*, 2006). For example, breathlessness may be due to the effects of the disease itself, the treatment, concurrent medical conditions (these can be related or unrelated to having cancer) or a combination of factors (Moore *et al.*, 2006). Table 5.1 shows causes of breathlessness in patients with cancer.

Causes of breathlessness in patients with cancer

Cancer-related	Treatment-related
Obstruction/compression by tumour	Radiation damage to lung, eg fibrosis,
Lung metastases	pneumonitis
Lung or airway collapse	Chemotherapy damage, e.g. drug-induced
Hilar or mediastinal lymphadenopathy	pneumonitis, cardiomyopathy
Lymphangitis carcinomatosa	Effects of surgery reducing lung capacity, e.g.
Superior vena cava obstruction	pneumonectomy/lobectomy
Pleural effusion	**Concurrent medical conditions**
Consolidation	Ischaemic heart disease
Pneumothorax	Cardiac failure
Aspiration pneumonia	Asthma
Tracheo-oesophageal fistula	COPD (chronic obstructive pulmonary disease)
	Anaemia
	Anxiety
	Obesity

Table 5.1   Causes of breathlessness in patients with cancer (Moore *et al.*, 2006: 509)

Causes identified by patients

> ... if I talk too much I get out of breath, if I walk too much I get out of breath, if I walk to the shop or lift anything I lose my breath, or if I get cross or emotional ... Shopping – by the time I get to the check out, I have had enough – I hold on to the trolley for support ... Dressing is a bit of a bind, getting out of the bath, going upstairs – I'm breathless at the top ... housework – I need to rest between activities and I don't do any hard housework ...
>
> Quote from a patient: O'Driscoll *et al.* (1999: 40–1)

The most common causes of breathlessness identified by patients in O'Driscoll and colleagues' (1999) study included exertion, walking and walking up the stairs. Other daily activities could trigger attacks, as could strong emotions and extremes of weather.

Emotions such as anger, fear, frustration, excitement and anxiety (see Chapter 4) can cause attacks, as can expressions of emotions such as crying and laughing. Unfortunately, the negative emotions are compounded by the experience of breathlessness, resulting in a vicious circle (Figure 5.1).

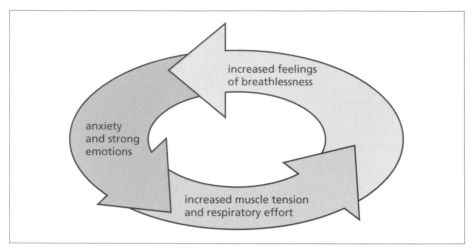

Figure 5.1 Psychological factors in breathlessness

Activity 2: The causes of breathlessness

Discuss the possible causes of breathlessness in patients in your clinical area with other members of your team. You may wish to review patients' notes in order to do this exercise thoroughly. Then briefly identify the problems associated with breathlessness that you have encountered in these patients, such as lack of mobility, fatigue, sleeplessness, decreased appetite, anxiety, etc.

Feedback

The causes of breathlessness may be varied and complex, and there may also be differences in the patient's experience of breathlessness, depending on the different causative conditions as well as other possible symptoms they may be experiencing. Considering the causes of breathlessness and the complexity of problems associated with breathlessness should have made you start thinking about the different ways in which the symptom can be managed. We will look at the management of breathlessness later on in this chapter.

The pathophysiology of breathlessness

> The assessment of dyspnoea in palliative care should be aimed much more to its characterization as a symptom than to the understanding of the functional and gas-exchange abnormalities.
>
> Ripamonti and Bruera (1997: 220)

It may be helpful to have a basic knowledge of the pathophysiology of breathlessness in order to understand something about the complexity of the symptom. However, according to Ripamonti and Bruera (1997), the pathophysiology of breathlessness is complex and not very well understood. Breathlessness is frequently associated with abnormalities in the mechanisms that regulate normal breathing (Ripamonti and Bruera, 1997), as well as psychological and social factors interacting with physiological ones to generate the sensation of breathlessness (Mosenthal and Lee, 2002). Factors that may contribute to the problem of breathlessness include:

- Mechanical factors – e.g. an increase in respiratory effort to overcome a certain load (for example a tumour, pulmonary embolus, pleural effusion);
- Chemical factors – breathing patterns alter as changes in blood levels of carbon dioxide and oxygen stimulate the respiratory centre in the brainstem;
- Emotional factors – feelings such as rage, fear or sadness – all have the potential of changing the rhythm and depth of breathing (Moore *et al.*, 2006).

If you would like to learn more about the pathophysiology of breathlessness in detail, read the following papers:

Ripamonti, C. and Bruera, E. (1997) 'Dyspnea: pathophysiology and assessment'. *Journal of Pain and Symptom Management*, 13(4), pp.220–232.

Ahmedzai, S. (1998) 'Palliation of respiratory symptoms', in Doyle, D., Hanks, G.W. and MacDonald, N. (editors) *Oxford textbook of palliative medicine* (2nd Ed.). Oxford: Oxford University Press, pp.583–616.

At this stage of your learning it may be more useful to understand the mechanisms of normal breathing, so that when we come to consider coping strategies, you will understand why it might be helpful to teach a patient how to use breathing re-training exercises. The following activity is aimed at helping you to review the mechanism of breathing.

Activity 3: The mechanism of normal breathing

For this activity you will need your copy of the CD-ROM *A breath of fresh air* (Interactive Education Unit at The Institute of Cancer Research, 2007). (We gave details in the Preparation activity at the beginning of the chapter on how to obtain it.)

Go to the 'Anatomy and physiology' section of the CD-ROM, select 'Structure and function of the lung' and then review the respiratory system.

Review the anatomy of the lung.

- What are the conducting and respiratory zones?

Review the physiology of normal breathing.

- How does stress affect breathing?

Review the cycle of normal breathing.

- What are the two main types of breathing?

Describe the factors that affect breathing.

Feedback

The process of breathing is so fundamental to life that it is mainly under involuntary control. However, it can be influenced by a variety of physiological and psychological factors. When caring for a patient who is breathless, it may be helpful to have a basic knowledge of the anatomy and physiology of breathing so you can feel more confident in addressing problems.

You also need to remain alert to other factors that influence breathlessness, such as the patient's understanding of the disease, emotions/anxiety, depression, frustration, environment, exercise and so on, many of which we have already mentioned. Furthermore, the longer a symptom continues, the more likely it is that psychological factors such as fear, depression, anxiety and frustration will influence the perception and intensity of breathlessness. See Chapter 4 for details of the causes and management of anxiety and depression.

THE IMPACT OF BREATHLESSNESS ON QUALITY OF LIFE

> . . . I didn't think I would be able to catch my breath again, I didn't think I'd be OK, I was frightened, anxious, worried and scared.
> Quote from a patient: O'Driscoll *et al.* (1999: 39)

Breathlessness affects every aspect of a patient's life. It can also be frightening for the family, who may feel helpless when watching someone they love struggling for breath. Fear, anxiety, loss of control, loss of independence, immobility and lowered self-esteem are all features of the experience of breathlessness that can impact quality of life.

> . . . can't manage very well or at all, can't manage the housework or cooking, walking hills, can't dance anymore, get out of breath, can't

manage the hill with the wind against me, older people were passing me by, can't do a lot of things used to . . .

Quote from a patient: O'Driscoll *et al.* (1999: 41)

O'Driscoll *et al.* (1999), reviewing the experience of breathlessness in 52 patients with lung cancer, identified the most common physical sensations associated with breathlessness as shortness of breath (n = 38), inability to take a deep breath (n = 11) or to get enough air (n = 11). The emotions most commonly associated with breathlessness were panic (n = 21), feeling of impending death (n = 16), fear/fright (n = 16) and anxiety (n = 12).

The impact of breathlessness on a person facing a life-threatening illness may be profound. It is likely to increase their fear of breathlessness, because patients commonly perceive the symptom as a threat to life itself. The following quote illustrates this:

I panic a bit sometimes, because deep down I know that [this breath] could be my last one . . . It's an awful feeling.

Quote from a patient: Roberts *et al.* (1993: 314)

Actions or emotions that cause breathlessness are then also seen as threats to life and unsurprisingly patients attempt to manage their breathlessness by avoiding activities that trigger breathlessness (Table 5.2).

The restrictions imposed by breathlessness have further effects on the patient's quality of life (Figure 5.2). For example, an inability to work is likely to lead to financial hardship, which in turn is likely to impact on relationships within the family. This can then cause emotional distress leading to further episodes of breathlessness.

To summarise – breathlessness impacts on every aspect of patients' lives, restricting their activities and reducing their world in many different ways: socially, physically, emotionally and spiritually. Sometimes patients feel reluctant to talk about the obvious impact breathlessness may have on their day-to-day living, because they feel a loss of self-esteem in acknowledging that they are not able to do the most basic things. The speed at which breathlessness can develop as a problem gives little time to adjust and often patients feel that they *should* be managing and coping despite breathlessness. Thus they may attempt to carry on regardless, not perhaps realising that there are strategies they can learn that might ease the restrictions of breathlessness and help them function once more.

Restrictions imposed by breathlessness

Around the house:
- difficulty with doing the ironing;
- difficulty with hanging out washing;
- difficulty with using the Hoover;
- difficulty getting washed/dried/dressed;
- breathlessness going to the toilet;
- breathlessness preparing/eating meals;
- breathlessness answering the phone.

Outside the house:
- difficulty with driving;
- difficulty with usual run of things;
- unable to run business/work;
- difficulty with going for a walk outside the house;
- can't manage walking round the shops;
- difficulty with gardening.

Social activities:
- difficulty going out in the evening;
- difficulty with dancing/standing;
- can't manage recreational activities;
- social life adversely affected;
- difficulty with reading;
- difficulty with sport.

Implications on personal life and self:
- difficulty in maintaining sexual relations;
- difficulty with fulfilling usual role within the family;
- hopelessness/uncertainty about the future;
- doesn't want to continue living like this;
- fear of breathlessness prevents one from doing things;
- can't do what you want to do.

O'Driscoll *et al.* (1999: 41)

Table 5.2   Restrictions imposed by breathlessness

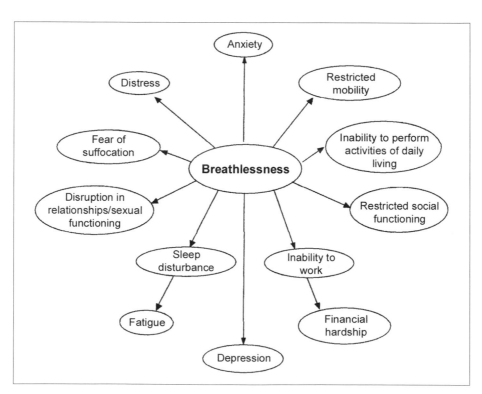

Figure 5.2   Effects of breathlessness on quality of life (adapted from Interactive Education Unit at The Institute of Cancer Research, 2001)

Finding out in detail about every aspect of a patient's life and being able to make what may seem an obvious suggestion – such as having a chair nearby so they can sit down for a rest while doing a chore – might make the difference between coping and not coping. In order to do this, however, we need to begin by listening to the patient – finding out exactly how breathlessness is impacting on their life and their family's lives. The following activity is designed to help you begin this process.

Activity 4: The impact of breathlessness

In this activity it would be good if you could find firstly a patient and, secondly, a family member who is prepared to talk with you about the impact of breathlessness on their life. Prepare them initially by telling them why you want to talk to them, what questions you are hoping to ask and agree with them how long it should take. The family member you talk with doesn't need to be a family member of the patient you talk with. Out of courtesy, the patient whose family member will be talking with you should be consulted about the discussion. It is best to find a family member of a patient who is happy for them to talk with you.

You may also need to ensure that you cannot be disturbed and remind them that you can stop at any time if they want to. If you cannot speak directly to a patient or family member, you could reflect on previous conversations with patients and their families. Try to identify the impact of breathlessness on aspects of their lives, which may include the following:

- physical;
- social;
- psychological;
- spiritual;
- cultural.

Compare your notes with those from Activity 2, which focused on the patient's perspective. Are there differences/similarities between the problems you have identified and those your patients identified?

Feedback

Listening carefully to patients describing their experiences of breathlessness will tell you about how they are coping/not coping. The language they use might tell you about what breathlessness means to them. For example, they might describe breathlessness in physical terms such as 'tiring, heavy or a tight sensation' or they might use emotional descriptions such as 'frightening, frustrating, helpless or suffocation'. You may be surprised by how far-reaching some of the effects felt by family members may be. Finding out the impact of breathlessness on the different aspects of people's lives will help you to think about the needs/problems of patients and family members, and how you might help them to begin to address them. We will be looking at how you can involve the families of patients with breathlessness in the management of breathlessness towards the end of this chapter. You will probably find that some of the work you have done in this activity will be useful background work for Activity 14.

THE ASSESSMENT OF BREATHLESSNESS

Assessment is a very important first step in managing breathlessness. It is also worth remembering at the outset that it may take time to build up a relationship with the patient where they feel safe enough to disclose difficult feelings and fears. Assessment should therefore be an ongoing part of the work. For example, if you are caring for a patient who finds it difficult to talk about emotional issues, you may need to start by asking them about the practical problems. When there is a rapport and trust between you, you may feel it is appropriate to move on and address some of the other issues affecting their breathlessness. During the screening assessment (see Chapter 3) the following patient details may have been collected:

- disease, stage and treatment;
- understanding of their illness;
- social circumstances – family background, social support, work and domestic situation;
- current concerns and goals.

The assessment should also cover the patient's sleep patterns, which may have been disturbed. Patients with breathlessness often lie awake at night, afraid that if they go to sleep they will just stop breathing.

In your focused assessment (see Chapter 3), you might gather information about:

- how the patient describes their breathlessness and the meaning it holds for them;
- their emotional response to breathlessness;
- the effect breathlessness has on the different aspects of their lives;
- what helps breathlessness;
- what makes it feel worse;
- the severity and pattern of breathlessness;
- any self-help strategies they have found helpful;
- the practical and social implications for the patient and their family of managing breathlessness.

Bredin (2003) also suggests that it is important to identify significant anxiety and depression or other significant factors (physical and emotional) that might necessitate referral on to members of the multi-professional team. (See also Chapter 4.)

Another valuable part of the assessment process is to enable the patient to 'tell their story', which may be therapeutic, since it gives them an opportunity to unburden themselves of material they may have previously been unable to talk about. It also gives you an opportunity to find out about their world of living with breathlessness – how they experience and cope with it. The more information you gather at this stage the better able you will be to respond therapeutically.

Tools for measuring breathlessness

There is a variety of tools for measuring breathlessness in advanced cancer but, because many of them have been designed for clinical trials, they are not appropriate in the palliative care setting. We will look at a tool that uses the visual analogue scale (VAS – we introduced this in Chapter 3) and at a tool designed specifically for use in palliative care – Corner and O'Driscoll's (1999) assessment guide.

The VAS has also been used as part of an assessment tool in two studies by Corner *et al.*, 1995 and Bredin *et al.*, 1999. It includes three scales, each headed: 'Please rate how breathless you have felt in the last week'.

- Scale 1 gives a vertical VAS and asks the patient to indicate how breathless they felt when their breathing was at its best.
- Scale 2 gives a vertical VAS and asks the patient to indicate how breathless they felt when their breathing was at its worst.
- Scale 3 gives a vertical VAS to measure distress, with 10 = Extreme distress and 0 = No distress. The patient is asked how much distress their breathlessness has caused them.

These scales are shown in Figure 5.5, and you can also obtain a copy of them from the assessment guide in the 'Resources' section of the CD-ROM *A breath of fresh air* (Interactive Education Unit at The Institute of Cancer Research, 2007).

Activity 5: Measurement of breathlessness

What tool (if any) is used for the measurement of breathlessness in your clinical area?

If you do not currently use a tool, perhaps you could try the VAS tool with patients whose breathlessness you wish to assess over time. If this is the case, discuss whether you can do this with your manager and how you might go about introducing such a tool in your workplace. You may already have used this tool for patients with other symptoms or have other tools to measure symptoms. It is important to discuss with your colleagues what they feel about using such tools and when they are appropriate and for whom.

The questions on the VAS measure the patient's breathing at its best, its worst, and the level of distress breathlessness causes. What other information do you currently gather? Why might you ask for this particular information? Are there any other questions that you think it would be helpful to ask? Discuss these issues with your colleagues.

Feedback

Measuring breathlessness with an appropriate tool may be useful, particularly when you need to assess changes in breathlessness over time or the impact of a particular intervention for breathlessness. Sometimes patients find it hard to talk about the distress breathlessness causes and at such times the VAS scale can be useful. For example, you will find if you ask a patient to imagine on a scale of 1–10 how much distress they are experiencing, they can usually give you an answer immediately, and this then gives you a starting point to assess changes. There will also be some patients who are simply too tired or unwell to comply with this kind of exercise – it is essential to assess carefully with whom it is appropriate to use this tool.

A breathlessness assessment guide for use in palliative care

Corner and O'Driscoll (1999) developed a breathlessness assessment guide for use in palliative care. It aims to encourage nurses and other members of the team who might use it to address breathlessness as a multidimensional problem. A more recent version of the breathlessness assessment guide is shown in Figures 5.3, 5.4 and 5.5. If you wish to use the breathlessness assessment guide shown in Figures 5.3, 5.4 and 5.5, you can do so by obtaining a copy from the 'Resources' section of the CD-ROM *A breath of fresh air* (Interactive Education Unit at The Institute of Cancer Research, 2007). Or you may prefer to draw up your own assessment tool in collaboration with your colleagues.

Activity 6: Creating your own assessment tool

Read through the breathlessness assessment guide shown in Figures 5.3, 5.4 and 5.5. What do you think about it and could you imagine using it with patients in your care?

Compare the information gathered in the assessment tool with the information that you currently gather. What are the differences and similarities?

Discuss with your colleagues what you want from an assessment tool for breathlessness.

Considering the different factors that may affect breathlessness, what questions do you and your colleagues consider it important to ask patients?

On the basis of your discussions, draw up your own assessment tool. You might like to include some of the points shown on Figures 5.3 and 5.4, or a selection of VASs, as shown in Figure 5.5, to measure changes in breathlessness over time as well – as any extra questions that you think are useful.

Feedback

Your new assessment tool should enable you to gather enough useful information to be able to identify how breathlessness is impacting on patients' quality of life. It can also be used as a tool to evaluate your interventions. For example, if you are using a VAS to measure a patient's distress and you use it repeatedly over time, you will see how the patient's scores change. Assessment tools are meant only as guides, so choose or develop one that it is meaningful to you and your team and bear in mind that the more you work with it, the more likely you are to find it of benefit in managing breathlessness.

BREATHLESSNESS ASSESSMENT GUIDE

Patient name: Occupation:

Date of initial assessment:

Diagnosis: Date of diagnosis:

Treatment and history:

Current medications:

UNDERLYING PATHOLOGY:
Pulmonary embolism
Pleural effusion
Chest infection
COAD / COPD
Pneumothorax
Superior vena cava obstruction

CURRENT RESPIRATORY SYMPTOMS [Please tick]

Symptom	None	Mild	Moderate	Severe	Additional comments
Cough					
Chest pain					
Sputum					
Haemoptysis					

Shortness of breath	Yes/No	Additional comments
Climbs hills or stairs without breathlessness		
Walks any distance on flat without breathlessness		
Walks greater than 100 yards without breathlessness		
Breathless walking less than 100 yards		
Breathless on mild exertion, e.g. undressing		
Breathless at rest		

Other symptoms (please specify)

Figure 5.3 Breathlessness assessment guide, page 1 (Macmillan Practice Development Unit,*
Centre for Cancer & Palliative Care Studies, at The Institute of Cancer Research)
*The MPDU relocated to the University of Southampton in 2002.

Housing/Social/Domestic situation (living arrangements, family, supportive others, stairs, bath/shower, windows, lifts)

Breathlessness frequency:

Most/all the time ☐   Several times a day ☐   Once or twice a day ☐

Several times a week ☐   Once a week ☐   Less than once a week ☐

Other (please specify):

Timing of breathlessness:

Continuous ☐

Intermittent ☐   Morning ☐   Evening ☐   Night ☐

WHAT THINGS MAKE YOU BREATHLESS?

Walking, hills/slopes/stairs, carrying heavy items, bending, washing, dressing, drying oneself, housework, weather, emotions, activities, everything.

WHAT DO YOU DO TO IMPROVE YOUR BREATHLESSNESS?

Pacing, slowing down, resting, nothing helps, gasp, pant, relaxation, not over exerting, massage, teamwork, oxygen, nebulisers, inhalers, opening window, using a fan, not worry about it, positive thinking, talking, visualisation, fighting it.

WHAT DO YOU FEEL YOU ARE UNABLE TO DO AS A RESULT OF YOUR BREATHLESSNESS?

Around the house – housework, meal preparation, answering the phone. Outside the house – gardening, shopping, driving, work. Social life, recreational activities, dancing, sport. Implications on personal life and self – difficulty maintaining sexual relationships, can't do anything, can't fulfil usual role within family.

WHEN YOU EXPERIENCE A SENSATION OF BREATHLESSNESS, CAN YOU DESCRIBE IN YOUR OWN WORDS HOW IT MAKES YOU FEEL?

Frightened, panic, anger, fear, lonely, impending death, claustrophobia, choking, tightness, loss of control, inability to get enough air or breath, suffocation, tired, exhaustion, gasping, panting.

MANAGEMENT STRATEGIES:

(Include management on ward at the present time and if appropriate referral to palliative care team, physio and occupational therapist.)

Issues that need clarification or need to be revisited at next visit:

Assessment completed by: Date of next meeting:

© Centre for Cancer & Palliative Care Studies, at The Institute of Cancer Research

Figure 5.4 Breathlessness assessment guide, page 2 (Macmillan Practice Development Unit,* Centre for Cancer & Palliative Care Studies, at The Institute of Cancer Research
*The MPDU relocated to the University of Southampton in 2002.

Please rate how breathless you have felt in the last 24 hours		
When your breathing has been at its best	When your breathing has been at its worst	In general how much distress does your breathlessness cause you?
10 (Extreme Breathlessness)	10 (Extreme breathlessness)	10 (Extreme distress)
9	9	9
8	8	8
7	7	7
6	6	6
5	5	5
4	4	4
3	3	3
2	2	2
1	1	1
0 (No breathlessness)	0 (No breathlessness)	0 (No distress)

© Centre for Cancer & Palliative Care Studies, at The Institute of Cancer Research

Figure 5.5 Breathlessness assessment guide, page 3 (Macmillan Practice Development Unit,* Centre for Cancer & Palliative Care Studies, at The Institute of Cancer Research)
*The MPDU relocated to the University of Southampton in 2002.

THE MEDICAL MANAGEMENT OF BREATHLESSNESS

Much of current practice in the palliative management of breathlessness is based on custom and practice, rather than a rigorously developed evidence base. While interventions used therapeutically may be based on rational principles, the evidence for their use is in most instances lacking . . . There is also evidence that breathlessness is a symptom which remains unrelieved in many instances despite the use of standard palliative interventions.

The extent of the difficulty over evidence for the management of breathlessness has almost reached a crisis point and, undoubtedly, new thinking needs to emerge as to the future direction for research and therapeutic intervention.

Corner *et al.* (1997: 1)

As well as being based on custom and practice, rather than a sound evidence base, the current medical management of breathlessness tends to focus on treating the causes of the breathlessness (such as cancer) instead of on managing it. Cowcher and Hanks (1990) emphasise the importance of alleviating breathlessness from its very first appearance. They suggest that the symptomatic treatment of breathlessness can be successfully performed alongside specific therapy measures aimed at reversing the underlying disease process causing the breathlessness. Dunlop (1998) agrees that the treatment of breathlessness should not be withheld until treatment of the underlying disease process is complete. Cowcher and Hanks (1990) also stress that the symptomatic treatment of breathlessness should be appropriate to the patient at that time and tailored to the individual.

When the causes of breathlessness cannot be reversed, especially for patients receiving palliative care, or near the end of life, treatment is mainly pharmacological. However, breathlessness presents nurses with a significant challenge because it remains largely *resistant* to pharmacological interventions (Krishnasamy *et al.*, 2001). Furthermore, drug treatments do not address the problem of living and coping with breathlessness, because they are not aimed at the functional and emotional aspects of the experience that remain difficult to manage and may be overwhelming for the patient. Given the problems in treating breathlessness, Corner *et al.* (1997) suggest that a philosophy of palliative care is necessary that offers support and gives people experiencing breathlessness active strategies for managing the symptom themselves (Corner *et al.*, 1997). We will look at these strategies later on in 'Nursing strategies for managing breathlessness'. First we will consider treatments for underlying disease and the symptomatic treatment of breathlessness.

Treatment aimed at reversing the underlying disease process

Corner *et al.* (1997) state that cause-directed treatments should be used to their greatest possible benefit, but should be used appropriately for the patient. Such treatments may include:

- chemotherapy;
- radiotherapy;
- hormonal therapy;
- treatment of infections;
- drainage of effusions;
- correction of anaemia;
- endobronchial techniques;
- identification and treatment of non-cancer-related causes of breathlessness.

However, as the evidence for the effectiveness of many of these in the treatment of breathlessness is either unavailable or equivocal, ongoing repeated treatments (e.g. drainage of pleural effusion) should be given only where a clear symptom benefit has been demonstrated for the individual undergoing treatment.

Symptomatic treatment of breathlessness

Pharmacological treatments

Currently there is little evidence to guide drug therapy in breathlessness (Corner *et al.*, 1997). A trial of therapy is the best way to determine the effectiveness of drug treatment for each individual (Corner *et al.*, 1997). Teams would need to agree how to conduct the trial and how to evaluate the results. (We look at quality assurance in Chapter 8.) Drugs currently used to control breathlessness include:

- **Opioids** – are traditionally the treatment of choice. Although widely used in palliative care, there is a lack of controlled data to prove their efficacy. A recent Cochrane review of studies exploring the benefits of opioids in relieving breathlessness in terminal illness concluded that there is evidence to support the use of oral or parental opioids to palliate breathlessness (Jennings *et al.*, 2003). However, the authors recommend that further research with larger numbers of patients using standardised protocols and quality of life measures is needed (Jennings *et al.*, 2003).
- **Steroids** – may be useful in breathlessness caused by endobronchial disease, lymphangitis carcinomatosis or radiation pneumonitis. Cowcher and Hanks (1990) recommend a five-day therapeutic trial.
- **Nebulised therapies** – bronchodilators should be used with patients who have reversible airway obstructions and nebulised saline may help patients with viscid secretions, but there is no scientific evidence to support the use of nebulised opioids (Jennings *et al.*, 2003).
- **Benzodiazepines** – are commonly used to treat anxiety, but their use remains controversial. They have a place when used subcutaneously in end-stage/terminal breathlessness. They may be useful in episodic breathlessness at an earlier stage but no evidence exists for their use.
- **Diuretics** – have a specific role in relieving breathlessness associated with heart failure. Patients with lymphangitis may respond dramatically to diuretics and some patients whose breathlessness is associated with peripheral oedema may also benefit.
- **Anxiolytics** – usually result in sedation and may therefore not be appropriate. Buspirone is a non-sedating partial seratonin agonist and may increase capacity in patients with COPD, but has a slow onset time and may therefore not be appropriate in palliative care.
- **Nabilone** – is a synthetic cannabinoid. It has anti-emetic, anxiolytic and bronchodilator effects. However, it also has anticholinergic and psychotropic effects. Its use should only be considered in patients with breathlessness which is getting rapidly worse and which doesn't respond to anything else.

Non-pharmacological treatments

These include:

- **Oxygen** – may help some people but, again, although widely used there are no studies confirming its benefit in the absence of hypoxia (Moore *et al.*, 2006). A recent report from a working group of the Scientific Committee for the Association of Palliative Medicine recommended that short-term oxygen therapy may be used for patients with advanced cancer to relieve breathlessness (Booth *et al.*, 2004). However, some patients may develop a psychological dependency on it, which, in turn, causes additional problems such as reduced mobility and heightened anxiety for fear of being unable to breathe without it (Bredin, 2003). Therefore, patients need to be assessed thoroughly on an individual basis following an agreed trial period and the use of oxygen should only be continued if there is obvious benefit (Corner *et al.*, 1997, Booth *et al.*, 2004). Studies suggest that a draught of cool air from a fan may be just as effective (Booth *et al.*, 1996; Bruera *et al.*, 1993; Schwartzstein *et al.*, 1987).
- **Laser treatment** – where high-energy laser beams are directed at tumours during bronchoscopy, can be used to improve symptoms but it is limited by the requirement for bronchoscopy and the cost of the treatment.
- **Stents** – have been used to maintain patency of bronchi. An expandable wire stent or silastic tube can be placed during bronchoscopy. However, the complication rate is relatively high, with up to 10 per cent mortality being reported due to infection or haemorrhage. In a patient with cancer, tumours may grow over the end of the stent. Expandable wire stents are also being used for patients with superior vena caval obstruction (SVCO), where immediate relief of symptoms is usual, but reocclusion occurs in 10–20 per cent of cases (Dunlop, 1998).
- **Physiotherapy** – can be used to help clear bronchial secretions and make breathing more efficient. However, some of these techniques may be too aggressive for patients with advanced disease pathology (Heyse-Moore, 1993). Gentle breathing exercises such as breathing re-training may be more beneficial to patients when used as part of an integrated approach to managing breathlessness. (We look at breathing re-training later in this chapter.)

Activity 7: The medical management of breathlessness

The aim of this activity is to make you think critically about the medical treatments used to manage breathlessness and consider their effectiveness in terms of *how they benefit patients* in your care.

Make brief notes on the different types of medical treatments (pharmacological/non-pharmacological) that are used to manage breathlessness in your clinical area. Consider:

- how each treatment works to relieve breathlessness;
- the indications for a given treatment (i.e. when breathlessness is mild/moderate/severe);
- the side effects/contraindications;
- the effects of any given treatment on individual patients you have cared for.

Then discuss with your colleagues what they feel are the merits/drawbacks of each given treatment. What is the evidence base for each treatment used? If there is no evidence base, what is the justification for their use?

Feedback

If it is not possible to reverse the cause of breathlessness, drug therapy is often seen as the primary means of alleviating the symptom. It is important to be familiar with the treatments patients may receive – and the evidence base for these. When patients are receiving a treatment that is palliative, weighing up the pros and cons of a particular therapy in terms of an improvement in quality of life will be paramount. Using our own knowledge and understanding of available treatments and the evidence base for them, we can assist patients and their families to make more informed choices.

NURSING STRATEGIES FOR MANAGING BREATHLESSNESS

In this final part of the chapter we will introduce two concepts of breathlessness and its treatment – the integrative model and the breathlessness model. We will go on to consider the importance of therapeutic working and then look at several behavioural strategies for managing breathlessness. Finally, we will examine how to help patients manage panic attacks, how to involve the family in the management of breathlessness and how best to help patients experiencing breathlessness during the last few days or hours of their lives (end-stage breathlessness).

The integrative model of breathlessness

In order to make sense of breathlessness, it may be helpful to consider using a model to illustrate aspects of the experience, which we now understand is influenced by a variety of physiological, psycho/emotional, social and spiritual factors. A number of models have been used to describe the experience of breathlessness, including Steele and Shaver (1992) and Corner *et al.* (1995).

Steele and Shaver (1992) suggest a bio-psychosocial model of breathlessness, in which psychological, social and behavioural factors are considered important aspects of the experience. According to Corner *et al.* (1995), while this model is of value, factors such as anxiety are treated as separate from the physical causes of the symptom, requiring separate interventions. Corner *et al.* (1995) take the Steele and Shaver (1992) model one step further and suggest an integrative model of breathlessness, where breathlessness is 'viewed holistically in the context of the individual's life, illness experience and its meaning' (Corner *et al.*, 1995: 6).

The integrative model of breathlessness (Figure 5.6) shows the emotional experience of breathlessness as inseparable from its physical experience. The integrative model argues that separating out the physical and emotional aspects of breathlessness will have little meaning to the person experiencing breathlessness, because anxiety and breathlessness are often indistinguishable (Corner *et al.*, 1995). Care in this model is aimed at enabling individuals to manage breathlessness for themselves, helping them gain a sense of control once more, as well as addressing the 'existential impact of living and dying with breathlessness' (Krishnasamy *et al.*, 2001: 105). This model sits alongside the traditional biomedical model, which is characterised by a focus on pathophysiology and in which the therapeutic aim is to isolate the causes of breathlessness in order to bring about cure or remove the sensation of breathlessness (Krishnasamy *et al.*, 2001). In contrast, Corner *et al.*'s model is intended to 'complement' medical approaches, so that patients are able to receive the best of all professional skills (Krishnasamy *et al.*, 2001).

We believe Corner *et al.*'s (1995) model is the most appropriate one to use within a palliative care setting, because it is holistic and it enables both patients and their carers to address the problem of living and dying with breathlessness. It also values the importance of the patient's perspective – understanding the *patient's experience* and *what breathlessness means to them* – as being central to being able to intervene therapeutically (Bailey, 1995).

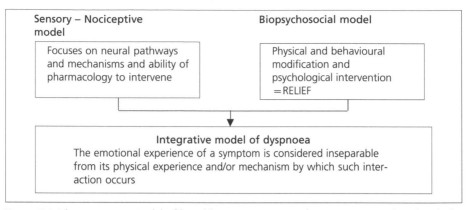

Figure 5.6 The integrative model of breathlessness (Corner *et al.*, 1995: 6), reproduced with the permission of MA Healthcare Ltd. **http://www.ijpn.co.uk** (site accessed 30/6/08).

The breathlessness intervention

Despite the use of medical and pharmacological interventions, it would seem that breathlessness remains difficult to treat and there is evidence to suggest that patients receive little professional help or advice on ways of managing the symptom (Roberts *et al.*, 1993; Higginson and Mc-Carthy, 1989). In response, researchers at the Macmillan Practice Development Unit, Centre for Cancer and Palliative Care Studies, The Institute of Cancer Research, London, developed a nurse-led intervention (Figure 5.7) for the management of breathlessness in patients with lung cancer (Corner *et al.*, 1995; Corner *et al.*, 1996; Bailey, 1995; Bredin *et al.*, 1999). (In 2002, the Macmillan Practice Development Unit relocated to the University of Southampton.) The intervention was evaluated in two research studies: the first, a small pilot study that involved 20 patients, indicated the potential value of the intervention in managing breathlessness (Corner at al., 1996). The second was a multi-centre randomised control trial, which evaluated the intervention using a larger

- Detailed assessment of breathlessness and factors that ameliorate or exacerbate it.

- Advice and support for patients and families on ways of managing breathlessness.

- Exploration of the meaning of breathlessness, their disease and feelings about the future.

- Training in breathing control techniques, progressive muscle relaxation and distraction exercises.

- Goal setting to complement breathing and relaxation techniques, to help in the management of functional and social activities and to support the development and adoption of coping strategies.

- Early recognition of problems warranting pharmacological or medical intervention.

Bredin *et al.* (1999: 902)

Figure 5.7 The intervention

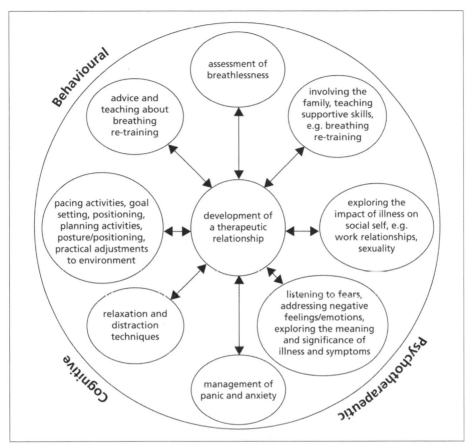

Figure 5.8 The breathlessness intervention (adapted from Interactive Education Unit at The Institute of Cancer Research, 2001)

more diverse patient sample (Bredin *et al.*, 1999). 119 patients with lung cancer from six centres around the UK were recruited into the study. Patients receiving the intervention were invited to attend a nursing clinic once a week for up to eight weeks, where they received a range of strategies aimed at assisting them to cope with breathlessness (Figure 5.8). Patients allocated to the control group received their usual standard care. Both groups completed a range of measurements at base, four and eight weeks. The results of the study showed a significant improvement for the intervention group in breathlessness, performance status and physical and emotional states compared to the control patients (Bredin *et al.*, 1999).

More recently a study by Hately *et al.* (2003) replicated the intervention in a specialist palliative care setting and confirmed the findings of the two earlier studies, reporting significant improvements in patients' breathlessness, functional capacity, activity and distress levels.

Although this research has specifically focused on breathlessness in patients with lung cancer, the work may be of relevance to patients with breathlessness due to other conditions, because the strategies used are intended to empower patients to manage breathlessness for themselves, regardless of their diagnosis. Since the dissemination of the research nationally and internationally over the past few years, the intervention has been refined and extended in a number of ways. Currently the strategies that comprise the intervention are being used by nurses, occupational therapists and physiotherapists, within a variety of clinic and palliative care settings, for patients with cancer as well as for patients who have breathlessness due to other causes.

Psychotherapeutic working – the therapeutic relationship

Nursing when it is therapeutic concentrates on the task of maintaining and supporting the expression of normal emotion. It assists people facing cancer and its treatment to maintain some sense of normal equilibrium, it helps to contain the excesses of the situation people find themselves in.

(Corner *et al.*, 1995: 178)

Figure 5.8 shows that the therapeutic relationship between practitioner and patient is at the core of the breathlessness work – it is this relationship that underpins all the other strategies offered to patients. Bailey (1995) found evidence of the importance of the therapeutic relationship while researching the development and evaluation of a psychosocial intervention for breathlessness in patients with lung cancer. He suggested that the essence of what was therapeutic was the nurse's ability to listen to the patient, acting as a 'container' and 'holding' the patient's distress, making it more tolerable.

. . . if they feel they need to, or talk about how bad it is, what's happening, to actually show you can take it, if you know what I mean, you can hold it, say it's alright . . .

Quote from nurse-researcher: Bailey (1995: 189)

Bailey (1995: 188) draws on psychodynamic theory to describe the act of being there for the patient as 'a maternal function', similar to the way in which a mother contains and manages the infant's distress. Over time, this kind of relationship can help a patient learn to tolerate profoundly difficult feelings (Judd, 1993).

You are never quite sure about how far to take it with patients because sometimes it is sort of in the air and it is unsaid and you have to name it. Mentioning dying can be quite important.

Quote from nurse-researcher: Plant and Bredin (2001: 9)

As well as containing fears, psychotherapeutic working involves acknowledging the losses – big and small – that come about as a result of having a symptom such as breathlessness:

> . . . and part of what is therapeutic [in that] is simply acknowledging the losses and allowing for the grief for those losses. There's things that would be hoped for but are no longer going to be.
>
> Quote from nurse-researcher: Plant and Bredin (2001: 9)

Psychotherapeutic working is also about exploring the impact of the patient's illness in other areas of the patient's life, such as on their family, relationships, work, sexuality and social life. For example, many patients will be reluctant to talk about the restrictions breathlessness imposes on their relationships and sexuality – and it can be challenging for the practitioner to address such problems. All too often, we feel unsure of how to respond, and may avoid talking about these important issues. However, if we are prepared to listen and show we are interested, we can encourage patients to unburden themselves of their concerns. It can be a relief to talk about the problem and often making a simple suggestion or helping the patient to reflect on the problem in a different way can be enough to help them cope once more.

So how do nurses create a relationship that is therapeutic? Basically, it takes time, effort and a willingness to enter into the patient's world of living with breathlessness (Plant and Bredin, 2001). This kind of relationship has been described as a partnership between patient and practitioner where the qualities of reciprocity and mutuality are required (Krishnasamy *et al.*, 2001). Plant and Bredin (2001) also highlight certain other key qualities of this relationship such as acceptance, genuineness, sensitivity and empathy. They also suggest that there are a number of important features that underpin successful therapeutic intervention, which may include the practitioner's ability to:

- create a sense of trust and safety within the relationship;
- listen, contain and be with the patient's/family's distress;
- pay attention to her or his own feelings/intuition;
- obtain appropriate support and supervision.

We will now go on to look at these abilities in more detail.

Creating a sense of trust and safety

Plant and Bredin (2001) suggest that in order to create a sense of trust and safety so that feelings and problems can be talked about, we need to work within a framework. This framework is about setting down the boundaries that define the nature of the relationship between practitioner and patient. For example, you may need to consider the environment that you work in with patients: ideally this would be a space that is quiet, comfortable and free from interruptions. Obviously, this is an ideal that for many nurses is simply not possible but it can be something to aim for.

Professionally, you may need to think of creating boundaries for yourself and your patients by considering such issues as confidentiality and setting the framework for how you are actually going to work with patients, i.e. when, where, how often, how long, what are the shared goals and what are the aims of our interventions?

On a personal level, you may need to pay attention to your own behaviour, thoughts, feelings and attitudes. You may need to consider such issues as personal disclosure and the way in which you communicate with patients. If you can stay open, calm and confident, patients are more likely to be able to talk and share with you. You also need to have the self-belief that you can make a difference – even if you feel daunted by the problems you are addressing. Finally, you need to be able to reflect on the implications of working with seriously ill people and recognise your own limits. This is much easier to do when you work within your own framework of support and supervision – we will come back to this later in the chapter.

Listening, containing and being with the patient's/family's distress

> There were some days with patients where I really felt I haven't done anything for these people, I really wasn't sure if I had been any help at all you know, but at the end of the session they're like 'I feel so much better now'. 'You've been such a great help.
>
> Quote from nurse-researcher: Plant and Bredin (2001: 13)

We often underrate just how valuable a skill listening can be as, all too often, the pressures of work make us feel guilty if we are not seen to be 'doing' something – and it can be difficult to ignore these pressures. As you listen it will be important to be open to whatever material the patient and family brings. One way of showing that you are listening is to reflect back what you hear, as this gives a person a sense of being heard and understood. It can be important too, to avoid the temptation to rush in and say too much – allow for space and silence – the person can then take their time and find their own unique way of saying what needs to be said. We often feel as we are listening that there must be something we should do or say in reply to make the person feel better – often it is simply enough to trust and listen. In order to help the person who is talking feel as safe as possible, as we have already mentioned, you may also need to consider the environment in which you hold the conversation. You may need to warn colleagues beforehand of what you are planning to do (although of course you may not always be able to), and you will need to be firm with them and other members of staff that they cannot interrupt.

Sometimes, because of the intolerable nature of the patient's distress and the seeming relentlessness of the symptom of breathlessness, you may well feel challenged to the limit of your capabilities. If you then feel helpless or uncertain about what to do or say, you may find yourself avoiding (sometimes unconsciously) the patient's distress. That is why it will be important to work within a supervised network of support, where you in turn can be held and have a chance to offload.

Activity 8: Listening exercise

This exercise is designed to help you consider the value of listening.

Find a colleague willing to do this exercise with you.

Take about 20 minutes.

Person 1: You have five minutes to talk uninterrupted about an experience you have had recently where you felt challenged by your work in some way. Recount your story in detail: when, where, who and what took place. What were the difficulties for you and what was the outcome?

Person 2: Sit and listen to Person 1 speaking without interrupting for five minutes. Listen with all your senses. Note how you are feeling as they talk. What seems important to you about their story?

Swap places and do the exercise again, i.e. Person 1: listening and Person 2: talking.

Take five minutes each at the end to swap your experiences: how did it feel to be listened to without interruption? How did you feel having told your story? How did it feel to be the listener? Was anything helpful/unhelpful about the listening? What elements of the listening felt important? Did anything change for you both as a result of telling your stories?

Feedback

One of the most underrated but valuable skills we have to offer is the ability to 'listen' both to our patients and their families – as ourselves. Developing a trusting relationship, in which the patient can be listened to and encouraged to talk about the problems of living with and managing their breathlessness, is vital if the primary aim of breathlessness management is about counteracting isolation and helplessness, addressing anxieties and fears and understanding the meaning of breathlessness for the patient.

Pay attention to your own feelings/intuition

> The being side of you has to be very conscious when you are entering into the clinic because you really don't know what people are going to bring. You are going to use your antenna which have to be really out on stalks and you have to be very present to do that.
>
> Quote from nurse-researcher: Plant and Bredin (2001: 8)

Not only is it important to be 'present' when working with patients, but you also need to be able to listen to your own feelings and intuition about what is happening between yourself and those you are caring for. Often people who are struggling with powerful bodily feelings and distress – such as not being able to breathe properly – may also find it impossible to put their experience into words. By paying attention to what breathlessness evokes in you, you can sometimes gain a sense of what is going on for the patient. For example, you may have noticed how you are left feeling after a conversation or interaction with a patient – and that the feeling you come away with was not there before your conversation. This is because at times, if we are open, we can receive powerful feelings of *what is not being expressed* by those around us. If this is the case, stop, listen to yourself – ask yourself whether this feeling is in any way connected to the work you have been doing with your patient. Can you use this information to tell you something about what is going on in your patient's world? Maybe you might want to draw attention to this kind of communication in your reflection time with colleagues, which we will come to next.

Obtaining appropriate support and supervision

> The process of understanding what is being contained is emotionally demanding for the practitioner. It requires an ability to be able to 'think about', accept and respond to whatever material the patient brings into the relationship. In order to do this effectively, the practitioner must work within a framework of support that allows them to acknowledge and process their own feelings, reactions and experiences arising from their encounters with patients.
>
> (Interactive Education Unit at The Institute of Cancer Research, 2001)

As we have already highlighted, entering into a therapeutic relationship can at times be demanding and emotionally exhausting. In order to be able to support patients, nurses must also feel supported by co-workers and the organisation for which they work (Bailey, 1995). It takes time to develop a support network and, though we care for others, it may well be that we are less good at taking care of ourselves. Support and supervision are an issue for the whole team, since the better supported we are in a recognised professional context, the more capable we will be of functioning as part of a team and managing other people's demands, both physical and emotional. The first step is to recognise that this endeavour is as vital as any other aspect of your clinical work. Next, it may be important to raise this issue with your manager as well as your team, and together consider the most appropriate ways of developing support/supervision systems for yourselves (if this is not already happening). However, you may need to take matters into your own hands and initiate your own support system. Bear in mind developing a support network takes motivation: one solution may be to set up a system of peer supervision (time set aside with a colleague to debrief, listen and reflect on your work with patients) so that you can receive appropriate support.

Activity 9: Obtaining appropriate support

It is most likely that in your work you spend a certain amount of time supporting patients – and their families – who are feeling frightened, anxious and distressed.

Although your support brings relief for the patient and their family, at times it may be emotionally exhausting and distressing for you as well. You may also have little opportunity to address this aspect of your work, because of the sheer enormity of your workload and the lack of time and space provided for such reflection and support. So to whom can you turn for support?

It may be some or any of the following people:

- your manager;
- nurse colleagues in your clinical area;
- members of the health care team;
- family and friends;
- a critical companion, clinical supervisor, peer supervisor;
- psychologist, chaplain, counsellor, occupational health department;
- members of your AL set/your AL set facilitator.

Write down whom you can turn to for support and why. Are you happy that you have a reasonable support network around you? Or do you need to network a bit more to ensure that you have appropriate people available to offer you the support you need? Discuss this issue with your team/manager and agree on what support (formal or informal) would be helpful to you in this work.

Feedback

Just like our patients, we all need opportunities to talk, reflect, feel heard and understood, and it is important that we do so within a safe, confidential space. Working in the frontline with seriously ill people is challenging no matter how experienced the practitioner and, at times, it is bound to touch us in ways we are unprepared for. Most days you can go home and forget all about work – however, there will be times you can't. It may be inappropriate to share with family or friends, no matter how supportive they are. Likewise, finding a colleague who can listen may not be so easy, particularly if they are busy or emotionally drained themselves. Therefore, we would encourage you to develop a system of regular supervision/peer support for yourself, where you can debrief and reflect on your work and be professionally supported. This is not only essential for your personal wellbeing, but is also very much a necessary part of your professional responsibility to yourself, your team and your patients.

Behavioural strategies

Being breathless is not only frightening but can leave patients feeling helpless with little control over what they are experiencing. The behavioural component of the intervention aims to restore a sense of control and encourage a positive attitude to achieving personal goals. Patients can be taught techniques that they can use at home, such as breathing re-training, relaxation, distraction exercises, activity pacing, positioning and energy conservation.

Breathing re-training

In normal breathing, the muscles of the upper chest and shoulders relax, the diaphragm contracts and the lower ribs and upper abdomen expand. This is called abdominal or diaphragmatic breathing. This is illustrated in Figures 5.9–5.12.

Patients who are breathless tend to breathe with the upper chest and shoulders. This leads to rapid, shallow and less efficient breaths and can be immensely tiring – and it may also trigger panic attacks. We look at the management of panic later in this chapter. It can also increase tension in the upper body, which can cause a change in body posture, making normal breathing even harder. Breathing re-training (also sometimes referred to as breathing control) is about promoting a normal, gentle, breathing pattern. This technique can be used with breathless patients, but it must be emphasised that it will *not* alter lung pathology. Bailey (1995) identifies the aims of breathing re-training as being to:

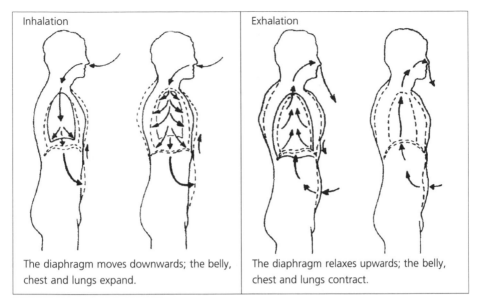

Figure 5.9 Inhalation (side view)   **Figure 5.10** Exhalation (side view)

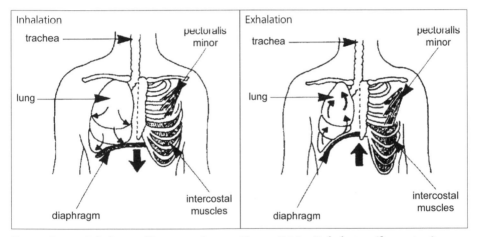

Figure 5.11 Inhalation (front view)   **Figure 5.12** Exhalation (front view)

Source for Figures 5.9 and 5.10: Lewis (1997:102); source for Figures 5.11 and 5.12: Lewis (1997: 32). Reproduced by kind permission of Rodmell Press, www.rodmellpress.com (Site accessed 30/6/08)

- promote a relaxed and gentle breathing pattern;
- minimise the work of breathing;
- establish a sense of control;
- improve ventilation at the base of the lungs;
- increase the strength, co-ordination and efficiency of the respiratory muscles;
- maintain mobility of the thoracic cage;
- promote a sense of wellbeing.

Breathing re-training may also involve the following:

- teaching diaphragmatic/lower chest breathing – we explain this in more detail below;
- slowing breathing or breathing more gently;
- pursed lip breathing – i.e. breathing out through pursed lips;
- relaxing the shoulders and upper chest, possibly by getting someone to apply a gentle downward pressure on the patient's shoulders or applying downward strokes to the patient's back;
- managing attacks of breathlessness;
- breathing while performing activities;
- distraction/relaxation techniques.

There are a number of important steps that need to be covered before teaching breathing re-training to a patient, including:

- establishing a good rapport with the patient by taking time to listen – finding out about what affects the patient's breathing, how they are coping, and the fears they may have;
- observing the patient's posture and breathing rate/pattern;
- explaining about the most efficient way to breathe;
- drawing attention to the patient's breathing pattern and explaining how breathing re-training can help restore a sense of control;
- taking time to find a position that is comfortable and relaxing.

(Interactive Education Unit at The Institute of Cancer Research, 2001)

You also need to consider the patient's willingness and ability to learn the technique. If the patient finds breathing re-training helpful, they can be encouraged to use it while performing activities. This will be discussed later under 'Activity pacing'. We also suggest that you have a go and practise this technique for yourself so that you can have a sense of what is meant by breathing with your diaphragm. The next activity will explain how you can do this.

Activity 10: Practising breathing re-training

In order to help your patients develop their confidence and skill in breathing re-training, it would be good if you were to have a sense of how it feels on yourself first.

Allow 30 minutes to complete the exercise. If possible this exercise will be easier to do if you practise with a partner – one reading while the other listens and tries it out. Then swap and do the exercise again. If done carefully, you will both feel the benefit of calm, relaxed breathing. To start with, find a quiet place where you will not be disturbed and make yourselves comfortable, then read through Steps 1–5 below and try them out.

Person doing the exercise – start by making sure you are sitting or lying (at least partially upright) in a comfortable position with your back well supported. The person reading through the exercise will also need to do so in a calm, relaxed manner, taking time not to rush.

1 Become aware of your body: feel your feet against the floor, drop your shoulders and soften the muscles in your face and around the stomach area. Relax like this for a few minutes.
2 Slowly place your hand flat on your stomach (just under your ribcage) and become aware of that part of your body.
3 Give a little cough and, as you do so, you will feel your diaphragm move.
4 Now become aware of your breath. As you breathe in softly and slowly, feel your hand being pushed out gently by the diaphragm and then, as you breathe out, feel your hand move in again as the diaphragm relaxes.
5 Repeat this exercise two or three times, until you get a sense of your hand moving – out on your in-breath as your ribcage expands and in on your out-breath as the diaphragm relaxes once more.
6 Continue to do this for a few minutes and check you are still relaxed. If it helps, concentrate on breathing slowly in through your nose and out through your mouth, making your out-breath slightly longer than your in-breath.

When you have both had a go, practise the exercise again. At the end, take some time to consider:

- How did you feel being the 'patient'?
- Could you feel your diaphragm move out as you gently breathed in?
- Do you feel different from when you began?
- How did it feel to be the practitioner?
- As the practitioner, what did you learn?
- Could you imagine teaching this to some of the patients you encounter in your work area?
- What other information/support might help you to feel more confident in learning this technique? (For example, reading other books/listening to breathing or relaxation tapes/talking to or observing colleagues who may already have these skills.)

Finally, now you have got a sense of breathing with your diaphragm, observe yourself in the next week or so and notice how you breathe. Do you hold your breath when you are tense or upset? What is your posture like? Can you notice where you hold any tension in your body? Practise breathing with your diaphragm in the next few days when you can remember – and notice how it feels.

Feedback

It is unlikely that you will feel confident to teach breathing re-training exercises to patients straight away, since it takes time and expertise to develop this skill. At this stage it is best to get a 'sense' of what we mean by diaphragmatic breathing and practise with colleagues. You can also discuss with your team leader how you might develop these skills. For example, you could seek advice from physiotherapists and occupational therapists or more senior nurse practitioners working with breathless patients. For a more detailed description of breathing re-training, see the CD-ROM *A breath of fresh air* (Interactive Education Unit at The Institute of Cancer Research, 2007). There is a video demonstration of a patient being taught diaphragmatic breathing in the 'Video gallery' of the 'Intervention' section of the CD-ROM.

Relaxation

Relaxation is a technique that can benefit patients who are breathless because it helps restore a sense of calm and wellbeing. This is because the relaxation response is the opposite of the body's stress response, and cuts through the vicious circle of fear and tension, which can all too often make breathlessness worse (Figure 5.1). It can be helpful too for patients who may be prone to panic attacks – they can use it as part of a self-help strategy to manage breathlessness attacks and break the cycle of anxiety and panic (Moore *et al.*, 2006). We look at the management of anxiety in Chapter 4 and at the management of panic later in this chapter.

Literature that endorses relaxation as a useful strategy for breathlessness comes mainly from work with patients who have breathlessness as a result of chronic respiratory diseases (Janson-Bjerklie and Clarke, 1982; Renfroe, 1988; Gift *et al.*, 1992). However, studies by Corner *et al.* (1995), Bredin *et al.* (1999) and Hately *et al.* (2003) used relaxation as part of a nursing intervention for patients with lung cancer. More research is needed to identify the benefits of individual strategies, but these results are promising and indicate that relaxation, used in conjunction with other strategies, may be of benefit to patients with breathlessness regardless of the underlying disease pathology.

Like the breathing exercises, relaxation is something that needs to be learned consciously and practised regularly for it to be helpful. Patients benefit most from being taught relaxation techniques over a number of sessions in comfortable surroundings, free from distractions (Moore *et al.*, 2006). The length of time needed to practise relaxation can vary from a short five-minute relaxation to a longer 20-minute session, depending on the patient's needs. There are a number of ways you can help patients to get started in using this worthwhile coping strategy.

- Firstly, you might explain why relaxation may be helpful in terms of managing breathlessness, i.e. relaxation helps calm both body and mind and relieves tension and stress, which in turn can help patients to manage their breathlessness more effectively.

- You could suggest that patients or their family buy a relaxation tape and practise by themselves (see the 'Resources for relaxation and visualisation' section at the end of this chapter for more information on where to buy tapes/CDs for relaxation).
- There might be a tape-recorder/CD player in your work area and a set of tapes that you could offer patients.
- You might want to contact the occupational therapy department and find out whether they offer group relaxation classes or whether an OT or physiotherapist could assist you in working with patients.
- Finally, you could have a go and teach relaxation yourself. It is not that difficult to do – it just needs a bit of time and confidence to build up your skills!

If you decide that relaxation is something you would like to offer to patients, then one way of getting started is to practise again either by yourself or with a colleague. Follow the relaxation exercise below – 'Script of a simple relaxation' – also available in the 'Resources' section of the CD-ROM *A breath of fresh air* (Interactive Education Unit at The Institute of Cancer Research, 2007), or try a different one suggested in the 'Resources for relaxation and visualisation' section at the end of this chapter. Before you begin it is important to remember the following points:

- Relaxation should be enjoyable.
- Relaxation can send you to sleep.
- There are different ways to relax – talking a person through a relaxation script is just one method.
- Make sure that your patient/partner is comfortable and warm and that you cannot be disturbed.
- Explain briefly what you are going to do, give your partner permission to move during the relaxation (if they need to) and tell them they can stop at any time.
- Remember to keep your voice calm and relaxed during the session and speak slowly.

When working with someone, remember to stay relaxed yourself. If you believe in what you are doing and remain relaxed, your partner/patient will experience your calmness and respond similarly.

At the end of the session it is important to let the person relaxing rest quietly for a few minutes. If they are awake, gently suggest that, in their own time, they become aware of the room once more, the sounds they can hear and slowly have a stretch or a yawn and open their eyes.

Finally, when we are working with someone who cannot get their breath, all too often we feel helpless – and very often patients are too exhausted or too anxious to speak. It is equally unhelpful to give advice such as 'stay calm' or 'slow your breathing down' – they would if they could. However, taking patients away from their thoughts and breathing, bringing them to an awareness of their body through simple relaxation techniques, can help them to slow down naturally. It can often be a first step to helping them regain a sense of control and calm once more.

Script of a simple relaxation

Notice what is going on around you ... look up at the ceiling and take in your surroundings ... then release your attention to them and gently, when you are ready, close your eyes. Listen to any sounds you can hear ... in this room or outside ... notice them, then release your attention to them.

Become aware of how you feel physically, where you feel comfortable or uncomfortable – you may not necessarily feel anything – then release your attention to that. Become aware of your thoughts ... what is uppermost in your mind? Notice your thoughts ... allow yourself to watch them, follow them ... then let them go ... as you take this precious time for yourself ...

Bring your awareness to the here and now, releasing all that is past just a moment ago ... and all that is to come in the rest of the day ... and just say to yourself silently ... 'I am preparing to relax' ...

Repeat: ... 'I am preparing to relax' ...

Slowly, we are going to take our awareness down through the body. As sensations in your body become noticeable, observe the sense of soft presence wherever your awareness is focused.

Beginning with the head, allow it to sink a little deeper into the pillow behind you and become a little heavier ... let the muscles of the face soften ... feel your forehead becoming a little wider and smoother ... let your eyes soften, muscles relaxing ... check your jaw ... feel it loosen, slacken, drop slightly, teeth parted, your lips soft and hardly touching ... any tension slowly draining away ...

Bring your awareness to your neck and shoulders ... let your neck become a little looser and a little longer ... let your shoulders become heavy ... the distance between your jaw and shoulders becoming a little wider ... as you let go and relax ...

Then coming to your arms, focus the mind down through the arms to your hands and fingers . . . allow the fingers to soften and the arms to feel heavy, limp and soft . . .

Now bring your attention to your chest and focus a moment on your breathing . . . feel the soft sensation of your chest rise and fall, gently, slowly . . . allow the breath to flow peacefully throughout the whole of your body . . . and if you like, silently say to yourself as you breathe out, the word 'calm' . . . 'calm' . . .

Coming to the area around the stomach, let the muscles slacken, loosen and soften . . . like taking off a tight belt, feel the tension fading away . . .

Notice your back and spine . . . allow the back muscles to soften and become heavy as you sink a little deeper into the chair . . .

Then moving down the body, relax the buttocks and thighs . . . let your legs gently roll outwards as the hips widen, all the muscles becoming easy, heavy, soft and loose . . . with no effort . . .

Bringing your awareness to your legs, let them feel heavy too . . . all the tension just draining softly away . . .

Finally, notice your feet and toes, maybe wiggle your toes slightly then stop – feel the feet soften, becoming heavy and limp . . .

Now as you begin to relax fully, gently become aware of the whole of your body . . . how does it feel? . . . Is there anywhere that still feels tense? . . . If so, go to that place and give it permission to relax . . . tension fading . . . dissolving away . . .

If you want to, come back to your breathing . . . feel the gentle rhythm and flow of air, soft and easy . . . if you like, say that word 'calm' again to yourself . . .

Allow that calm and peace to soak through the whole of your body as you continue to let go . . . now I am going to leave you to relax quietly for a few minutes . . .

When you are ready . . . slowly in your own time become aware of the sounds in the room once more, begin to move gently, open your eyes and stretch . . .

Activity 11: Learning about and practising relaxation

If you have not worked with relaxation techniques before, start by reading some of the literature. It helps to understand the physiology of stress, the 'fight or flight' response and what is meant by 'conscious relaxation'. We would recommend that you read one or both of the following:

- Naifeh, K.H. (1994) 'Functions of the autonomic nervous system', in Timmons, B. and Ley, R. (editors) *Behavioural and psychological approaches to breathing disorders.* New York: Plenum Press, pp.42–4 of Chapter 1, 'Basic anatomy and physiology of the respiratory system and the autonomic nervous system'.
- Woodham, A. and Peters, D. (1997) 'Relaxation and breathing', in *The encyclopedia of complementary medicine.* London: Dorling Kindersley, pp.170–3.

Find a written relaxation script that you like and think others would find relaxing if you were to read it to them or use the one we have provided. Read it to yourself a few times and then find a colleague who is prepared to help you, and who may also be interested in relaxation techniques. Arrange to meet in a quiet room for a 15-minute practice relaxation session. Read through the relaxation script together and then agree who will read the script and who will relax.

The 'patient' should take off their shoes and rest comfortably in a chair or lying down. The 'practitioner' should dim the lights and then quietly and slowly read or talk through the relaxation script.

At the end just sit together quietly relaxing for five minutes.

After the session discuss the following questions with your colleague:

- What was it like to be the 'patient'?
- What was it like to be the 'practitioner'?
- Were you able to relax?
- If not, why not?
- How could the session be made more relaxing?

Arrange another session, but this time swap roles. Discuss the session as before.

Feedback

Relaxation techniques can be straightforward for patients to learn, although often we feel daunted at the prospect of teaching them to others. However, they can be of real benefit to patients – and staff! Your colleague may be prepared to try out different relaxation scripts with you or listen to tapes or music to relax to. The more you practise relaxation techniques with colleagues, the easier it will be to use them with patients.

Distraction techniques

You can use distraction techniques such as visualisation and guided imagery to help patients in a number of ways, by suggesting they visualise/imagine:

- relief of the symptom, e.g. imagine taking a deep breath and it spreading throughout the body, all the way down to the toes;
- a 'video' of a time when they felt a certain way, e.g. relaxed and calm, to help them feel that way again;
- a situation in the future, making the pictures positive and how you want them to be, e.g. getting into a shower breathing easily, feeling calm, pacing yourself.

Activity 12: Visualisation

Spend some time creating an image for yourself that you might find useful in your work. For example, think of an image that you find soothing and calming, such as being in a beautiful place (this might be a garden, a beach, a mountain, a beautiful room – whatever pleases you).

Close your eyes for a few minutes and conjure up the images this place evokes in you and then write them down. Think about all your senses – what smells are in this place, textures, colours and sounds, etc.

Over the next few days spend ten minutes or so each day relaxing (you could put on some music too), get comfortable, close your eyes and take yourself off to your calm beautiful image – dwell in it and enjoy it. Each time you finish, note how you feel. As your image becomes more familiar, you may find it easier to conjure up and easier to think of when you want to feel calm and peaceful. Notice how you feel when using a visualisation – does it give you a sense of how this strategy could help patients?

If you don't feel confident to work with imagery/visualisation with patients immediately, get in some practice. Write out a script, remember the importance of preparation and, when you feel ready, practise on yourself and then on a colleague.

Feedback

Even in as short a time span as three or four days you should notice that the visualisation has an overall calming effect. You should be able to slip into it more quickly each day and to call it up when you need it in times of stress. Visualisation should help patients in the same way as it has helped you, with the added benefits of managing breathlessness and panic attacks too. Practising this strategy by yourself and with a colleague should give you the confidence to work with visualisation and imagery with your patients. It is important to allow patients to choose their own soothing image. For example, you may find the image of a beach soothing but a patient who has a fear of water may not find it so. We look at other ways of managing panic later in this chapter.

Activity pacing

Activity pacing is a technique used to help patients slow down, plan and pace their activities. Used in conjunction with breathing re-training it can help patients to manage their breathlessness and feel more in control (Corner *et al.*, 1995). Patients who are breathless often stop all activity for fear of becoming breathless but this has a negative impact on their quality of life. Helping patients (and their families) plan and modify the way they carry out activities can help rebuild confidence and prevent inactivity.

The aims of activity pacing, therefore, are to decrease anxiety, increase activity and fitness, and improve wellbeing (Interactive Education Unit at The Institute of Cancer Research, 2001). There are several stages involved in teaching activity pacing, including:

- Assessing and analysing the problem – i.e. what does breathlessness prevent this patient from doing? What difficulties do they experience in carrying out a particular activity and why? What advice and adjustments need to be made?
- Setting realistic goals – it is important to mutually agree on one or two *achievable* goals. This gives the patient/family something to aim for and helps build confidence.
- Assessment of the environment – how does the patient presently function in their environment? What changes might need to be made so they can accomplish their goals?
- Planning activities – this involves thinking/talking through with the patient how they can plan a given activity. Things to consider might include frequency and timing of activity, organising and simplifying tasks and energy conservation. For example, perhaps a patient wants to go out for a walk in the garden. Planning might include talking through the timing, i.e. the best time of the day to go out (when energy levels are highest). Then discussing how to go about the activity (considering aids that might make the task easier, resting places to sit and recover breath, moving/changing around the environment to make it simpler to function). Finally talking through how to pace and slow down, i.e. walking a few steps stopping and resting, then walking a bit further, stopping and resting, and so on.
- Using activity pacing in conjunction with breathing re-training exercises. If a patient has mastered breathing re-training, you may be able to teach them to pace an activity and use breathing re-training

exercises, thereby increasing their chances of successfully completing a task. For example, perhaps a patient wants to be able to climb the stairs. You can teach the patient to walk up a couple of stairs, then stop, practise breathing re-training exercises and then, when they have recovered their breath, walk up a couple more stairs, stop (before getting out of breath) breathe and recover – then move, stop, breathe, recover, etc. (Interactive Education Unit at The Institute of Cancer Research, 2001). You can find a good example of how to work with activity pacing in the 'Video gallery' of the 'Intervention' section of the CD-ROM *A breath of fresh air* (Interactive Education Unit at The Institute of Cancer Research, 2007).

Positioning

Positioning can play a part in the vicious circle shown in Figure 5.1. Tense positioning creates more tension by sending continuous information that the body is prepared for a 'flight or fight' response. Messages are then continually sent to muscles to accentuate their tension. This tension is therefore self-perpetuating and adds to the anxiety that the patient feels. Paying attention to a patient's position and posture seems so obvious and yet can be overlooked by health care professionals who do not always make this activity a priority. Offering advice on how to alter posture and positioning in order to minimise the work of breathing can make a very real difference to the patient's wellbeing.

Conservation of energy

Breathlessness as a symptom in patients with advanced disease is often severe and patients have often had little time to learn how to cope with it. They frequently try to carry on as they have always done, which often leads to frustration and failure when things go wrong. Therefore, alongside activity pacing, it can help to talk with patients about 'energy conservation'. By this we mean thinking about the balance between the amount of energy expended and the amount of energy available. Sometimes it helps to use the analogy of 'the bank account', e.g.:

- You only have so much in your account and no more.
- How are you going to spend your energy?
- Where can you save energy?
- What is important/not so important to achieve?
- What can be achieved today/tomorrow or the next day?

Thinking this way helps patients to be realistic, prioritise and set achievable goals.

There is a very useful section about conserving energy ('Modifying the activities of daily living to conserve energy') in Chapter 6 on fatigue.

Management of panic

> ... that it is a frightened feeling where you don't think you'll get another breath and because it is accompanied by fear and panic and feeling tight, you can actually feel that tightening feeling of fear in your chest and mind ...
>
> Quote from a patient: O'Driscoll *et al.* (1999: 39)

Within the integrative model a cognitive approach is used to manage panic and anxiety, and address patients' beliefs about their illness/breathlessness:

> A patient's perception of their illness and symptoms and the meaning they attribute to these feelings will influence how they adjust and cope. For example, anxiety and breathlessness are likely to be exacerbated in patients whose predominant belief is that they may die during a panic attack. A cognitive approach can be used to help patients examine their beliefs and 'reframe' them so that they appear less threatening. This might involve helping the patient understand how their beliefs (fear of dying) might affect their emotions (increasing anxiety), which in turn may worsen their breathlessness. By separating these issues rationally – fear of death from breathlessness – the patient can then be offered ways in which to manage or improve their symptoms.
>
> Interactive Education Unit at The Institute of Cancer Research (2001)

Panic attacks are not only a big problem for patients with severe breathlessness – they can also be frightening for those close to the patient to witness. It can be challenging too for the practitioner to know how best to approach the problem since there can be both physical and psychological triggers to each attack. However, there is much that can be done to help patients and their families, and patients may find some of the following strategies useful.

- Listening to fears and exploring beliefs such as the fear of dying during an attack. This is a common fear. Telling patients that breathlessness itself is not harmful and that it is highly unlikely that they would die from a panic attack can be reassuring.
- Educating patients about the vicious circle of fear and panic (Figure 5.1). Explaining, for example, how fear increases anxiety, which then increases physical tension, which increases breathlessness further.

Once patients understand this cycle, they can be taught strategies such as breathing re-training that can help to break it.

- Examining behaviours, i.e. what are the physical/emotional triggers behind an attack and how does the patient/family respond? For example, a patient might be more prone to having panic attacks at night, when they are on their own. Exploring why this is happening and making suggestions to interrupt the cycle of panic/anxiety might help the patient to feel more in control and therefore less likely to panic. (We look at helping patients experiencing anxiety in Chapter 4.)
- Teaching coping strategies, e.g. pacing, positioning, relaxation, breathing re-training, etc.
- Involving the family so that they understand what is happening and can help the patient work through the strategies outlined above.

You may find this next activity quite emotionally demanding and so make sure you make full use of the support offered by your AL set and facilitator. Read through the activity – it is a role-play – and then discuss any issues that it raises for you with the members of your AL set.

Some participants may choose not to do the role-play or may not be able to maintain it for long. When you have completed the role-play, discuss what happened, how you felt and why, with the members of your AL set, or, if you prefer to discuss it on a one-to-one basis, discuss it with your facilitator.

Activity 13: Role-play

Find a partner and carry out this exercise, taking it in turns to be the patient or the nurse. Practise for 15 minutes, then stop and discuss your experiences. Make sure that your feedback is constructive.

Patient – you have recently been admitted to a palliative care unit. You are breathless and frightened, as so far you have had little advice about how to cope with your breathlessness. You are afraid to move because you are frightened of bringing on an attack. You have asked the nurse to give you some advice about how to prevent a breathlessness attack and maintain your mobility, as you live on your own at home and want to be independent for as long as possible.

Nurse – your job is to listen to the patient's concerns, identify problems and plan two or three goals with the patient. Consider what advice you might offer and what strategies you could suggest to help alleviate a breathlessness attack, e.g. activity pacing, breathing re-training exercises, relaxation, etc. Find out about their home environment – what do they find easy/difficult to do at home? What other suggestions can you make for adjusting activities/behaviours to maintain independence when they return home?

Feedback

Role-play can be challenging, but it can teach you a great deal. First, it can help you to think about how it feels to be the patient. Second, it can help you to think about what skills you already have as a nurse in terms of helping patients and where you may need to gain more experience/learn new skills. If you feel uncertain about teaching a particular strategy such as activity pacing, who else in the team might be able to help? You could also refer to the 'Recommended sources of information' at the end of the chapter for ways to improve your knowledge.

INVOLVING THE FAMILY

We know from earlier on in this chapter that breathlessness affects not just the patient but those close to them as well. Often family/friends will also be feeling at a loss to know how to help. Therefore an important aspect of working with patients who are breathless will be involving the family. There are a number of ways you can do this.

- With the patient's permission, encourage family members to be present when you are talking with a patient about their breathlessness and offering advice on the ways in which it can be managed.
- Teach the family the same coping strategies you have taught the patient, such as breathing re-training, activity pacing and relaxation. In this way patient and family can practise together and support each other more fully. Furthermore, if family members can remain calm when breathlessness is severe, the patient will feel less panicked and anxious.
- Encourage family members to talk about their own fears and anxieties and acknowledge their feelings.
- Provide written advice and information about coping with breathlessness (see the information on breathlessness booklets in the 'Recommended sources of information' at the end of this chapter) to allay fears and to reinforce verbal support.
- Consider who else within your team the family could talk to or receive advice from, such as occupational therapists, physiotherapists, etc.

Activity 14 – Involving the family

In this activity we want you to consider how you can involve the patient's family.

Find a family member/close friend who you think would be willing to talk with you. Check that the patient is comfortable with the idea.

Prepare them by explaining that you would like to find out about their experience of living with someone who is breathless.

Explore how they and/or other members of the family have been affected personally by the experience of living with someone who is breathless:

- How do they cope?
- What would help them to cope better?
- What, if anything, has helped them so far?
- What information might be helpful to them to enable them to support their loved one?
- What kind of support do they feel they need in order for them to be able to support their loved one better?

Feedback

Having talked to a family member/close friend, you may have a different perspective on how people cope and manage when being around someone who is experiencing breathlessness. As a result of this exercise, you might want to review the information that your team gives out to people/families caring for someone who is breathless. The information you gather now will help you begin this review and consider in more depth how you might support those who care for someone who is breathless.

END-STAGE BREATHLESSNESS – STRATEGIES FOR THE LAST DAYS OF LIFE

Patients who are breathless in the last few days or hours of their life will require the appropriate palliative care to ease their suffering and distress (Interactive Education Unit at The Institute of Cancer Research, 2007). Breathlessness at this stage may be difficult to treat with non-pharmacological strategies such as breathing re-training exercises or relaxation, since these strategies will require the patient to do the work, and all too often patients are too ill or exhausted to respond. However, because anxiety is likely to remain a large component of the experience of breathlessness, it will be important for nurses to alleviate this by whatever means possible. Giving clear explanations of what is happening, involving the family, ensuring that the environment in which the patient is nursed is well ventilated, peaceful and free from clutter, will all be important in maintaining the patient's comfort and reducing their anxiety. The use of a fan by the bedside may also be helpful. The family will also require a great deal of support at this time, since it is distressing to observe someone who is dying with breathlessness. This anxiety may also be increased if they fear the patient might suffocate or choke – this can in turn exacerbate the sense of breathlessness for the patient (Mosenthal and Lee, 2002). Taking time to educate and support the family about what is happening regarding the patient's laboured breathing will be important, and reassuring them that, at this stage, breathlessness can often be more distressing to the observer than it is for the person who is breathless – unless they become anxious because others around them appear to be (Mosenthal and Lee, 2002).

It is likely at this stage that treatments for breathlessness such as oxygen, opioids and benzodiazepines will be more commonly used and even increased if they are found to reduce distress. However, routes of administration may need to be altered if patients can no longer take them orally (Interactive Education Unit at The Institute of Cancer Research, 2007). Be aware, however, that the administration of opioids and benzodiazepines can depress ventilation and lead to terminal sedation (Interactive Education Unit at The Institute of Cancer Research, 2007), although their use is legally sanctioned under the 'principle of double effect' as long as they are given with the intention of relieving suffering and not of hastening death (Interactive Education Unit at The Institute of Cancer Research, 2007). ('An act with [the] primary intention of doing good which produces a secondary effect that is harmful may be considered to have double effect', cited in Mosenthal and Lee, 2002: 383.)

Activity 15: Reflecting on breathlessness

In this activity we want you to consider and reflect on what you have learned in this chapter, so that you can develop your skills and understanding of managing patients who are breathless. It may be best if you carry out this activity with a colleague and discuss your responses with them. Then make brief notes of your discussion. You may find it helpful to use the model of reflective practice given in Chapter 2, or to use one with which you are already familiar.

Firstly take a few minutes to reflect on what you have learned in this chapter.

What information have you found:

- helpful?
- unhelpful?

How do you feel working through this chapter has increased your knowledge and understanding of breathlessness?

How do you feel now when approaching someone who is breathless compared to when you started this chapter?

What skills mentioned in this chapter do you feel comfortable using with patients?

What more do you want to do in terms of developing your skills in order for you to feel more comfortable in working with breathless patients and their families?

Can you identify other members of the multidisciplinary team that you would like to share/collaborate with in order to improve the service you offer to patients and their families in managing breathlessness?

Finally, if you have used any of your new skills with patients while working through this chapter, discuss with them the impact this new way of managing breathlessness has had on their quality of life. Once you have done this, and had time to reflect upon the patients' comments, review all of your answers to the above questions and make any changes you feel are necessary in light of the patients' comments.

Feedback

Now that you have reached the end of this challenging chapter, you may need some time to reflect on and consolidate your learning. The material we have provided is simply a starting point to help you to increase your skills and knowledge in managing this challenging symptom. Remember that simply 'being there' alongside patients and their families at a time when they feel vulnerable, anxious and fearful is therapeutic. The real experts are our patients – we can learn from them if we truly listen – so begin with where you are now, share your insights, interests and accomplishments and enjoy the rest of your learning.

SUMMARY

In this chapter we have focused on the impact of breathlessness on the patient's life and the importance of acknowledging the emotional as well as physical aspects of breathlessness. We have looked at the problems with the evidence base of much medical treatment and advanced an intervention that combines cognitive, behavioural and psychotherapeutic approaches. Having completed this chapter, you should be able to:

- explain the nature and causes of breathlessness;
- describe the impact of breathlessness on quality of life for patients and their families;
- clarify the importance of making a careful assessment of the patient's breathlessness;
- summarise the current medical treatments for breathlessness, the evidence base for them and the benefits and limitations of medical treatments alone, with special emphasis on the emotional and functional impact of breathlessness;

- describe current nursing strategies for managing breathlessness, emphasising the value of the integrative model for managing breathlessness and explaining the importance of the therapeutic relationship;
- describe how the successful management of breathlessness can improve the quality of life of patients receiving palliative care.

RECOMMENDED SOURCES OF INFORMATION

Titles followed by O/P are out of print – but you may be able to find library copies.

Interactive Education Unit at The Institute of Cancer Research (2001, 2007) *A breath of fresh air: an interactive guide to managing breathlessness in patients with lung cancer*. London: Interactive Education Unit at The Institute of Cancer Research. For more details see: **www.icr.ac.uk/ieu/ projects/Breathlessness Project/ConceptBens.htm** (Site accessed 13/5/08). The CD-ROM is available free of charge to health care professionals. A new and updated version of the CD-ROM was launched in July 2007 and is available from: **ieu@icr.ac.uk** or 0800 9177263.

Patient information booklets

Three useful information booklets for patients with breathlessness can be obtained in PDF format from the 'Resources' section of the CD-ROM *A breath of fresh air* (Interactive Education Unit at The Institute of Cancer Research, 2007). The booklets are designed for patients living at home but much of the information will be useful to you and your patients regardless of your setting. The booklets are:

- *Coping with breathlessness;*
- *Living with breathlessness;*
- *Managing breathlessness.*

Resources for relaxation and visualisation

A breath of fresh air

There are three relaxation/visualisation scripts in the 'Resources' section of the CD-ROM *A breath of fresh air* (Interactive Education Unit at The Institute of Cancer Research, 2007). There is also a video demonstrating relaxation with a patient in the 'Video gallery' of the 'Intervention' section of the CD-ROM.

Relax and breathe CD/audiotape

The Institute of Cancer Research in partnership with Macmillan Cancer Relief has developed a *Relax and breathe* resource for patients. Available in audiotape and CD format, it features practical guidance and relaxation exercises for patients and their carers. To order a copy, contact Macmillan Resources on 0800 500 800. A Relax and breathe professional resources pack is available from the same number, providing a CD version of the resource and guidance to practitioners for its use.

Stress, breathing and relaxation audiotapes can also be obtained from:

www.bhma.org Site accessed 13/5/08.

British Holistic Medical Association
PO Box 371
Bridgwater
Somerset
TA6 9BG
United Kingdom

On breathlessness

Ahmedzai, S. (1998) 'Palliation of respiratory symptoms', in Doyle, D., Hanks, G.W. and MacDonald, N. (editors) *Oxford textbook of palliative medicine* (2nd Ed.). Oxford: Oxford University Press, pp.583–616.

Bailey, C. (2001) 'Breathlessness', in Corner, J. and Bailey, C. (editors) *Cancer nursing: care in context*. Oxford: Blackwell Science, pp.367–75.

Birks, C. (1997) 'Pathophysiology and management of dyspnoea in palliative care and the evolving role of the nurse'. *International Journal of Palliative Nursing*, 3(5), pp.264–74.

Bredin, M. and Plant, H. (2001) 'The challenges of working with breathlessness: the nurse's experience'. Macmillan Practice Development Unit, Centre for Cancer and Palliative Care Studies, The Institute of Cancer Research (unpublished work).

Bredin, M., Corner, J., Krishnasamy, M., Plant, H., Bailey, C. and A'Hern. R. (1999) 'Multicentre randomised controlled trial of nursing intervention for breathlessness in patients with lung cancer'. *British Medical Journal*, 318, 3 April, pp.901–4.

Corner, J., Plant, H., A'Hern, R. and Bailey, C. (1996) 'Non-pharmacological intervention for breathlessness in lung cancer'. *Palliative Medicine*, 10(4), pp.299–305.

Gallo-Silver, L. and Pollack, B. (2000) 'Behavioural interventions for lung cancer-related breathlessness'. *Cancer Practice*, 8(6), pp.268–73.

Gift, A. (1990) 'Dyspnea'. *Nursing Clinics of North America*, 25(4), pp.955–65.

Heyes-Moore, L., Ross, V. and Mullee, M.A. (1991) 'How much of a problem is dyspnoea in advanced cancer?' *Palliative Medicine*, 5(1), pp.20–6.

Higginson, I. and McCarthy, M. (1989) 'Measuring symptoms in terminal cancer: are pain and dyspnoea controlled?' *Journal of the Royal Society of Medicine*, 82(5), pp.264–7.

Interactive Education Unit at The Institute of Cancer Research (2001, 2007) *A breath of fresh air: an interactive guide to managing breathlessness in patients with lung cancer.* London: Interactive Education Unit at The Institute of Cancer Research. For more details see: **www.icr.ac.uk/ieu/projects/Breathlessness Project/ConceptBens.htm** (Site accessed 13/5/08). The CD-ROM is available free of charge to health care professionals from the dedicated orderline: 0800 9177263. A new and updated version of the CD-ROM was launched in 2007.

Johnson, M. and Moore, S. (2003) 'Research into practice: the reality of implementing a non-pharmacological breathlessness intervention into clinical practice'. *European Journal of Oncology Nursing*, 7(1), pp.33–8.

Krishnasamy, M., Corner, J., Bredin, M., Plant, H. and Bailey, C. (2001) 'Cancer nursing practice development: understanding breathlessness'. *Journal of Clinical Nursing*, 10(1), pp.103–8.

Muers, M. (1993) 'Understanding breathlessness'. *Lancet*, 342, 13 November, pp.1190–1.

Pennel, M. and Corner, J. (2001) 'Palliative care and cancer', in Corner, J. and Bailey, C. (editors) *Cancer nursing: care in context.* Oxford: Blackwell Science, pp.517–34.

West, N. and Popkess-Vawter, S. (1994) 'The subjective and psychosocial nature of breathlessness'. *Journal of Advanced Nursing*, 20(4), pp.622–6.

On breathing and relaxation

Benson, H. (1975) *The relaxation response.* New York: Morrow.

Davis, M., McKay, M. and Eshelman, E.R. (2000) *The relaxation and stress reduction workbook* (4th Ed.). Oakland, CA: New Harbinger Publications Inc.

Donavan, M. (1980) 'Relaxation with guided imagery: a useful technique'. *Cancer Nursing*, 3(1), pp.27–32.

Gift, A., Moore, T. and Soeken, K. (1992) 'Relaxation to reduce dyspnea and anxiety in COPD patients'. *Nursing Research*, 41(4), pp.242–6.

Janson-Bjerklie, S. and Clarke, E. (1982) 'The effects of biofeedback training on bronchial diameter in asthma'. *Heart and Lung*, 11(3), pp.200–7.

Lehrer, P. and Woolfolk, R. (1994) 'Respiratory system involvement in western relaxation and self-regulation', in Timmons, B. and Ley, R. (editors) *Behavioural and psychological approaches to breathing disorders.* New York: Plenum Press, pp.191–200.

Lewis, D. (1997) *The tao of natural breathing.* San Francisco: Mountain Wind. Current publishing information: Lewis, D. (2006) *The tao of natural breathing.* Berkeley, CA: Rodmell Press, **www.rodmellpress. com** (site accessed 30/6/08).

Levine, S. (1986) *Who dies?* Bath: Gateway, pp.114–45.

Lum, L. (1977) 'Breathing exercises in the treatment of hyperventilation and chronic anxiety states'. *Chest, Heart and Stroke Journal,* 2, pp.6–11.

Mitchell, L. (1990) *Simple relaxation* (new Ed.). London: John Murray. O/P

Renfroe, K.L. (1988) 'Effect of progressive relaxation on dyspnea and state anxiety in patients with chronic obstructive pulmonary disease'. *Heart and Lung,* 17(4), pp.408–13.

Sims, S. (1987) 'Relaxation training as a technique for helping patients cope with the experience of cancer: a selective review of the literature'. *Journal of Advanced Nursing,* 12(5), pp.583–91.

Woodham, A. and Peters, D. (1997) *The encyclopedia of complementary medicine.* London: Dorling Kindersley, pp.170–3.

On the therapeutic relationship

Bailey, C. (1995) 'Nursing as therapy in the management of breathlessness in lung cancer'. *European Journal of Cancer Care,* 4(4), pp.184–90.

Corner, J. (1997) 'Beyond survival rates and side effects: cancer nursing as therapy'. *Cancer Nursing,* 20(1), pp.3–11.

Ersser, S. (1998) 'A search for the therapeutic dimensions of nurse-patient interaction', in McMahon, R. and Pearson, A. (editors) *Nursing as therapy* (2nd Ed.). Cheltenham: Thornes, pp.43–84. O/P

Ersser, S.J. (1997) 'The concept of nursing as therapy', in Ersser, S.J. *Nursing as a therapeutic activity: an ethnography.* Aldershot: Avebury. O/P

Froggatt, K. (1995) 'Nurses and involvement in palliative care work', in Richardson, A. and Wilson-Barnett, J. (editors) *Nursing research in cancer care.* London: Scutari, pp.151–64. O/P

Kleinman, A. (1998) *The illness narratives: suffering, healing and the human condition.* New York: Basic Books.

Lanceley, A. (2001) 'Therapeutic strategies in cancer care', in Corner, J. and Bailey, C. (editors) *Cancer nursing care in context.* Oxford: Blackwell Science, pp.120–38.

McMahon, R. and Pearson, A. (editors) (1998) *Nursing as therapy* (2nd Ed.). Cheltenham: Thornes.

Mitchell, A. (1995) 'The therapeutic relationship in health care: towards a model of the process of treatment'. *Journal of Interprofessional Care,* 9(1), pp.15–20.

Savage, J. (1995) *Nursing intimacy: an ethnographic approach to nurse-patient interaction.* Harrow: Scutari. O/P

Scholes, J. (1998) 'The therapeutic use of self: a component of advanced nursing practice', in Rolfe, G. and Fulbrook, P. (editors) *Advanced nursing practice.* Oxford: Butterworth-Heinemann, pp.257–70.

REFERENCES

Ahmedzai, S. (1998) 'Palliation of respiratory symptoms', in Doyle, D., Hanks, G.W. and MacDonald, N. (editors) *Oxford textbook of palliative medicine* (2nd Ed.). Oxford: Oxford University Press, pp.583–616.

Bailey, C. (1995) 'Nursing as therapy in the management of breathlessness in lung cancer'. *European Journal of Cancer Care*, 4(4), pp.184–90.

Booth, S., Kelly, M.J., Cox, N.P., Adams, L. and Guz, A. (1996) 'Does oxygen help dyspnea in patients with cancer?' *American Journal of Respiratory Critical Care Medicine*, 153(5), pp.1515–18.

Booth, S., Anderson, H., Swannick, M., Wade, R., Kite, S. and Johnson, M. (2004) 'The use of oxygen in the palliation of breathlessness. A report of the expert scientific committee of the Association of Palliative Medicine'. *Respiratory Medicine*, 98, pp.66–77.

Bredin, M. (2003) 'Breathlessness', in Aranda, S. and O'Connor, M. (editors) *Palliative care nursing: a guide to practice* (2nd Ed.). Melbourne: Ausmed Publications, Chapter 11: pp.116–34.

Bredin, M., Corner, J., Krishnasamy, M., Plant, H., Bailey, C. and A'Hern, R. (1999) 'Multicentre randomised controlled trial of nursing intervention for breathlessness in patients with lung cancer'. *British Medical Journal*, 318, 3 April, pp.901–4.

Bruera, E., de Stoutz, N., Velasco-Leiva, A., Schoeller, T. and Hanson, K. (1993) 'Effects of oxygen on dyspnoea in hypoxaemic terminal-cancer patients'. *Lancet*, 342, 3 July, pp.13–14.

Carrieri, V.K., Janson-Bjerklie, S. and Jacobs, S. (1984) 'The sensation of dyspnea: a review'. *Heart and Lung*, 13(4), pp.436–46.

Corner, J. and O'Driscoll, M. (1999) 'Development of a breathlessness assessment guide for use in palliative care'. *Palliative Medicine*, 13(5), pp.375–84.

Corner, J., Plant, H. and Warner, L. (1995) 'Developing a nursing approach to managing dyspnoea in lung cancer'. *International Journal of Palliative Nursing*, 1(1), pp.5–11.

Corner, J., Plant, H., A'Hern, R. and Bailey, C. (1996) 'Non-pharmacological intervention for breathlessness in lung cancer'. *Palliative Medicine*, 10(4), pp.299–305.

Corner, J., Book, S, Wilcock, A., Macleod, R., Ahmedzai, S. and Connolly M. (1997) 'Developing consensus on the palliative management of breathlessness: a draft consensus document' (unpublished work).

Cowcher, K. and Hanks, G.W. (1990) 'Long-term management of respiratory symptoms in advanced cancer'. *Journal of Pain and Symptom Management*, 5(5), pp.320–30.

Dunlop, R. (1998) *Cancer: palliative care*. London: Springer.

Gift, A., Moore, T. and Soeken, K. (1992) 'Relaxation to reduce dyspnea and anxiety in COPD patients'. *Nursing Research*, 41(4), pp.242–6.

Hately, J., Laurence, V., Scott, A., Baker, R. and Thomas, P. (2003) 'Breathlessness clinics within specialist palliative care settings can improve the quality of life and functional capacity of patients with lung cancer'. *Palliative Medicine*, 17, pp.410–17.

Heyse-Moore, L. (1993) 'Respiratory symptoms', in Saunders, C. and Sykes, N. (editors) *Management of terminal malignant disease* (3rd Ed.). London: Edward Arnold, pp.76–94.

Higginson, I. and McCarthy, M. (1989) 'Measuring symptoms in terminal cancer: are pain and dyspnoea controlled?' *Journal of the Royal Society of Medicine*, 82(5), pp.264–7.

Interactive Education Unit at The Institute of Cancer Research (2001, 2007) *A breath of fresh air: an interactive guide to managing breathlessness in patients with lung cancer*. London: Interactive Education Unit at The Institute of Cancer Research. For more details see: **www.icr.ac.uk/ieu/projects/Breathlessness Project/ConceptBens.htm** (Site accessed 13/5/08.) The CD-ROM is available free of charge to health care professionals from the dedicated orderline: 0800 9177263.

Janson-Bjerklie, S. and Clarke, E. (1982) 'The effects of biofeedback training on bronchial diameter in asthma'. *Heart and Lung*, 11(3), pp.200–7.

Jennings, A.L., Davies, A.N., Higgins, J.P.T. and Broadley, K. (2003) 'Opioids for the palliation of breathlessness in terminal illness (*Cochrane review*)', in The Cochrane Library 2003: Issue 3, Oxford: Update Software.

Judd, D. (1993) 'Life-threatening illness as psychic trauma: psychotherapy with adolescent patients', in Erskine, A. and Judd, D. (editors) *The imaginative body*. London: Whurr, pp.87–112.

Krishnasamy, M., Corner, J., Bredin, M., Plant, H. and Bailey, C. (2001) 'Cancer nursing practice development: understanding breathlessness'. *Journal of Clinical Nursing*, 10(1), pp.103–8.

Lewis, D. (1997) *The tao of natural breathing*. San Francisco: Mountain Wind. Current publishing information: Lewis, D. (2006) *The tao of natural breathing*. Berkeley, CA: Rodmell Press, **www.rodmellpress.com** (Site accessed 30/6/08.)

Moore, S., Plant, H. and Bredin, M. (2006) 'Management of breathlessness in people with cancer', in Kearney, N. and Richardson, A. (editors) *Nursing patients with cancer: principles and practice*. New York: Churchill Livingstone, pp.507–25.

Mosenthal, A. and Lee, F. (2002) 'Management of dyspnea at the end of life: relief for patients and surgeons'. *Journal of American College of Surgeons*, 194(3), pp.377–86.

Naifeh, K.H. (1994) 'Functions of the autonomic nervous system', in Timmons, B. and Ley, R. (editors) *Behavioural and psychological approaches to breathing disorders*. New York: Plenum Press, pp.42–4.

O'Driscoll, M., Corner, J. and Bailey, C. (1999) 'The experience of breathlessness in lung cancer'. *European Journal of Cancer Care*, 8(1), pp.37–43.

Plant, H. and Bredin, M. (2001) 'The challenges of working with breathlessness: the practitioner's experience'. [Unpublished interview data taken from nurses taking part in the multicentre study by Bredin *et al.*, 1999.]

Renfroe, K.L. (1988) 'Effect of progressive muscle relaxation on dyspnea and state anxiety in patients with chronic obstructive pulmonary disease'. *Heart and Lung*, 17(4), pp.408–13.

Reuben, D.B. and Mor, V. (1986) 'Dyspnea in terminally-ill cancer patients'. *Chest*, 89, pp.234–6.

Ripamonti, C. and Bruera, E. (1997) 'Dyspnea: pathophysiology and assessment'. *Journal of Pain and Symptom Management*, 13(4), pp.220–32.

Roberts, D., Thorne, S.E. and Pearson, C. (1993) 'The experience of dyspnea in late-stage cancer: patients' and nurses' perspectives'. *Cancer Nursing*, 16(4), pp.310–20.

Schwartzstein, R.M., Lahive, K., Pope, A., Weinberger, S.E. and Weiss, J.W. (1987) 'Cold facial stimulation reduces breathlessness induced in normal subjects'. *American Review of Respiratory Diseases*, 136(1), pp.58–61.

Steele, B. and Shaver, J. (1992) 'The dyspnea experience: nociceptive properties and a model for research and practice'. *Advances in Nursing Science*, 15(1), pp.64–76.

Twycross, R.G. and Lack, S.A. (1990a) *Therapeutics in terminal cancer* (2nd Ed.). Edinburgh: Churchill Livingstone.

Twycross, R.G. and Lack, S.A. (1990b) 'Respiratory symptoms', in Twycross, R.G. and Lack, S.A. *Therapeutics in terminal cancer* (2nd Ed.). Edinburgh: Churchill Livingstone, pp.123–36.

Woodham, A. and Peters, D. (1997) *Encyclopedia of complementary medicine*. London: Dorling Kindersley, pp.170–3.

Chapter 6

Fatigue

Emma Ream

INTRODUCTION

Fatigue has been defined as reduced capacity to sustain force or power output, reduced capacity to perform multiple tasks over time and simply a subjective experience of feeling exhausted, tired, weak or having lack of energy (Wessely, 1995). It can incorporate feelings ranging from tiredness to exhaustion and, in chronic illness, is typically unrelenting (Ream and Richardson, 1996). Patients find fatigue difficult to explain to others and often use metaphors to convey their experiences of it. They have likened it to having the 'stuffing taken out of them' and refer to how its impact reduces their 'zest for life' (Ream and Richardson, 1996: 48).

For most people, fatigue is a temporary condition – something you feel after strenuous exercise or because of mental stress. You know that after a rest, or a holiday, you'll feel better. It can serve a useful purpose in stopping you working or playing too hard or it can be a useful early indicator of disease. However, fatigue can also be a serious, sometimes chronic, medical condition, which can severely affect people's health and quality of life. Fatigue is the most prevalent symptom identified by cancer patients (Curt *et al.*, 2000) and in cancer patients is referred to as cancer-related fatigue (CRF). Fatigue is also a symptom of illnesses such as multiple sclerosis, motor neurone disease, HIV and rheumatoid arthritis. Fatigue is *different* when you have cancer or another chronic illness:

> CRF was found to be more rapid in onset, more energy draining, more intense, longer lasting, more severe, and more unrelenting when compared with 'typical' fatigue. CRF caused distress in the physical, social, spiritual, psychological, and cognitive domains of the participants' lives.
>
> Holley (2000: 87)

In one study (Stone *et al.*, 2000), over half (58 per cent) of patients with cancer reported that fatigue had affected them in the past month.

Patients felt that fatigue adversely affected their daily lives more than pain or nausea/vomiting (52 per cent vs. 11 per cent and 5 per cent) and also that fatigue was less well managed and controlled than pain or nausea/vomiting (33 per cent vs. 9 per cent and 7 per cent) (Stone *et al.*, 2000).

> I would rather do an activity with pain than be wiped out with fatigue. With the pain, I would cook the dinner and just find a different way to do it; with the fatigue, I couldn't even attempt it. I don't have any control.
>
> Patient, quoted in Tack (1990: 67)

Unfortunately, many cancer patients don't discuss their fatigue with the health care professionals who are caring for them, as they think that it is inevitable, it doesn't seem important enough to mention or they think that nothing can be done (Stone *et al.*, 2000). We will look at barriers to communication later on in the chapter.

Patients often misinterpret CRF as a sign that their cancer therapy isn't working or that the cancer is getting worse and may stop their therapy because of it. It is therefore important to reassure patients suffering from fatigue that it can be managed and that it may end when their treatment ends (although it may not). It is also important to help patients to understand that fatigue is a real and acknowledged phenomenon associated with their illness or the treatment for it:

> I think the fact that I recognised fatigue in my mind made me feel better because otherwise you are trying to fight against it . . . Before that I just carried on doing things. But here I said, 'Right, this is related to the illness, so you might as well sit down, take your time'.
>
> Patient, quoted in Ream (1995: 68)

An important part of the nurse's role is to help patients understand their symptoms and to help patients to learn how to make the most of life while allowing for their symptoms.

Preparation

Before Activity 1 you may like to read the following article (but you can do the activity without it):

Krishnasamy, M. (2000) 'Fatigue in advanced cancer: meaning before measurement?' *International Journal of Nursing Studies*, 37(5), pp.401–14.

Before Activity 5 you may like to read the following article (but you can do the activity without it):

Krishnasamy, M. (1997) 'Exploring the nature and impact of fatigue in advanced cancer'. *International Journal of Palliative Nursing*, 3(3), pp.126–31.

Activity 9 asks you to obtain and read the following article:

Ahlberg, K., Ekman, T., Gaston-Johansson, F. and Mock, V. (2003) 'Assessment and management of cancer-related fatigue in adults'. *The Lancet*, 362 (9384), August 23, pp.640–50.

Start looking into how you can get hold of it now so that you are prepared when you reach Activity 9.

Activity 9 also asks you to try out a selection of pain assessment tools. If you think you might like to use the Brief Fatigue Inventory (Figure 6.3), it is a good idea to begin the process of obtaining permission to use it now – it may take a month or more for the copyright holders to respond. If you wish to use the Brief Fatigue Inventory, you must not adapt it in any way and you must obtain permission from the University of Texas MD Anderson Cancer Center Department of Symptom Research **www.mdanderson.org/ departments/PRG** There is a simple permission request form to fill in: **www.mdanderson. org/departments/prg/display.cfm?id = 9FD3C2D8-77B9-11D5-812C00508B603A14& pn = 0EE78204-6646-11D5-812400508B603A14&method = displayfull**(sites accessed 30/6/08).

Activity 10 asks you to obtain and read the following article:

Porock, D., Kristjanson, L.J., Tinnelly, K., Duke, T. and Blight, J. (2000) 'An exercise intervention for advanced cancer patients experiencing fatigue: a pilot study'. *Journal of Palliative Care*, 16(3), pp.30–6.

Start looking into how you can get hold of it now so that you are prepared when you reach Activity 10.

Note that the evidence base for this chapter is taken from studies of populations of patients with cancer, as this is where the vast majority of research on the effects and management of fatigue and the experience of fatigue has occurred. However, it seems that the fatigue of chronic illness may be similar across illnesses, although the experience itself (or what people read into it/how they interpret it) may differ. Many of the fatigue management strategies that we suggest later in this chapter may therefore be helpful to patients regardless of the cause of their fatigue.

> **LEARNING OUTCOMES**
>
> When you have completed this chapter, you will be able to:
> - define fatigue and explain its impact on the lives of patients and their families;
> - compare and contrast the symptoms of fatigue, cancer-related fatigue and anaemia-related fatigue;
> - explain the factors that can cause or exacerbate fatigue;
> - identify ways of overcoming the barriers to dialogue about fatigue between patients and health care professionals;
> - outline the assessment of fatigue;
> - critically evaluate different approaches to the management of fatigue and the effectiveness of treatment on the patient's quality of life.

FATIGUE AND ITS IMPACT

A complication in the definition of fatigue is described by Brown (1999: 6):

> The term weakness is often used synonymously with fatigue by clinicians and patients alike and many consider them to be part of the same phenomenon.

However, weakness is generally considered to be primarily a physical experience, whereas fatigue is considered to be multidimensional, in that it affects all areas of a patient's life.

Activity 1: What is fatigue?

Think about times when you have been too exhausted to move and make brief notes on how you felt. Think about descriptions of fatigue you have heard from patients. Try to jot down notes on the most common descriptions of fatigue. From your notes, create a definition of fatigue. Share your definition with patients and other members of your team, and ask for their comments. Refine your definition and then compare it with the one we give below.

Feedback

The definition that we give is actually quite complex. We have analysed our definition below to draw out its full implications. Can you do something similar with your own definition?

Fatigue has been defined as:

> A subjective, unpleasant symptom which incorporates feelings ranging from tiredness to exhaustion, creating an unrelenting overall condition which interferes with individuals' ability to function to their normal capacity.
>
> Ream and Richardson (1997: 45)

By analysing the definition of fatigue given above, we can also identify some of the effects of fatigue on patients' lives (Table 6.1).

Attributes	Impact
Subjective	An experience that only the patient can accurately measure or describe to others. (We will look at the measurement of fatigue in 'The assessment of fatigue', later in this chapter.)
Unpleasant	In general, patients perceive fatigue to be unpleasant, although patients experience it and interpret it differently depending on their past experiences and outlook.
Range of feelings	It can vary in intensity from tiredness to exhaustion. It is dynamic and often changes unpredictably during the day or from one day to the next.
Unrelenting	Fatigue can prove difficult for patients to manage if they are not educated in appropriate methods to adopt for its relief or supported and coached in their endeavour to find the optimal approach.
Overall	It is a symptom that affects the entire person. Often patients report feeling fatigued physically, cognitively and emotionally.
Function	Fatigue is a multidimensional phenomenon and its combined effects have the potential to impact on all areas of individuals' daily lives.

Table 6.1 Attributes and impact of fatigue

We will look at the impact of fatigue on patients' lives in more detail in a moment but first we will consider the symptoms of fatigue.

SYMPTOMS OF FATIGUE

In this section we will look at the symptoms of fatigue and differentiate the symptoms of cancer-related fatigue from those of other forms of fatigue. We will identify the patterns of fatigue associated with various forms of cancer therapy, and highlight the additional symptoms that indicate that a patient is suffering from anaemia.

> It's like you've done something really physical like you know sort of walked from here to Brighton, and when you get there, all your arms and legs ached and you felt tired, and just wanted to collapse and sleep . . .
>
> Patient, quoted in Ream (1995: 48)

Physical symptoms of fatigue can include:

- tired eyes;
- tired legs;
- tired arms;
- lack of energy;
- lack of stamina/endurance;
- loss of strength;
- whole body tiredness;
- weakness.

Patients may identify other physical symptoms, such as dizziness or a change in appetite – eating more or less than usual. They may also identify cognitive symptoms, such as poor concentration, 'fuzzy thinking', forgetfulness, drowsiness/sleepiness, memory loss and shortened attention span. Emotional symptoms may include irritability, impatience, depression, a tendency to lack motivation or to become easily bored.

> That was the thing that went with it [the fatigue] was having poor concentration . . . my ability to connect ideas somehow, to sort of synthesise things, wasn't so good and I really got panicked [at work].
>
> With the feeling tired, you feel kind of depressed . . . you know, sometimes you think, 'What's the point?' like . . . 'Oh, what's the point of all this, taking all these pills and doing it, eh?' Hoping to get better. You know, and that's how you feel.
>
> Patients, quoted in Ream (1995: 62)

Cancer and fatigue

Holley (2000: 91–2) suggests that CRF is a unique problem, differing from other forms of fatigue in that it is:

- more rapid in onset;
- more intense;
- more energy draining;
- longer lasting;
- often unexpected.

CRF may be due to the effects of the cancer itself or to the treatments the patient is receiving. Fatigue associated with cancer therapy has a pattern dependent on the form of therapy.

Patterns of fatigue

Specific patterns of fatigue are associated with the following treatments for cancer:

- chemotherapy;
- surgery;
- radiotherapy;
- biotherapy.

The following details are taken from Davies (1996: 60–3). Note that although fatigue generally follows these patterns, you may find differences between individuals.

Chemotherapy

- Fatigue increases steadily with each cycle of chemotherapy.
- Patterns vary with disease type, duration and magnitude of therapy and with drug regimen.
- Fatigue is usually first reported three to four days following initiation of chemotherapy, and reaches its peak at around ten days into the treatment cycle; symptoms then improve until the next cycle.
- Fatigue is a frequent side effect of chemotherapy (50–96 per cent); sometimes it can be so severe as to result in discontinuation of therapy.

Surgery

- Many patients experience fatigue before surgery.
- Fatigue peaks at about seven days following surgery.
- Most patients return to the preoperative levels of fatigue after one month and experience no fatigue three months postoperatively.

Radiotherapy

- Fatigue is a frequent and significant side effect (35–100 per cent).
- Typically, fatigue worsens with each successive treatment cycle (or 'fraction of treatment').
- At weekends, when patients are not undergoing treatment, fatigue may be lessened.
- Fatigue may last three or more months after therapy ceases.

Biotherapy

Fatigue is a common side effect of most biotherapeutic agents, including interferon and tumour necrosis factor. Interleukin-2 is reported to cause severe fatigue, greater than that associated with other biological agents. Fatigue often increases with dose and duration of therapy and may be a dose-limiting side effect, reported as a constellation of flu-like symptoms.

Anaemia and fatigue

Patients may exhibit the general symptoms of fatigue, such as tiredness and exhaustion, dizziness and poor concentration, but be alert to the presence of the following additional symptoms:

- headaches;
- shortness of breath;
- rapid heartbeat;
- paleness of lips, skin and eyelids;
- loss of appetite;
- gastrointestinal disturbances – diarrhoea/constipation.

These symptoms may indicate that the patient is anaemic and the anaemia may be the cause of the fatigue. They may, however, be unrelated to anaemia and be symptoms of the patient's underlying condition. The level of haemoglobin in the patient's blood will indicate whether or not they are anaemic. We look at haemoglobin levels in 'Managing anaemia', later in the chapter.

Activity 2: Reflecting upon fatigue

Reflect upon the experience of fatigue of patients in your clinical setting. Think about one or two patients and how they described their experience of fatigue. Compare their descriptions of their symptoms with those we have described above. Make brief notes on:

- its physical manifestations and whether these changed with time (including the circadian rhythm/daily pattern);
- its cognitive and emotional manifestations;
- its behavioural manifestations;
- any indications that the fatigue was cancer related;
- any patterns that you noticed in the physical manifestations or other indications that the fatigue might be associated with cancer therapy;
- any indications that the fatigue experienced by patients was related to anaemia.

Feedback

If you knew little about fatigue before starting work on this chapter, you may have suddenly realised that patients you have worked with were suffering from fatigue for a variety of reasons, including cancer, cancer therapy, anaemia and other chronic illnesses.

Activity 3: Identifying fatigue symptoms

Now that you have reflected upon the experience of fatigue of patients in your clinical setting, identify one or two patients who are currently experiencing fatigue. Discuss their physical symptoms with them and compare them with those we have described above. Alternatively, you could reflect on similar conversations you have had with patients in the past. Make brief notes on:

- its physical manifestations and whether these change with time (including the circadian rhythm/daily pattern);
- its cognitive and emotional manifestations;
- its behavioural manifestations;
- any indications that the fatigue is cancer related;
- any patterns in the physical manifestations, or other indications that the fatigue might be associated with cancer therapy;
- any indications that the fatigue is related to anaemia.

It is likely that your patients will tell you about the effects of fatigue on other parts of their lives and not just give you the details of the physical symptoms. Make notes on what they tell you, as you can use the information in Activity 5.

Feedback

You should have been able to identify whether the fatigue experienced by your patients is due to cancer, cancer therapy, anaemia or some other cause. We will look at the causes of fatigue in the next section and at the management of fatigue later in the chapter.

Activity 4: Fatigue symptom checklist

You might like to create a couple of fact sheets to help other members of your team identify the symptoms of fatigue.

Create a fact sheet listing the symptoms of fatigue and anaemia (anaemia symptoms are those of fatigue plus the additional symptoms we have identified).

Create a fact sheet identifying the way in which CRF differs from other forms of fatigue (as identified by Holley, 2000), and showing the patterns of fatigue related to the different forms of cancer therapy.

Feedback

Your colleagues should find the fact sheets useful and, if you display them on a noticeboard in your clinical area, so may your patients.

IMPACT OF FATIGUE ON PATIENTS' LIVES

Energy crisis
At first I was energized
The diagnosis shocked me into action
The clutching fear galvanized me
The details demanded attention
The family's tears called for comfort
The decisions were made
The adrenaline flowed and I was energized
But one day all the energy was gone –
Physical, psychic, emotional –
The days turned into weeks
And the weeks into months
Now I search
Each cell of my body
Each corner of my mind
For
one tiny spark

Hjelmstad (1993), cited in Holley (2000: 87)

The physical effects of fatigue may cause many changes in all aspects of the patient's life, including changes in their:

- role/function in the family, and therefore family dynamics;
- economic status, if they are unable to perform paid work;
- self-esteem;
- coping ability (we looked at coping skills in Chapter 2);
- perceptions of the future.

Irrespective of the underlying illness, almost all patients with cancer report that fatigue is one of their most frequently experienced (sometimes daily), severe and troublesome symptoms. It has implications for the patient and for the entire family or supportive network. Carers may have to alter their working arrangements or cease work altogether, they may have to undertake additional or changed roles within the household and they may find the fatigued status of their loved one depressing and frustrating. The fatigue experienced by one family member often becomes a burden shared by all.

Patients suffering from fatigue often feel guilty, as they don't understand why they can no longer 'pull their weight' in the family, for example. They may also feel anxious because they feel they have lost control of their own bodies. They may not understand why napping/resting/sleeping still leaves them unrefreshed and expect to be able to get back to normal after a good rest.

For patients with cancer, many of these problems are based on not realising (or not being warned) how different CRF is from typical fatigue. Holley (2000: 91–2) found that CRF was:

- more rapid in onset – 'Suddenly you're down and out and don't know how you got there'.
- more intense – 'You're a lot more tired.'
- more energy draining – 'With this kind of fatigue, you can't even form it in your mind [to get up].'
- longer lasting – 'not having as much energy all day long, all the time'.
- often unexpected – 'they couldn't tell you how the fatigue was going to make you feel . . .'.

She also found that patients were affected in the physical, social, spiritual, psychological and cognitive domains of their lives.

> I want to take my loved one dancing and can't do it, and that bothers me.

> Normally I attended church three times a week, but I wanted to maintain my work schedule, so I decreased church going to once a week.

> Feelings like uncertainty, dread, powerlessness, loss of control, possible hopelessness, disease puts you into this frame of mind and gives you those feelings. The fatigue will highlight these feelings.
>
> Patients, quoted in Holley (2000: 92)

Activity 5: The impact of fatigue

Review the notes you made in Activity 3, or discuss the impact that fatigue has had on their life with one or two patients and with their families if possible. Alternatively, reflect on similar discussions you have had with patients in the past. Make notes on how fatigue has affected the patient:

- psychologically/emotionally;
- cognitively;
- socially;

- culturally;
- spiritually.

Also note down how the fatigue has impacted on their families.

Feedback

Fatigue affects all aspects of a patient's life and those of their family, and each aspect impacts upon another. An awareness that their mind is not as sharp as it was may make a patient impatient and frustrated, anxious or depressed. These feelings will affect their relationships with their family and friends. The physical or cognitive restrictions placed upon them by fatigue may mean that they are unable to pursue their hopes and goals, and may result in spiritual difficulties, especially if the fatigue is related to cancer or another life-threatening illness.

It's not just one thing, it's not just me lungs, or heart or me economic circumstances, or the way things are at home, or . . . it's the whole, everything . . .

Patient, quoted in Ream (1995: 53)

CAUSES OF FATIGUE

One of the causes of CRF is anaemia, which can be induced by chemotherapy, radiotherapy, blood loss or iron deficiency. Chemotherapy can lower the number of red blood cells in the blood. The red blood cells contain haemoglobin (Hb), which carries oxygen and transports it around the body. Oxygen is essential for the body's energy production so that muscles and organs work properly. When the number of red blood cells is depleted, patients may get tired even when they do something only mildly strenuous. Cancer treatment may also reduce the appetite, which reduces the energy available from food, and side effects such as vomiting and diarrhoea can further affect nutritional intake. CRF may also be caused by toxic substances released by dying cancer cells. Causes of fatigue (both CRF and non-cancer-related fatigue) may include:

- medication(s);
- the body using extra energy to repair tissue damage (e.g. after surgery or radiotherapy);
- infection;
- side effects of treatments, such as fever, nausea, vomiting, diarrhoea, pain, breathlessness;
- not eating enough, or not eating well enough (reduces the energy available from food, as do vomiting and diarrhoea);

- not sleeping enough, not sleeping properly, sleeping too much;
- inactivity/over-exertion;
- depression;
- electrolyte imbalance;
- dehydration.

Tack (1990) suggests that there is a strong relationship between the symptoms of fatigue and pain, as respondents to her interview schedule frequently related fatigue to pain:

> Constant pain is very fatiguing. When I'm fatigued, I can't cope as well with the pain.
>
> Patient, quoted in Tack (1990: 67)

We consider pain – its causes, manifestations, and management – in Chapter 7.

Emotional states such as depression, anxiety and fear can cause or exacerbate fatigue, and these may affect and be affected by the patient's physical and spiritual state, and social and cultural situation.

Diseases not related to cancer, such as chronic obstructive pulmonary disease (COPD, formerly known as chronic obstructive airways disease, COAD), rheumatoid arthritis, HIV, multiple sclerosis and motor neur-one disease, may cause fatigue.

Any one of the above factors (or more frequently a combination) can cause or exacerbate fatigue. The most sophisticated explanation of the manifestation of fatigue is provided by the Psychobiological-Entropy Model (Figure 6.1) (Winningham, 1992, Nail and Winningham, 1993, cited in Winningham *et al.*, 1994).

This model describes how any of the factors above give rise to a downward spiralling of inactivity, deconditioning and fatigue, until the individual reaches an endpoint characterised by disability.

You should warn patients if they are about to commence any treatment that could potentially cause or exacerbate fatigue. Without such preparation, patients may misinterpret its onset and perceive it as an ominous sign or an indication that their illness is progressing. The patterns of fatigue associated with cancer therapies, which we described earlier, are well established. When patients are about to undergo these therapies, you can therefore give them an idea of the fatigue they might experience.

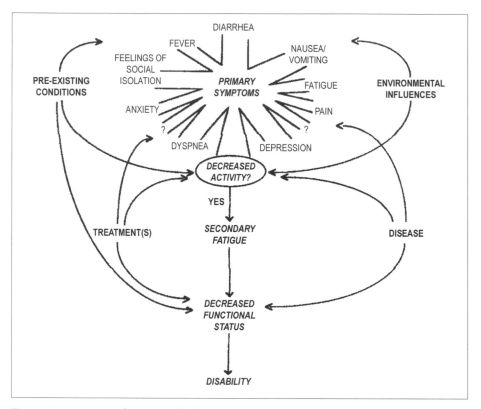

Figure 6.1 Winningham's Psychobiological-Entropy Model (Winningham *et al.*, 1994: 25). Republished with permission of the Oncology Nursing Society, from Winningham, M., Nail, L.M., Burke, M.B., Brophy, L., Cimprich, B., Jones, L.S., Pickard-Holley, S., Rhodes, V., St Pierre, B., Beck, S., Glass, E.C., Mock, V.L., Mooney, K.H. and Piper, B. (1994) 'Fatigue and the cancer experience: the state of the knowledge'. *Oncology Nursing Forum*, 21(1), pp.23–36; permission conveyed through Copyright Clearance Center, Inc. **www.ons.org** (site accessed 30/6/08)

Activity 6: Causes of fatigue

Review the patient details from Activities 3 and 5. If you didn't know, or were unsure of, the causes of fatigue in those patients, can you now identify those causes? Make brief notes on this.

Did the patients receive any advice on managing their fatigue, or treatment for it? If so, what advice/treatment did they receive? Did you feel it was effective? Did the patients feel it was effective? Make brief notes on this.

Feedback

We will look at the management of fatigue later in the chapter. Did you find that your opinion of the effectiveness of the management/treatment of fatigue matched those of your patients? You may have over- or under-estimated the patient's experience of fatigue. This may be because of communication problems. Patients often don't talk much – or at all – about their fatigue and we will look at barriers to dialogue about fatigue next.

BARRIERS TO DIALOGUE ABOUT FATIGUE

It's important for patients to discuss their fatigue with health care professionals and also with others suffering from fatigue. The former can help them obtain the information they need to manage their fatigue or treatments for it. The latter can help them feel that they are not alone. Unfortunately, it appears that there are barriers to effective communication between patients and health care professionals. Stone *et al.* (2000) found that just over half of patients (52 per cent) don't mention the fatigue they are experiencing to their hospital doctor. The most common reasons for failing to mention it included:

- 'I thought it was inevitable.'
- 'It didn't seem important enough to me.'
- 'I believed that nothing could be done.'
- 'My hospital doctor never raised it as an issue.'
- 'I hardly ever experienced it.'
- 'I didn't want to bother the hospital doctor with it.'

Cella *et al.* (1998) identify ten patient-related 'fatigue management barriers':

1. treatment futility;
2. fear of disease progression;
3. desire to be a 'good patient';
4. fear of distracting doctor;
5. lack of concern;
6. fear of stigma;
7. general medication concerns;
8. preference for non-medication interventions;
9. fear of jeopardising cancer/AIDS treatment;
10. lack of communication.

Even patients who have discussed their fatigue with medical staff may still have trouble coming to terms with it:

> I was flabbergasted. I saw one of Dr X's registrars last week and he said that some people don't get any side effects, this terrible fatigue, and I thought, 'I'm young, well relatively young, I'm 37 and healthy ... and I'm finding it very gruelling'. I felt as though I was doing

something wrong, that I'm feeling so ill, that I shouldn't be feeling so ill, I don't know. All I know is what I have experienced.

Patient, quoted in Ream (1995: 69)

Activity 7: Barriers to dialogue

Have you found that patients are reluctant to mention their fatigue? Are there particular types of health care professional in whom they seem more prepared to confide? What sort of difference does it make if you bring the subject up? What reasons do patients give for not mentioning their fatigue?

Feedback

You may have found that patients are more likely to discuss their fatigue with HCAs or with nurses, rather than with doctors, for example. You may find that your bringing the subject up is like giving permission to acknowledge fatigue as a problem – patients may suddenly be prepared or even eager to discuss it with you, especially once they realise that it may not be inevitable/interminable. The most common reason patients give for not mentioning their fatigue is that they believed it to be inevitable, but you may be able to give advice or recommend treatment that will help them manage their fatigue or even recover from it.

Unfortunately, there are health care professionals who are unaware of the significance of fatigue. Like many patients, some may believe that fatigue is inevitable or that nothing can be done about it or that it is unimportant compared with other problems. They may just not listen to patients when they try to tell them about their fatigue:

he [a doctor] has no idea . . . he doesn't listen to what it's like, really like to feel like this all the time, you see they don't take it seriously.

Patient, quoted in Krishnasamy (2000: 409)

Activity 8: Encouraging communication

Discuss barriers to dialogue about fatigue with your colleagues – not only from the patient's side but from the practitioner's side too. Find out what their views on fatigue are and what their feelings about patients experiencing fatigue are. Does it seem to you that your colleagues underestimate the significance of fatigue to patients? If so, discuss with them the importance of acknowledging fatigue's significance. Then go on to discuss how the team can encourage patients to acknowledge their fatigue.

Feedback

Another barrier to effective communication may be that practitioners don't ask patients about fatigue, or don't acknowledge it as a problem, because it is difficult to treat. Caring for a person with this very difficult symptom may make practitioners feel helpless and hopeless and some may unconsciously avoid patients experiencing fatigue.

Once you have made the other members of your team aware of the significance of fatigue, you can work together to encourage patients to talk about it. You can do this by bringing the subject up with patients and introducing the concept that fatigue may not be inevitable/interminable. It is important to acknowledge the patient's experience. 'Being there' for the patient – trying to understand their experience – is therapeutic and may help the patient feel less isolated.

Team members may find peer supervision or the use of a reflective (or learning) diary useful in learning to acknowledge their own feelings about fatigue and patients experiencing fatigue. They may therefore become better equipped to help their patients as they would have learned how to confront the problem rather than avoid it.

When you are talking to patients about fatigue, and discussing strategies for managing or treating fatigue, remember that fatigue includes symptoms such as poor concentration, forgetfulness, memory loss, short attention span, drowsiness/sleepiness, irritability, impatience, depression and a tendency to lack motivation or to become easily bored. You should therefore try to:

- use simple sentences and common words;
- explain unusual words;
- use a conversational style of speech.

Use your non-verbal and observational skills to optimise your communication with these patients.

Each patient's experience of fatigue is unique, and each patient will describe their symptoms differently. Remember that patients are likely to use colloquialisms when describing their experience of fatigue, such as 'knackered' or 'feel like I'm 90', as well as terms like 'lethargic' or 'exhausted'.

TOOLS FOR THE ASSESSMENT OF FATIGUE

> An understanding of which patients are more likely to experience significant fatigue can assist nurses and other healthcare providers to assess and manage fatigue, thereby improving patient outcomes.
>
> Sura *et al.* (2006: 1020)

As we mentioned in Chapter 3, assessment is a continuous process. You are continually checking the patient's state of health and quality of life, the appropriateness and effectiveness of any interventions and identifying what changes need to be made to improve the patient's quality of life. Before selecting a tool for the assessment of fatigue, you should consider the following questions:

- If the tool is intended for patient completion, will a patient experiencing fatigue have the physical and mental stamina to complete the tool?
- If the tool is intended as a prompt for the professional, how can you make the best use of it, without over-tiring the patient, when interviewing a patient experiencing fatigue?
- Is the tool I am considering appropriate for use with or by this individual at this time?
- What use will be made of the information I gather?

When patients make the effort to use assessment tools, it is important that they can see that the information you have obtained from them is going to be used properly.

Many of the instruments and/or questionnaires used to assess fatigue in research can be adapted and used in practice. Some, including the Piper Fatigue Scale (Piper *et al.*, 1998, see Figures 6.2a, 6.2b and 6.2c) and Brief Fatigue Inventory or BFI (Mendoza *et al.*, 1999, see Figure 6.3) are comprised of numerical rating scales or Visual Analogue Scales (VAS – we introduced these in Chapter 3). Such scales provide a sensitive record of patients' experiences in a manner which patients find both acceptable and quick to complete – particularly important with fatigue. The practitioner is faced with having to choose which VASs to include. Ahlberg *et al.* (2003) provide a useful discussion of the tools available to measure fatigue – you will be reading their article in Activity 9.

Activity 9 asks you to use an existing assessment tool or create your own. Please feel free to use the Piper Fatigue Scale (Figures 6.2a, 6.2b and 6.2c) or the Piper fatigue assessment guide (Figure 6.5). If you wish to adapt either of these tools, please specify what adaptations you have made and why and acknowledge Professor Piper as the original copyright

ID#_____   Date:_____

Page 1 of 3   Time:_____

PIPER FATIGUE SCALE©

Directions: Many individuals can experience a sense of <u>unusual</u> or <u>excessive</u> <u>tiredness</u> whenever they become ill or receive treatment for their illness. This unusual sense of tiredness is not usually relieved by either a good night's sleep or by rest. Some call this symptom "fatigue" to distinguish it from the usual sense of tiredness.

For each of the following questions, please circle the number which <u>best</u> describes the Fatigue you are experiencing <u>now</u> or for <u>today</u>. Please make every effort to answer each question to the best of your ability. If you are <u>not</u> experiencing fatigue now or for today, circle "0" for your responses. Thank you very much!

1. How long have you been feeling fatigued? *(Check one response only.)*
   a. _____ minutes
   b. _____ hours
   c. _____ days
   d. _____ weeks
   e. _____ months
   f. _____ other *(please describe)*:
   _____

2. To what degree is the fatigue you are feeling now causing you distress?

No distress   **A great deal of distress**
  0   1   2   3   4   5   6   7   8   9   10

3. To what degree is the fatigue you are feeling now interfering with your ability to complete your work or school activities?

None   **A great deal**
  0   1   2   3   4   5   6   7   8   9   10

4. To what degree is the fatigue you are feeling now interfering with your ability to visit or socialize with your friends?

None   **A great deal**
  0   1   2   3   4   5   6   7   8   9   10

5. To what degree is the fatigue you are feeling now interfering with your ability to engage in sexual activity?

None   **A great deal**
  0   1   2   3   4   5   6   7   8   9   10

6. Overall, how much is the fatigue which you are experiencing now interfering with your ability to engage in the kind of activities you enjoy doing?

None   **A great deal**
  0   1   2   3   4   5   6   7   8   9   10

© 1984; Revised 7/10/95; 5/98; 8/98

Figure 6.2a Piper fatigue scale page 1 (reproduced with permission from Professor Piper)

ID#_____   Date:_____
Page 2 of 3   Time:_____

PIPER FATIGUE SCALE©

7. How would you describe the degree of intensity or severity of the fatigue which you
   are experiencing now?

Mild   **Severe**
0   1   2   3   4   5   6   7   8   9   10

8. To what degree would you describe the fatigue which you are experiencing now as
   being:

Pleasant   **Unpleasant**
0   1   2   3   4   5   6   7   8   9   10

9. To what degree would you describe the fatigue which you are experiencing now as
   being:

Agreeable   **Disagreeable**
0   1   2   3   4   5   6   7   8   9   10

10. To what degree would you describe the fatigue which you are experiencing now as
    being:

Protective   **Destructive**
0   1   2   3   4   5   6   7   8   9   10

11. To what degree would you describe the fatigue which you are experiencing now as
    being:

Positive   **Negative**
0   1   2   3   4   5   6   7   8   9   10

12. To what degree would you describe the fatigue which you are experiencing now as
    being:

Normal   **Abnormal**
0   1   2   3   4   5   6   7   8   9   10

13. To what degree are you now feeling:

Strong   **Weak**
0   1   2   3   4   5   6   7   8   9   10

14. To what degree are you now feeling:

Awake   **Sleepy**
0   1   2   3   4   5   6   7   8   9   10

15. To what degree are you now feeling:

Lively   **Listless**
0   1   2   3   4   5   6   7   8   9   10

16. To what degree are you now feeling:

Refreshed   **Tired**
0   1   2   3   4   5   6   7   8   9   10

17. To what degree are you now feeling:

Energetic   **Unenergetic**
0   1   2   3   4   5   6   7   8   9   10

© 1984; Revised 7/10/95; 5/98; 8/98

Figure 6.2b Piper fatigue scale page 2 (reproduced with permission from
Professor Piper)

ID#_____

Page 3 of 3

Date:_____
Time:_____

PIPER FATIGUE SCALE©

18. To what degree are you now feeling:

Patient   **Impatient**

0   1   2   3   4   5   6   7   8   9   10

19. To what degree are you now feeling:

Relaxed   **Tense**

0   1   2   3   4   5   6   7   8   9   10

20. To what degree are you now feeling:

Exhilarated   **Depressed**

0   1   2   3   4   5   6   7   8   9   10

21. To what degree are you now feeling:

Able to concentrate   **Unable to concentrate**

0   1   2   3   4   5   6   7   8   9   10

22. To what degree are you now feeling:

Able to remember   **Unable to remember**

0   1   2   3   4   5   6   7   8   9   10

23. To what degree are you now feeling:

Able to think clearly   **Unable to think clearly**

0   1   2   3   4   5   6   7   8   9   10

24. Overall, what do you believe is most directly contributing to or causing your fatigue?

_____

_____

25. Overall, the best thing you have found to relieve your fatigue is: _____

_____

_____

26. Is there anything else you would like to add that would describe your fatigue better to us?

_____

_____

27. Are you experiencing any other symptoms right now? _____

_____

_____

© 1984; Revised 7/10/95; 5/98; 8/98

Figure 6.2c Piper fatigue scale page 3 (reproduced with permission from Professor Piper)

Brief Fatigue Inventory

STUDY ID# _____   HOSPITAL # _____

Date: _____ / _____ / _____   Time: _____

Name _____ _____ _____
              Last   First   Middle Initial

Throughout our lives, most of us have times when we feel very tired or fatigued.
Have you felt unusually tired or fatigued in the last week?   Yes [   ]   No [   ]

1. Please rate your fatigue (weariness, tiredness) by circling the one number
   that best describes your fatigue right NOW.

   0   1   2   3   4   5   6   7   8   9   10
   No   As bad as
   Fatigue   you can imagine

2. Please rate your fatigue (weariness, tiredness) by circling the one number that
   best describes your USUAL level of fatigue during past 24 hours.

   0   1   2   3   4   5   6   7   8   9   10
   No   As bad as
   Fatigue   you can imagine

3. Please rate your fatigue (weariness, tiredness) by circling the one number that
   best describes your WORST level of fatigue during past 24 hours.

   0   1   2   3   4   5   6   7   8   9   10
   No   As bad as
   Fatigue   you can imagine

4. Circle the one number that describes how, during the past 24 hours,
   fatigue has interfered with your:

   A. General activity
   0   1   2   3   4   5   6   7   8   9   10
   Does not interfere   Completely Interferes

   B. Mood
   0   1   2   3   4   5   6   7   8   9   10
   Does not interfere   Completely Interferes

   C. Walking ability
   0   1   2   3   4   5   6   7   8   9   10
   Does not interfere   Completely Interferes

   D. Normal work (includes both work outside the home and daily chores)
   0   1   2   3   4   5   6   7   8   9   10
   Does not interfere   Completely Interferes

   E. Relations with other people
   0   1   2   3   4   5   6   7   8   9   10
   Does not interfere   Completely Interferes

   F. Enjoyment of life
   0   1   2   3   4   5   6   7   8   9   10
   Does not interfere   Completely Interferes

Figure 6.3 Brief fatigue inventory (Mendoza *et al.*, 1999: 1189). Copyright Charles S. Cleeland, PhD, Pain Research Group. Used with permission.

	Not at all	A little bit	Some- what	Quite a bit	Very much
1. I feel fatigued	0	1	2	3	4
2. I feel weak all over	0	1	2	3	4
3. I feel listless ('washed out')	0	1	2	3	4
4. I feel tired	0	1	2	3	4
5. I have trouble starting things because I am tired	0	1	2	3	4
6. I have trouble finishing things because I am tired	0	1	2	3	4
7. I have energy	0	1	2	3	4
8. I am able to do my usual activities	0	1	2	3	4
9. I need to sleep during the day	0	1	2	3	4
10. I am too tired to eat	0	1	2	3	4
11. I need help doing my usual activities	0	1	2	3	4
12. I am frustrated by being too tired to do the things I want to do	0	1	2	3	4
13. I have to limit my social activity because I am tired	0	1	2	3	4

Figure 6.4 FACT-F (Cella, 1997: 15) Reprinted from *Seminars in Hematology*, 34(3 Supplement 2), July 1997, Cella, D. 'The Functional Assessment of Cancer Therapy – Anemia (FACT-An) scale: a new tool for the assessment of outcomes in cancer anemia and fatigue', pp.13–19. With permission from Elsevier **http://www.elsevier.com** (site accessed 30/6/08).

holder. Professor Piper would appreciate it if you could e-mail her with your adaptations and rationale and if you have any questions or need any help with it, she would be very pleased to help you. You can contact her at: **bpiper@nursing.arizona.edu**

Other questionnaires, such as the FACT-F (Functional assessment of cancer therapy – fatigue, Yellen *et al.*, 1997 (see Figure 6.4), are comprised of Likert Scales (introduced in Chapter 3) where patients indicate how much they agree with each item. Once more, patients generally find such scales acceptable.

Interview schedules that allow patients to vocalise their experiences have also been developed for different groups of patients, including those with cancer and rheumatoid arthritis. These can prove useful where patients are too debilitated to complete a questionnaire by hand or where a conversational approach is preferred. (See the examples in Figures 6.5 and 6.6.)

It is important that you ask enough questions about the areas of life in which patients are affected. By assessing fatigue in this way, you will be

---

Are you fatigued now?

How intense/severe is your fatigue now? (1–10)

Circadian pattern?

Onset and duration?

Pattern

☐ Brief ☐ Momentary ☐ Acute transient ☐ Intermittent
☐ Seldom ☐ Infrequent ☐ Often ☐ Frequent
☐ Constant ☐ Continuous ☐ Chronic

How does your current level/pattern of fatigue compare to before your illness?

Signs/symptoms of fatigue

☐ Tired eyes ☐ Tired legs ☐ Tired arms ☐ Whole body tiredness

☐ Lack of energy ☐ Lack of stamina/endurance ☐ Weakness
☐ Loss of strength ☐ Other

Are you experiencing other symptoms right now?
  How intense/severe are these symptoms? (0–10)

What increases your fatigue?

What decreases your fatigue?

How has fatigue affected your:

☐ Ability to concentrate ☐ Ability to direct attention/attention span ☐ Memory
☐ Ability to think clearly ☐ Drowsiness/sleepiness ☐ Alertness

How has fatigue affected your moods?

☐ Irritable ☐ Impatient ☐ Depressed ☐ Lack motivation
☐ Become easily bored

How distressing is the fatigue for you?

Does the fatigue have any special meaning for you?

☐ Normal ☐ Abnormal ☐ Usual ☐ Unusual ☐ Other

How has fatigue affected your usual routines/activities of daily living?

Significant findings from the:

☐ Medical history ☐ Physical examination ☐ Laboratory data
☐ Radiology ☐ Other

Source: Davies (1996)

Figure 6.5 Piper Fatigue Assessment Guide (reproduced with permission from Professor Piper). © Barbara F. Piper, DNSc, RN, AOCN, FAAN, Professor and Chair of Nursing Research, The University of Arizona College of Nursing.

better able to promote suitable self-care strategies. However, the questionnaire must be quick to complete, as patients may find lengthy questionnaires too tiring.

Background

Brief history of individual
1. Age
2. Gender
3. Cultural/lifestyle orientation
4. Role expectations
   • Occupation
   • Home
   • Social
   • Economic (insurance coverage)
   • Breadwinner?
   • Living with? Responsible for?
5. Normal activity patterns
6. Normal sleep patterns
7. Preexisting conditions
8. Diagnosis
9. Treatment regimen

Functional Work Output

Focus on changes
1. Are routine tasks getting harder?
2. Have you slowed down?
3. Have you stopped doing some things because of fatigue or any other symptom?

Changes in everyday activities
1. Are you capable of complete self-care?
2. Have you changed your bedtime? How much time do you spend in bed, resting, napping?
3. Are your activity-rest patterns changing?
4. Are you able to participate in family activities?
5. Are you making occupation-related changes?
6. Have you changed your social activities?
7. Have you changed your eating habits? Drinking habits?
8. Do you have any other health problems? Anything that affects your activity? (Consider need for referrals.)

Impairment/Pathophysiology

Diagnostic and laboratory tests
1. Decreased hemoglobin?
2. Hydration status?
3. Electrolyte imbalance? (potassium and magnesium!)

Preexisting conditions or disabilities?

Physical assessment–look for changes in:
1. Alertness and focus? Confusion, irritability, or short attention span?
2. Posture (slumped or erect)?
3. Gait, coordination, and balance (shuffle? steady pace? moving slowly and deliberately?)
4. Ability to arise from seated position?
   • Needs to use hands?
   • Able to rise rapidly from seated to standing position and keep balance?

Feelings Related to Fatigue

Describe sensation of fatigue
1. Ask specifically about no energy, tiredness, or exhaustion.
2. Ask about other symptoms (weakness, depression, dyspnea, pain, etc.).

Establish symptom burden
1. Check intensity of fatigue and related symptoms (get rating on fatigue and other prominent symptoms such as dyspnea, depression, weakness, pain).

0   10
| | | | | | | | | | |

Patterns of fatigue (ask to see patient diary or chart).

Evaluate meaning of perceived symptom burden.

How do any of the above affect your quality of life?

Figure 6.6 Clinical assessment guide for fatigue and functioning (Winningham, 1996: Table 5–2). From Groenwald, S., Frogge, M., Goodman, M. and Yarbro, C. (editors) *Cancer symptom management*, 1996: Jones and Bartlett Publishers, Sudbury, MA. **www.jbpub.com** reprinted with permission (site accessed 30/6/08).

Keeping a fatigue diary

Patients may like to complete a diary, as this can help to delineate their experiences over time and provide a reference point for communication with their informal caregivers and health care team about this somewhat nebulous symptom. Encourage patients to keep a fatigue diary – day of the week, treatment cycles, activities and time of day may all be important. Explain to them how to use a VAS, or encourage them to write descriptions of how their fatigue feels ('tired', 'exhausted', 'wrung out', 'knackered', etc.). This will help to identify which activities make them fatigued and which seem to relieve their fatigue. It can be used to identify any rhythms or patterns to the fatigue. It can also be used to record behavioural changes (e.g. mood swings) that accompany episodes of fatigue or changes to the patient's cognitive abilities.

Activity 9: Assessing fatigue

Read the following article:

Ahlberg, K., Ekman, T., Gaston-Johansson, F. and Mock, V. (2003) 'Assessment and management of cancer-related fatigue in adults'. *The Lancet*, 362 (9384), August 23, pp.640–50.

Bear in mind the complexities of assessing fatigue identified in the article while working through the rest of this activity.

What tool do you currently use to assess fatigue (if any)?

Compare it with the examples we have shown you and identify what aspects of each tool would be most useful to you and your patients.

Create your own fatigue assessment tool based on the aspects you identified above or obtain permission to use one of the ones we have shown you.

Discuss the tool with your colleagues. Also discuss it with patients, if possible, or reflect upon patients' reactions to it when you have used it in the past. Remember that it's important that patients feel both physically and cognitively capable of completing it, so it shouldn't be too long or too complex.

Feedback

Even the most simple assessment tool can be useful for recording the symptoms and helping to identify the causes of fatigue. The next step is to identify how best to manage the patient's fatigue.

THE MANAGEMENT OF FATIGUE

Cella *et al.* (1998: 375) suggest the following fatigue management strategies.

Treating underlying causes of fatigue:

- Anaemia;
- Depression;
- Dehydration/malnutrition;
- Centrally-acting medications (e.g. opioids).

Treating fatigue directly

- Energy conservation and restoration;
- Sleep hygiene;
- Exercise;
- Pharmacological intervention (e.g. psychostimulants, steroids).

Managing consequences of fatigue

- Maintain important activities;
- Facilitate adjustment to limitations;
- Restructure goals and expectations;
- Sustain sense of meaningfulness.

In this section we look primarily at treating fatigue directly and briefly at managing the consequences of fatigue. There is, however, a subsection on the treatment of anaemia and one on nutrition. The management of depression is addressed in Chapter 4.

The mechanisms of fatigue are currently unclear and without this knowledge it is generally not possible to block the processes that lead to fatigue. Therefore interventions should be realistic and aim to:

- control the factors that can exacerbate fatigue;
- reduce the distress associated with fatigue;
- facilitate patients' engagement in pastimes that they enjoy and value;
- enable patients to live more effectively with fatigue.

In this section we look at non-pharmacological and pharmacological strategies for managing fatigue, although bear in mind that recent reviews have critiqued and synthesised both pharmacological and non-pharmacological interventions for fatigue (Ahlberg *et al.*, 2003; Wagner and Cella, 2004). We also look at strategies for managing anaemia (as anaemia may be the cause of the fatigue) and at ways in which you can help patients to manage the consequences of fatigue.

Non-pharmacological strategies for the relief of fatigue

When health care professionals leave patients to find their own way of managing fatigue, and do not advise them on effective methods for its relief, patients follow their common-sense and turn to actions that they used before the onset of their illness. These tend to be sedentary and typically include:

- resting and sleeping during the day;
- curtailing active pastimes;
- reducing activities outside the home;
- reading.

Instead of *alleviating* fatigue, these strategies can often *aggravate* it, largely by reducing exercise tolerance and capacity.

Education is therefore a fundamental aspect in the management of fatigue. Patients are better able to understand, adapt to and manage fatigue when they are educated about it. For example, activities that prove more effective in the relief of fatigue may be those that at first appear counterintuitive, such as exercise. However, remember that fatigue results in the following symptoms: 'fuzzy' thinking, poor concentration, forgetfulness, memory loss and shortened attention spans. Part of the nurse's role is to assess what is appropriate for each individual, so you should take these symptoms into account when advising patients on how to manage their fatigue.

A summary of suitable self-care strategies for the relief of fatigue is presented below (Figure 6.7).

Unfortunately, as the patient's disease progresses, it is likely that the self-care strategies given in Figure 6.7 will prove increasingly less effective. You therefore need to help patients to adapt to living with fatigue.

Exercise

Research evidence (Dimeo *et al.*, 1997a and 1997b; Mock *et al.*, 1997; Winningham *et al.*, 1989; MacVicar *et al.*, 1989) identifies exercise as a beneficial strategy to counteract fatigue in chronic and terminal illness. Recent reviews have usefully critiqued and synthesised these and other studies (Oldervoll *et al.*, 2004; Galvão and Newton, 2005).

Although this will necessarily become less active or strenuous as patients' disease progresses, and they become increasingly debilitated, activities

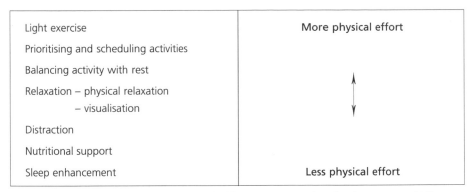

Light exercise	More physical effort
Prioritising and scheduling activities	
Balancing activity with rest	
Relaxation – physical relaxation – visualisation	
Distraction	
Nutritional support	
Sleep enhancement	Less physical effort

Figure 6.7 Self-care strategies for the relief of fatigue (Ream and Richardson, 1999: 1298). Republished with permission of the Oncology Nursing Society, from Ream, E. and Richardson, A. (1999) 'From theory to practice: designing interventions to reduce fatigue in patients with cancer'. *Oncology Nursing Forum*, 26(8), pp.1295–1305; permission conveyed through Copyright Clearance Center, Inc. **www.ons.org** (site accessed 30/6/08).

including arm exercises using resistance and marching on the spot can prove energising and suitable for this population of patients (Porock *et al.*, 2000).

However, patients with the following symptoms should not perform exercise (Davies, 1996: 97):

- irregular pulse or resting pulse above 100 beats/minute;
- recurring leg pain or cramps;
- chest pain;
- nausea or vomiting before or during exercise;
- disorientation/confusion;
- dizziness/blurred vision/faintness;
- bone, back or neck pain of recent origin;
- fever;
- sudden onset of breathlessness, muscular weakness or unusual fatigue.

Patients who have intravenous therapy should not exercise until 24 hours have passed since therapy.

Activity 10: Exercise for fatigue

Read the following article:

Porock, D., Kristjanson, L.J., Tinnelly, K., Duke, T. and Blight, J. (2000) 'An exercise intervention for advanced cancer patients experiencing fatigue: a pilot study'. *Journal of Palliative Care*, 16(3), pp.30–6.

Identify what exercises might be useful for patients suffering from fatigue in your clinical area. Discuss your intended exercise regime with your manager and the other members of your team – especially the physiotherapist if there is one – and make sure that the activities are suitable for the patients you intend to invite to participate. Discuss the idea with the patients and explain the benefits of exercise (patients may take some convincing).

NB: Before encouraging a patient to embark on any exercise regime, ensure that they do not have any of the contraindications we have listed.

After three to five days, discuss with patients whether they think the exercise has been beneficial. Increase/decrease exercise as appropriate to their feedback or suggest that they maintain the existing programme.

Feedback

Any exercise should be carefully tailored to the individual and regularly assessed. This is particularly important if a patient is suffering from fatigue that is worsening (perhaps because of an underlying and progressive disease), as the over-exertion of the exercise may make the fatigue worse. In this situation, exercise should be modified as the fatigue worsens.

Exercise intensity and duration should also be reduced if the patient experiences a worsening of any other symptom, such as pain or nausea/vomiting. For some patients, keeping active may be more useful and feasible than exercising.

Modifying the activities of daily living to conserve energy

Every activity a person performs uses energy and some activities obviously use far more energy than others.

Activity 11: Daily activities

Read through the list below, and then attempt to rate the activities in ascending order of energy output:

- conversation;
- dressing and undressing;
- grooming;
- showering;
- eating a meal;
- standing (relaxed);
- sitting;
- walking slowly (2.6 mile/hour);

- walking moderately fast (3.75 miles/hour);
- walking downstairs;
- walking upstairs.

Feedback

Unsurprisingly, walking upstairs is the most energetic activity and sitting is the least – it requires more than 60 times as much energy to climb the stairs as to sit in a chair. (Even sitting in a chair causes a 17–25 per cent increase over metabolic rate.) The full order is: sitting, eating a meal, grooming, conversation, standing (relaxed), dressing and undressing, walking slowly, walking moderately fast, walking downstairs and walking upstairs. Showering depends on the individual, but is normally somewhere between walking slowly and walking upstairs.

As patients suffering from fatigue may have very little energy, it is important that they prioritise and schedule their activities carefully. If a patient keeps a fatigue diary, they will be aware of the times in the day when their energy is at its peak and when it is at its lowest. They can identify the things that they really want to do, or the things that they must do that require a lot of energy, and schedule those things in for times when they know they will feel relatively energetic. This strategy treats energy as if it were a kind of reserve, using it only when necessary and making the most of it when it's full. One of the easiest ways of maintaining or topping up the level of energy you have in reserve is to conserve energy while performing the activities of daily living.

The suggestions below on how to modify the activities of daily living to conserve energy are a small subset of the many available suggestions and cover some aspects of bathing, grooming and personal hygiene, dressing and mobility. The following booklet contains more guidance on conserving energy while performing these and other activities: *Fatigue*. Available from Cancerbackup, 3 Bath Place, Rivington Street, London EC2A 3JR Tel: 020 7696 9003. Available online at: **www.cancer backup.org.uk/resourcessupport/Symptomssideeffects/Fatigue** (site accessed 30/6/08).

Bathing

Wash your hair in the shower, not over the sink. If possible, use the following items for your safety and comfort: a grab rail, a stool and/or a rubberised suction mat. Use a shower organiser over the showerhead to minimise bending and reaching. Use a long-handled sponge or brush to reach your feet or back. Wear a bathrobe to dry off in rather than rubbing yourself with a towel.

Grooming and personal hygiene

Sit down for these tasks and rest your elbows on the counter or dressing table. Use long-handled brushes or combs to avoid holding your arms over your head.

Dressing

Lay out your clothes before you start dressing. Wear loose-fitting clothes and slip-on shoes. Use a long-handled shoehorn and a sock aid. Wear clothes that fasten at the front, such as shirts/blouses, cardigans, etc., rather than items you have to put on over your head, such as pullovers. If you wear a bra, fasten it at the front and turn it round before pulling the straps up over your arms, or wear front-fastening bras.

Mobility

Wear low-heeled shoes with shock-absorbent sole or insole. Use a wheelchair for long trips.

Getting to sleep at night

Create a bedtime routine and follow it as closely as you can every night. Your mind and body will learn that the steps in your routine lead to going to bed and so you may find that you fall asleep more easily. You may find it helpful to have a warm bath, listen to soothing music, read a book or drink warm milk. We will look at more ways of maximising the benefit of sleep a bit later.

Activity 12: Daily activities – conserving energy

You might like to prepare a series of advice sheets for patients on how to conserve energy while performing the activities of daily living.

Base the sheets on the advice we have given. Your occupational therapist may be able to help you and will also be able to tell you about aids and equipment for the above strategies.

Feedback

Patients should notice an increase in their energy reserve if they can follow all the advice you have supplied. They may also have strategies of their own which may prove useful for other patients. Ask about the patient's own strategies when discussing the ones you have identified, and amend your advice sheets as necessary.

Distraction

Distraction activities that enable patients to focus on something other than their condition and their worries regarding the future can reduce stress and the fatigue that frequently accompanies it. These include activities such as listening to music, socialising or performing formal relaxation techniques. (We looked at relaxation techniques in Chapter 5, 'Breathlessness'.) Distraction techniques can also help to reduce the cognitive aspects of fatigue and enable patients to focus their attention more easily (Cimprich and Ronis, 2003).

We looked at simple craft activities in Chapter 4, and patients suffering from fatigue may enjoy some of them, such as jigsaws, crosswords and simple games like cards and dominoes.

Patients who maintain their sense of humour also maintain their morale and psychological wellbeing. You can use humour to establish a warm and therapeutic relationship with patients and to improve communication. Humour can reduce anxiety and tension, and enhance hope ('lift the spirits'). It may also have health benefits for the respiratory, cardiovascular, musculoskeletal, endocrine and immune systems.

Activity 13: Distraction

What distraction activities can you provide for patients suffering from fatigue in your clinical area?

If you don't have suitable resources, discuss with your colleagues how you might go about obtaining some. For example, art therapy is a useful form of diversion and relaxation but you may not have all the necessary materials.

Feedback

Find out if any volunteers who help out in your area can collect art supplies, musical instruments, or supply other items such as jigsaws, etc.

You could also contact the following for help: self-help groups, community groups that provide lunch clubs, etc., for example Crossroads, local day hospice, information services such as Cancerbackup, Breast Cancer Care, the Stroke Association, Macmillan Cancer Relief (which also provides some grants, but also provides benefit support thereby helping people access benefits to which they are entitled), and the local palliative care team.

Nutritional support

Patients should have a well-balanced diet, but may find that eating smaller meals more often is less tiring. Patients should be offered high energy foods and foods that they enjoy. Patients may feel less tired after lunch if they can eat more protein, such as fish and meat, instead of carbohydrates like bread, potatoes or pasta. Nuts and beans are good sources of vegetable protein, but patients may be too tired to chew nuts. Patients should drink at least eight glasses of liquid a day.

Activity 14: Diet

Is there a dietician on your team? If so, ask them what sorts of diets they would offer to patients suffering from fatigue.

Feedback

Dieticians will usually recommend a diet similar to the one below (Davies, 1996: 67), depending on the situation of each individual.

- Eat frequent small meals.
- Eat a well-balanced breakfast.
- Eat high protein foods, such as milkshake, yoghurt, eggnog and puddings, as snacks between meals.
- For extra calories, use gravy and sauces, and add cream or butter to foods where possible.
- Eat dairy products, meat, fish, peanut butter and eggs regularly, to boost the protein content of the diet.
- Eat grains, pasta, fruit and vegetables for their carbohydrate content, which provides energy for long periods.
- Drink at least eight glasses of liquid each day, to avoid dehydration and eliminate toxic waste products from the system. This can include soups. Patients may find it less daunting if you say they need to drink half a glass or three-quarters of a glass every hour rather than eight glasses a day.
- Moderate exercise before a meal can stimulate appetite.

Remember, however, that some patients may not wish to eat some of the items listed above, for moral, religious or cultural reasons, or because of allergies. Furthermore, some patients may be too ill to follow these suggestions. Also remember that patients who are very fatigued, or who have other physical symptoms or disabilities, may need practical help as well as encouragement to eat and drink.

Sleep

Davies (1996: 110–11) recommends the following steps to maximise the benefits of sleep.

- Sleep should be just long enough so that the patient wakes up refreshed; more sleep than is necessary can actually increase feelings of fatigue.
- A regular wake-up time in the morning strengthens the circadian rhythm and encourages regular times of sleep onset; this routine should be kept even at weekends.
- Reduce noise: loud noises may disturb sleep, even if the patient does not wake; sound attenuation of the bedroom may be advisable for those who sleep close to loud noise.
- Room temperature should be comfortably warm – not too warm and not too cold.
- A bedtime snack (particularly a warm milky drink) may help a patient to sleep; hunger can prevent or disturb sleep.
- Daytime naps can help or inhibit sleep at night; patients should learn how naps can affect sleep patterns.
- Stimulants that contain caffeine should be avoided, as it takes approximately eight hours to metabolise caffeine; poor sleepers are often sensitive to stimulants and should avoid stimulant drinks (such as coffee, tea and cola) after lunchtime.
- Alcohol intake should be limited; although an alcoholic drink before bedtime can help tense people fall asleep, the ensuing sleep is often fragmented.
- If falling asleep proves difficult, rather than getting angry, frustrated and tense, it may be better to give up trying, switch on the light and do something else.
- A steady, daily amount of exercise probably deepens sleep over time, but occasional exercise may not have a direct effect on sleep.

Other useful suggestions are:

- Take steroids, if prescribed, before 6 p.m., as they can cause restlessness if taken late in the day.
- Use sedatives, if prescribed. If the patient is unhappy with the idea of sedatives, suggest that they discuss possible herbal/homeopathic remedies with their GP or hospital doctor. It is important that, before taking any such remedies, they have consulted a doctor to ensure that there will be no adverse interactions with any prescribed medicine that they are taking.

Activity 15: Sleep

Identify which of the suggestions given above can be successfully implemented for patients suffering from fatigue in your clinical area.

Feedback

Unfortunately, many of these suggestions may not be possible in the hospital environment, for example, but those that can be implemented may still help patients with the management of their fatigue.

Pharmacological management of fatigue

Relatively little research evidence has evaluated the efficacy of different classes of drugs for the relief of fatigue. Anecdotal evidence suggests that steroids may have a role in the management of fatigue. These are often administered for their non-specific effects on appetite, mood and energy. Thus, they are often the drug of choice in practice. Some research evidence supports their benefits for reducing fatigue (Bruera *et al.*, 1985) but, given the side effects commonly associated with them, more research needs to be conducted to determine the optimal dosage that should be administered.

Progestational steroids may be indicated to boost appetite where patients are anorexic. Antidepressants may be required if the patient's anorexia and/or fatigue is linked to depression/negative mental affect.

Activity 16: The pharmacological management of fatigue

Reflect on the pharmacological management of fatigue in patients in your clinical setting. Make brief notes on:

- the strategies that you or other members of your team suggest to the patients;
- the success of these approaches.

Feedback

Often fatigue proves difficult to manage and it may take a period of trial and error before the optimal approach is found. If steroids don't appear to work within a week, or if antidepressants (according to type) don't appear to work within three to four weeks, withdraw them. This is important as the side effects can worsen the patient's overall wellbeing. Polypharmacy can be quite a problem for many patients.

Managing anaemia

Anaemia is often an unavoidable side effect of cancer and its treatment. It is frequently mild and does not require specific treatment, but sometimes it is more marked and needs treatment. Anaemia commonly contributes to fatigue.

In anaemia there is a reduced number of circulating red blood cells. These contain haemoglobin (Hb), which carries oxygen to the tissues. The level of haemoglobin is normally 130–180 g/l in men and 115–160 g/l in women. Small reductions in haemoglobin don't usually cause problems but, when levels are below 100 g/l, symptoms of fatigue, lack of energy and sometimes breathlessness can cause problems.

There is a widely held belief that iron is needed to treat anaemia but in cancer patients the anaemia is not due to a lack of iron, it mostly results from the effects of the cancer or its treatment. Similarly there is no need to take lots of special vitamins to try to help anaemia in cancer. A good balanced diet will provide all the substances necessary for blood formation and is also an important part of general self-care. Specific iron or vitamin supplements for anaemia should only be taken on medical advice, especially as iron supplements may cause uncomfortable side effects.

Anaemia can be caused or worsened by treatments for cancer and corrects itself once treatment is finished. However, as treatment effects can last a few weeks or months, anaemia may need to be treated during this time to optimise the patient's quality of life. Treatment options for anaemia include:

- no active treatment;
- red cell transfusion;
- erythropoietin.

No active treatment

It is quite acceptable not to attempt to improve the Hb level for mild forms of anaemia. (Furthermore, there are no simple, practical, inexpensive or risk-free methods by which this can be done.)

Red cell transfusion

Red cells can be replaced in the circulation by transfusion from donated blood. Blood is given through an intravenous drip and a typical transfusion will take 4–8 hours on a hospital day ward. This is a quick and effective means of dealing with anaemic symptoms, but its effect is temporary, lasting only a few weeks. Some patients may need only a single transfusion, but some may need several transfusions, depending on the clinical situation and the Hb level.

There are inconveniences for the patient and a small degree of risk involved, including transfusion reactions, transfusion-transmitted infections, immunosuppression and alloimmunisation. Other practical problems include shortages in the availability of blood products.

Erythropoietin

Another way of maintaining or increasing the number of red blood cells is to stimulate the bone marrow to produce more, by giving patients regular injections of recombinant human erythropoietin (EPO). EPO occurs naturally in the body and is a special hormone that stimulates the production of red blood cells. EPO can be manufactured using recombinant DNA technology. It is biologically indistinguishable from endogenous erythropoietin. It stimulates committed stem cells to increase erythroid (red blood cell) precursors, and results in an increased number of red blood cells entering the circulation with a resulting increase in Hb.

Injecting EPO is a very effective treatment for some types of anaemia where there is a lack of EPO or where extra high levels are needed to overcome a block to the action of the hormone. EPO is simpler than blood transfusions and can be used over longer periods to treat mild to moderate anaemia. There is a growing body of evidence (Abels, 1993; Demetri *et al.*, 1998; Glaspy *et al.*, 1997) supporting the benefits of EPO in managing anaemia in patients receiving chemotherapy and describing its impact on fatigue and overall quality of life. Marketed tradenames for EPO include EPREX®, ERYPO®, NeoRecormon® and Procrit®.

Activity 17: The management of anaemia-related fatigue

Discuss the three treatment options for anaemia with members of your AL set and with your colleagues.

Review the treatment (if any) of two or three of your patients who have had anaemia-related fatigue. Was the most appropriate treatment option chosen in each case? If not, what do you think should have been done and why?

Feedback

Discuss your thoughts on the treatment of anaemia-related fatigue with members of your AL set and your colleagues.

For all sorts of useful information on anaemia, and also cancer-related fatigue, visit the following website: **www.eprex.com** (site accessed 30/6/08).

MANAGING THE CONSEQUENCES OF FATIGUE

Cella *et al.* (1998: 376) suggest the following management strategies for reducing the potentially negative consequences of fatigue on the patient's general quality of life:

- assist the patient in maintaining important activities that are still possible;
- facilitate adjustment to the limitations imposed by the fatigue;
- help with restructuring goals and expectations to allow the patient to continue to feel that life contains important sources of meaning and pleasure, even if these are different from the sources prior to the illness.

Note, however, that the very unpredictability of fatigue can make planning difficult:

> the goal planning and things become almost impossible because it's so unpredictable. Some days are not so bad and others are awful, some mornings are bad and then the afternoon's better, it's all so short term.
>
> District nurse, quoted in Krishnasamy (1997: 130)

Cella *et al.* (1998) suggest that these strategies can be used in conjunction with management strategies for treating the underlying cause of the fatigue and the fatigue itself, and even when these strategies don't seem to be working. They also suggest that energy conservation, patient and family education, stress reduction, support groups and referral to a psychologist or social worker for coping assistance and psychotherapy may be helpful. (We looked at coping strategies in Chapter 2.)

In Chapter 5, 'Breathlessness', we stress the importance of the therapeutic relationship in supporting patients experiencing breathlessness. In a study designed to explore the nature and impact of fatigue, Krishnasamy (2000: 412) found that:

> a research approach that provided participants with an opportunity to talk about their fatigue was greatly valued by the patients who took part, stating that they felt heard and acknowledged.

Once again, 'being there' and 'listening' may be important parts of any nursing intervention. Krishnasamy (1997: 131) identifies the three core elements of a nursing intervention aimed at minimising the impact of fatigue in advanced cancer as:

- facilitating its expression through in-depth assessment of the phenomenon;
- supporting patients and carers as they struggle to find meaning in something so inherently disabling;
- shifting the focus of patients and lay and professional carers from managing the 'symptom of fatigue' to facilitating the process of living with the fatigue of dying.

Until patients and relatives can be supported to explore the existential meanings of the fatigue of advanced cancer, individuals will be left to experience the isolation and distress caused by this phenomenon.

Krishnasamy (1997: 131)

Activity 18: Helping a patient to manage fatigue

Read the case studies below and consider the patients' reactions to their fatigue. Then go on to identify the best ways to help Susan and David to live with their fatigue.

1. Susan

Susan was a lady in her mid-60s who had advanced ovarian cancer that had spread locally to her bowel. She was undergoing a course of palliative chemotherapy in an attempt to slow the progress of her disease. A proud lady, who had raised a family of four children and worked part-time throughout her adult years, she felt very distressed when her treatment impacted on her energy levels. By the end of her second course of treatment she was wondering what the value of her chemotherapy was. She was very surprised by how the chemotherapy had affected her. She had not expected to feel so exhausted.

She had spent the last few weeks wondering what was wrong with her. It took all her energy to get up in the morning, to have a bath and dress. She found this very difficult to come to terms with. After all, no one had warned her that she would feel like this. In fact, some people she knew from the hospital had sailed through treatment without feeling anything like the tiredness she felt. The medical staff had explained that it is quite possible to continue working during treatment. Although she had not worked since her illness, Susan could not imagine being able to work at all. Furthermore, she was unable to keep her house neat and tidy as she had done all her married years. Although her husband was tolerant of this, Susan felt guilty because she could not perform her usual duties in the house. Her husband, Mick, had even had to do the cooking. Furthermore, Susan had little energy for the pastimes that she really enjoyed such as singing in the local church choir.

2. David

David, a gentleman in his late 60s, has been living with chronic obstructive pulmonary disease for 12 years. He lives alone and reports that he suffers both dyspnoea and fatigue. However, he considers fatigue to be the more problematic of the two symptoms. He sleeps poorly and believes that this is one of the main factors giving rise to the fatigue that he experiences on a daily basis. He complains that he wakes in the night and, although not unduly breathless at this time, cannot get back to sleep afterwards. He lies awake feeling both lonely and scared. He has few hobbies and pastimes and refers to how he is becoming increasingly isolated as he seldom leaves his house – mainly because he is scared that he may become both fatigued and breathless while out.

Feedback

1. Susan

We would suggest that Susan could have been better prepared for her treatment and the fatigue to which it gave rise. It's important to supply accurate and realistic preparatory information that can facilitate patients' preparation for and adaptation to fatigue. You can support Susan by 'being there' for her, talking to her and listening to her. For example, while Susan's feelings of guilt about her inability to do everything she used to be able to do may remain, they may be reduced if you reassure her by confirming that fatigue is a valid and normal symptom experienced by many with cancer, and especially when having treatment. It is not a failing.

The best way to help Susan to live with her fatigue includes helping her to prioritise activities so that she can conserve energy for those that are really important to her. Start by finding out what she considers important – don't make assumptions. If cooking supper and managing some of the household tasks are important to her (in addition to singing in the church choir), find ways of helping her so that she is able to do them.

2. David

We would suggest that care for David should begin with a detailed assessment of both his physical and psychological status. This should allow time for exploration of how his symptoms are affecting him and of the anxiety that they are creating. Feelings of anxiety, sadness and isolation are not unusual in people like David, not least as he lives alone and may be fearful of what the future holds. The best way to help David manage fatigue better is three-fold – through his sleep, nutrition and exercise habits.

Attention must be paid to what he perceives to be at the root of his fatigue – lack of sleep. His sleep routine should be assessed and the bedroom environment reviewed. Factors including light, temperature and noise should be considered and altered if necessary (or possible). His positioning and support in bed should be reviewed. David mentions that returning to sleep is difficult because worrying thoughts enter his mind once he's awake. He may like to try some progressive muscle relaxation in bed – gentle and rhythmic tensing and relaxing of different muscle groups for a 10–15 minute period. This may help to induce sleep, as may visualisation exercises where he could concentrate on happy events and scenes and replay them in his head. These are just two examples of activities that could be used to help him relax and take his mind away from anxious thoughts.

It would be wise to check David's nutritional status. His nutritional intake may be insufficient and he could require nutritional support or referral to a dietician.

Finally, you could review his exercise capacity. You will need to determine how physically active he is and whether it could be possible for him to undertake some gentle exercise. This would help to maintain or improve his exercise capacity. Further, if he is physically tired when he goes to bed, he is more likely to sleep.

Reprioritising essential activities, reorganising daily tasks and setting goals can help patients to feel more in control of their lives and can enable them to manage fatigue more effectively.

SUMMARY

Although fatigue is a frequently occurring symptom of chronic and terminal illness, communication between patients and health care professionals about fatigue is frequently poor. Patients report that they find it distressing and that it is a factor that significantly impacts on the quality of their lives.

Fatigue needs to be regularly assessed in clinical practice and the management of fatigue needs to be improved. Patients should be discouraged from using sedentary methods for the relief of fatigue and may need encouragement to adopt innovative approaches to its relief. These may include a combination of different strategies tailored to the individual.

Some classes of drugs may prove beneficial to patients with fatigue. These should be prescribed with care, with the lowest possible doses administered to patients to provide relief.

Having completed this chapter, you should be able to:

- define fatigue and explain its impact on the lives of patients and their families;
- compare and contrast the symptoms of fatigue, cancer-related fatigue and anaemia-related fatigue;
- explain the factors that can cause or exacerbate fatigue;
- identify ways of overcoming the barriers to dialogue about fatigue between patients and health care professionals;
- outline the assessment of fatigue;
- critically evaluate different approaches to the management of fatigue and the effectiveness of treatment on the patient's quality of life.

USEFUL WEBSITES

www.eprex.com

This website provides information on what anaemia is and on how it can be managed. Site accessed 13/5/08.

www.cancer.gov/cancertopics/pdq/supportivecare/fatigue/patient

The National Cancer Institute (NCI) co-ordinates the National Cancer Program in the USA. It 'conducts and supports research, training, health information dissemination and other programs with respect to the cause, diagnosis, prevention and treatment of cancer, rehabilitation from cancer and the continuing care of cancer patients and the families of cancer patients.' This page provides links to details of the causes, assessment and treatment of fatigue. It is intended for patients, although there is a corresponding one for health professionals. Site accessed 30/5/08.

www.cancer.gov/cancertopics/pdq/supportivecare/fatigue/healthprofessional

PDQ is the NCI's comprehensive cancer information database. Most of the information contained in PDQ is available online at NCI's website. Both sites accessed 13/5/08.

www.cancerbackup.org.uk

This is the website of 'Europe's leading cancer information charity, with over 4,500 pages of up-to-date cancer information, practical advice and support for cancer patients, their families and carers.' Site accessed 13/5/08. It provides 'access [to] information on all aspects of cancer, written specifically for cancer patients, their families and carers, plus over 1,000 cancer questions and answers available online.' It runs 'local centres [that] provide face to face information and support for anybody affected by cancer, including cancer patients, their families and friends. They are usually based in a hospital providing cancer services.'

www.cancersymptoms.org

This website is designed for patients and caregivers by the Oncology Nursing Society in the USA to provide information on learning about and managing ten common cancer treatment symptoms, including fatigue. There is a link to pages on fatigue. Site accessed 13/5/08.

REFERENCES

Abels, R. (1993) 'Erythropoietin for anaemia in cancer patients'. *European Journal of Cancer*, 29A (Supplement 2), pp.S2–S8.

Ahlberg, K., Ekman, T., Gaston-Johansson, F. and Mock, V. (2003) 'Assessment and management of cancer-related fatigue in adults'. *The Lancet*, 362 (9384), August 23, pp.640–50.

Brown, D.J.F. (1999) 'The problem of weakness in patients with advanced cancer'. *International Journal of Palliative Nursing*, 5(1), pp.6–12.

Bruera, E., Roca, E., Cedaro, L., Carraro, S. and Chacon, R. (1985) 'Action of oral methylprednisolone in terminal cancer patients: a prospective randomized double-blind study'. *Cancer Treatment Reports*, 69(7/8), pp.751–4.

Cella, D. (1997) 'The Functional Assessment of Cancer Therapy – Anemia (FACT-An) scale: a new tool for the assessment of outcomes in cancer anemia and fatigue'. *Seminars in Hematology*, 34(3 Supplement 2), July, pp.13–19.

Cella, D., Peterman, A., Passik, S., Jacobsen, P. and Breitbart, W. (1998) 'Progress toward guidelines for the management of fatigue'. *Oncology*, 12(11A), pp.369–77.

Cimprich, B. and Ronis, D.L. (2003) 'An environmental intervention to restore attention in women with newly diagnosed breast cancer'. *Cancer Nursing*, 26(4), August, pp.284–92.

Curt, G.A., Breitbart, W., Cella, D., Groopman, J.E., Horning, S.J., Itri, L.M., Johnson, D.H., Miaskowski, C., Scherr, S.L., Portenoy, R.K. and Vogelzang, N.J. (2000) 'Impact of cancer-related fatigue on the lives of patients: new findings from the Fatigue Coalition'. *The Oncologist*, 5(5), pp.353–60.

Davies, J. (1996) *Action on fatigue: a European educational and research initiative for oncology nurses*. Amsterdam: Excerpta Medica.

Demetri, G.D., Kris, M., Wade, J., Degos, L. and Cella, D. (1998) 'Quality-of-life benefit in chemotherapy patients treated with epoetin alfa is independent of disease response or tumor type: results from a prospective community oncology study'. *Journal of Clinical Oncology*, 16(10), pp.3412–25.

Dimeo, F., Tilmann, M.H., Bertz, H., Kanz, I., Mertelsmann, R. and Keul, J. (1997a) 'Aerobic exercise in the rehabilitation of cancer patients after high dose chemotherapy and autologous peripheral stem cell transplantation'. *Cancer*, 79(9), pp.1717–22.

Dimeo, F., Steiglitz, R.D., Novelli-Fischer, U., Fetscher, S., Mertelsmann, R. and Keul, J. (1997b) 'Correlation between physical performance and fatigue in cancer patients'. *Annals of Oncology*, 8(12), pp.1251–5.

Galvão, D.A. and Newton, R.U. (2005) 'Review of exercise intervention studies in cancer patients'. *Journal of Clinical Oncology*, 23(4), pp.899–909.

Glaspy, J., Bukowski, R., Steinberg, D., Taylor, C., Tchekmedyian, S. and Vadhan-Raj, S. (1997) 'Impact of therapy with epoetin alfa on clinical outcomes in patients with nonmyeloid malignancies during cancer chemotherapy in community oncology practice'. *Journal of Clinical Oncology*, 15(3), pp.1218–34.

Groenwald, S., Frogge, M., Goodman, M. and Yarbo, C. (editors) (1996) *Cancer sympton management*. Boston: Jones and Bartlett.

Hjelmstad, L. (1993) *Fine black lines: reflection on facing cancer, fear, and loneliness*. Denver: Mulberry Hill Press.

Holley, S. (2000) 'Cancer-related fatigue: suffering a *different* fatigue'. *Cancer Practice*, 8(2), pp.87–95.

Krishnasamy, M. (1997) 'Exploring the nature and impact of fatigue in advanced cancer'. *International Journal of Palliative Nursing*, 3(3), pp.126–31.

Krishnasamy, M. (2000) 'Fatigue in advanced cancer: meaning before measurement?' *International Journal of Nursing Studies*, 37(5), pp.401–14.

MacVicar, M., Winningham, M. and Nickel, J. (1989) 'Effects of aerobic interval training on cancer patients' functional capacity'. *Nursing Research*, 38(6), pp.348–51.

Mendoza, T.R., Wang, X.S., Cleeland, C.S., Morrissey, M., Johnson, B.A., Wendt, J.K. and Huber, S.L. (1999) 'The rapid assessment of fatigue severity in cancer patients: use of the Brief Fatigue Inventory'. *Cancer*, 85(5), pp.1186–96.

Mock, V., Dow, K., Meares, C.J., Grimm, P.M., Dienemann, J.A., Haisfield-Wolfe, M.E., Quitasol, W., Mitchell, S., Chakravarthy, A. and Gage, I. (1997) 'Effects of exercise on fatigue, physical functioning, and emotional distress during radiotherapy for breast cancer'. *Oncology Nursing Forum*, 24(6), pp.991–1000.

Nail, L. and Winningham, M. (1993) 'Fatigue', in Groenwald, S.L., Frogge, M., Goodman, M. and Yarbro, C. (editors) *Cancer nursing: principles and practice* (3rd Ed.). Boston: Jones and Bartlett, pp.608–19.

Oldervoll, L.M., Kaasa, S., Hjermstad, M.J., Lund, J. and Loge, J.H. (2004) 'Physical exercise results in the improved subjective well-being of a few or is effective rehabilitation for all cancer patients?' *European Journal of Cancer*, 40, pp.951–62.

Piper, B.F., Dibble, S.L., Dodd, M.J., Weiss, M.C., Slaughter, R.E. and Paul, S.M. (1998) 'The revised Piper Fatigue Scale: psychometric evaluation in women with breast cancer'. *Oncology Nursing Forum*, 25(4), pp.677–84.

Porock, D., Kristjanson, L.J., Tinnelly, K., Duke, T. and Blight, J. (2000) 'An exercise intervention for advanced cancer patients experiencing fatigue: a pilot study'. *Journal of Palliative Care*, 16(3), pp.30–6.

Ream, E. (1995) *An exploration of the concept of fatigue in patients with cancer and chronic obstructive pulmonary disease*. MSc Thesis, King's College, University of London.

Ream, E. and Richardson, A. (1996) 'Fatigue: a concept analysis'. *International Journal of Nursing Studies*, 33(5), pp.519–29.

Ream, E. and Richardson, A. (1997) 'Fatigue in patients with cancer and chronic obstructive airways disease: a phenomenological enquiry'. *International Journal of Nursing Studies*, 34(1), pp.44–53.

Ream, E. and Richardson, A. (1999) 'From theory to practice: designing interventions to reduce fatigue in patients with cancer'. *Oncology Nursing Forum*, Sept., 26(8), pp.1295–305.

Stone, P., Richardson, A., Ream, E., Smith, A.G., Kerr, D.J. and Kearney, A. (2000) 'Cancer-related fatigue: inevitable, unimportant and untreatable? Results of a multi-centre patient survey'. *Annals of Oncology*, 11(8), pp.971–5.

Sura, W., Murphy, S.O. and Gonzales, I. (2006) 'Level of fatigue in women receiving dose-dense versus standard chemotherapy for breast cancer: a pilot study'. *Oncology Nursing Forum*, 33(5), pp.1015–21.

Tack, B. (1990) 'Fatigue in rheumatoid arthritis: conditions, strategies, and consequences'. *Arthritis Care and Research*, 3(2), pp.65–70.

Wagner, L. and Cella, D. (2004) 'Fatigue and cancer: causes, prevalence and treatment approaches'. *British Journal of Cancer*, 91, pp.822–8.

Wessely, S. (1995) 'The epidemiology of chronic fatigue syndrome'. *Epidemiologic Reviews*, 17(1), pp.139–51.

Winningham, M. (1992) 'The role of exercise in cancer therapy', in Watson, R. and Eisinger, M. (editors) *Exercise and disease*. Boca Raton: CRC Press, pp.63–70.

Winningham, M. (1996) 'Fatigue', in Groenwald, S., Frogge, M., Goodman, M. and Yarbro, C. (editors) *Cancer symptom management*. Boston: Jones and Bartlett, pp.42–59.

Winningham, M., MacVicar, M., Bondoc, M., Anderson, J. and Minton, J. (1989) 'Effect of aerobic exercise on body weight and composition in patients with breast cancer on adjuvant chemotherapy'. *Oncology Nursing Forum*, 16(5), pp.683–9.

Winningham, M., Nail, L.M., Burke, M.B., Brophy, L., Cimprich, B., Jones, L.S., Pickard-Holley, S., Rhodes, V., St Pierre, B., Beck, S., Glass, E.C., Mock, V.L., Mooney, K.H. and Piper, B. (1994) 'Fatigue and the cancer experience: the state of the knowledge'. *Oncology Nursing Forum*, Jan.–Feb., 21(1), pp.23–36.

Yellen, S.B., Cella, D.F., Webster, K., Blendowski, C. and Kaplan, E. (1997) 'Measuring fatigue and other anemia-related symptoms with the functional assessment of cancer therapy (FACT) measurement system'. *Journal of Pain and Symptom Management*, 13(2), pp.63–74.

Chapter 7

Pain

Linda Kerr

INTRODUCTION

Pain has plagued humanity since the beginning of time – it is one of the universal human experiences. Pain probably disables more people than any other symptom. It is an unpleasant physical and emotional experience that disturbs comfort, thought, sleep and normal daily activity.

Twycross and Wilcock (2001) suggest that around one-third of patients with cancer do not experience *severe* pain. Of the two-thirds who do experience severe pain, most (95 per cent) can and should have their pain relieved by conventional therapies, including analgesics and radiotherapy. Similarly, we believe that most patients, whatever the cause of their pain, can and should have their pain adequately controlled or managed. However, there is evidence of poor pain control in around one-third of patients in general palliative care settings (Addington-Hall and McCarthy, 1995).

One of the most important factors in effective treatment for patients experiencing pain, particularly chronic pain, is that the patient is believed about the nature of their pain (McCaffery, 1980; Seers and Friedli, 1996). However, Seers and Goodman's (1987) research on pain assessment by nurses discovered that they greatly underestimated the pain that patients experienced after surgery. Current anecdotal evidence seems to support this. The importance of being believed is illustrated in the following two extracts, which are taken from a study of patients' experiences of their chronic non-malignant pain (Seers and Friedli, 1996: 1162):

> I had something [chronic pain] that was medically unacceptable. The GP labelled me as neurotic because they couldn't find anything wrong. Their dismissive 'unlistening' attitude to my mysterious pain almost amounts, in my opinion, to mental cruelty.

> Most important thing is someone thinks the pain is not in my head and acknowledges it as real. KF has been the first person I've spoken

to about the pain who hasn't been dismissive. Means the pain is seen as real, when it is acknowledged as such you feel better about it.

Much of the literature available about pain is about physical pain. However, as in the rest of the book, we will be taking a holistic approach to pain, its assessment and management, and we will introduce the concept of 'total pain', which encompasses all areas of patients' lives.

You may find it difficult and challenging to work with patients in pain, particularly those who have chronic non-malignant pain. Remember that the other members of your team can help you with the assessment and management of pain. Your manager and members of your AL set will also be able to offer you support. If terms are used in this chapter with which you are unfamiliar, check the glossary at the end of the book for details.

Preparation

Teamwork and communication are essential aspects of assessing and managing pain. You may find it helpful to read through your work on those topics in Chapter 2 before beginning the pain assessment and pain management parts of this chapter.

For Activities 2 and 10, you will need a copy of:

Fordham, M. and Dunn, V. (1994) *Alongside the person in pain: holistic care and nursing practice*. London: Baillière Tindall. This title is currently out of print, but you may be able to find library copies or second-hand copies.

You can, however, do Activity 2 without a copy, but you will need a copy for Activity 10.

For Activity 6 you will need access to Section 9 of:

Doyle, D., Hanks, G. and MacDonald, N. (editors) (1998) *Oxford textbook of palliative medicine* (2nd Ed.). Oxford: Oxford University Press.

Activity 16 asks you to read the following article:

Livneh, J., Garber, A. and Shaevich, E. (1998) 'Assessment and documentation of pain in oncology patients'. *International Journal of Palliative Nursing*, 4(4), pp.169–75.

Start researching how you can obtain a copy so that you are prepared when you reach the activity.

Activity 18 asks you to try out a selection of pain assessment tools. If you think you might like to use the Brief Pain Inventory (short form) (Figures 7.6 and 7.7), it is a good idea to begin the process of obtaining permission to use it now – it may take a month or more for the copyright holders to respond. If you wish to use the Brief Pain Inventory (short form), you must not adapt it in any way and you must obtain permission from the University of Texas MD Anderson Cancer Center Department of Symptom Research **www.mdanderson.org/departments/PRG** There is a simple permission request form to fill in: **www.mdanderson.org/departments/prg/display.cfm?id = 9FD3C2D8-77B9-11 D5-812C00508B603A14&pn = 0EE78204-6646-11D5-812400508B603A14&method = displayfull** Sites accessed 13/5/08.

For Activity 23, you may find it useful to have a copy of the following document:

Finlay, I.G., Bowdler, J.M. and Tebbit, P. (2000) *Are cancer pain guidelines good enough? Benchmarking review of locally derived guidelines on control of cancer pain.* London: National Council for Hospice and Specialist Palliative Care Services (now the National Council for Palliative Care). You can order it from the National Council's website: **www.ncpc.org.uk/publications/pubs_list2.html** Site accessed 7/7/08.

In the section on the assessment of pain, and in later sections, we often refer to the SIGN Guidelines – *Control of pain in patients with cancer: a national clinical guideline.* These are available free from the website: **www.sign.ac.uk/guidelines/published/index.html** site accessed 13/5/08. We recommend that you obtain a copy of these guidelines, as they are currently (May 2008) the most up-to-date guidelines in this area. Note, however, that they have been under review and will be replaced by revised guidelines. If you visit the website, you will see that the status of the standards is helpfully indicated by an icon (currently 'Recommendations being updated').

This chapter is quite long and contains a lot of complex information. It is therefore divided into two main sections. The first section considers what we mean by pain, possible causes of pain, the nurse's role in working with patients experiencing pain, and the assessment of pain. The second section deals with the management of pain.

LEARNING OUTCOMES

When you have completed this chapter, you will be able to:
- describe the components and complexities of pain;
- outline the possible causes of pain;
- summarise the nurse's role in working with patients experiencing pain;
- list the aspects of the patient's pain experience that should be assessed;
- justify the introduction of a pain assessment process in your workplace;

- summarise the relative merits of the tools that can be used to assess pain in your patients;
- compare the different approaches that can be taken to the management of pain in your practice setting;
- discuss the following aspects of the pharmacological management of pain:
  - the WHO analgesic ladder;
  - the side effects of analgesics;
  - oral and non-oral routes of drug administration;
- outline non-pharmacological methods of managing pain, including medical and complementary approaches;
- critically evaluate how the management of pain can impact on the quality of life of patients receiving palliative care.

SECTION 1: PAIN AND ITS ASSESSMENT

What is pain?

The word 'pain' comes from the Latin word *poena*, which means penalty, implying that it is a punishment of some sort. The International Association for the Study of Pain (IASP) offers the following definition:

> an unpleasant sensory and emotional experience associated with actual or potential tissue damage, or described in terms of such damage.
>
> Merskey and Bogduk (1994: 210)

However, bearing in mind the need of the patient experiencing pain to be believed, and the tendency of some health care professionals to doubt patients' reporting of pain, we favour the following widely-accepted definition:

> Pain is what the experiencing person says it is, existing whenever he says it does.
>
> McCaffery (1972)

Activity 1: What is pain?

Think about the last time you experienced significant pain. Perhaps you sprained your ankle badly or hurt your back by lifting something that was far too heavy. Perhaps you suffer from migraines or some constant nagging pain. Write a description of the incident or injury, together with as detailed a description of the pain as you can manage. Think not only about the physical effect of the pain, but also about what difference it made to your mood.

Feedback

Your own pain experience is unique, as is that of every individual. You may have used words like 'agony' or 'excruciating'. Pains are often described as shooting, stabbing, burning, aching or throbbing. Pain may make you angry if it restricts your movement. Pain may make you depressed and withdrawn if it is excruciating and/or goes on for a long time without relief.

Note that patients may not use the word 'pain' to describe their pain experience. It is important to be aware that words such as discomfort, uncomfortable, sore, hurting and aching may be easier for patients to articulate.

Theories of pain

A knowledge of how physical pain is perceived is essential for the accurate assessment and management of pain. Fordham and Dunn (1994) state that pain research has focused on four theoretical positions, which can be expressed as follows. Pain is experienced as if:

- there is a direct, dedicated nerve 'hot line' from the site of injury to the brain – specificity theory;
- a summation of nerve impulses occurs over time and/or space in non-specific nerves – pattern theories;
- a modifiable open/closed mechanism exists in the nervous system (spinal cord) – gate control theory;
- a continuously active nervous system modifies input and output, reception and response – post gate control theories.

Fordham and Dunn (1994) suggest that these theories reflect a progression in knowledge, and that all have (or have had) partial explanatory value or apply to different pain phenomena. We will look briefly at gate control theory, before asking you to investigate all four theories.

According to gate control theory, the sequence that occurs in neural pathways to produce the sensation of pain is illustrated in Figure 7.1.

Nociception is the detection of noxious stimuli by specialised nerve endings known as nociceptors. We perceive nociceptive pain when nociceptors are stimulated by mechanical, thermal or chemical means. Nerve fibres are classified as A, B or C fibres, with alpha (α), beta (β), gamma (γ) and delta (δ) subcategories.

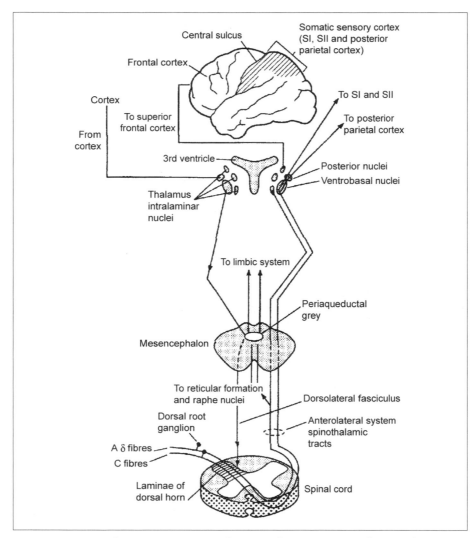

Figure 7.1 Central nervous system, pathways and structures (Fordham and Dunn, 1994: 30). Reprinted from Fordham, M. and Dunn, V. (1994) *Alongside the person in pain: holistic care and nursing practice*, with permission from Elsevier **www.elsivier.com** (site accessed 30/6/08).

Three types of nerve fibre have a role in pain perception:

- A-delta fibres, which respond to pricking, squeezing or pinching and lead to the sharp pain of an injury;
- C fibres, which respond to many noxious stimuli to produce throbbing or more diffuse pain;
- A-beta fibres may inhibit transmission of the painful stimulus to the brain – this is known as gate control.

The pain signal is transferred by the A-delta and C fibres to the dorsal horn of the spinal cord and, from there, via ascending spinal pathways, to the brain. Opioid receptors occur throughout the spinal cord and in many areas of the brain. When opioids combine with opioid receptors they produce analgesic effects.

Descending inhibitory neural pathways from the brain to the spinal cord involve the neurotransmitters serotonin and noradrenaline. This is the probable site of action of many adjuvant analgesics. Adjuvant analgesics are drugs that are not analgesics in their own right but can produce analgesia in certain situations. They are also referred to as secondary analgesics and co-analgesics. We will consider the use of non-opioid, opioid and adjuvant analgesics for pain relief in 'The management of pain' in Section 2 of this chapter.

Activity 2: Pain theories

Find out about the four theories mentioned above:

- specificity theory;
- pattern theories;
- gate control theory;
- post gate control theories.

You may find it helpful to read through pp.27–32 of the following book:

Fordham, M. and Dunn, V. (1994) *Alongside the person in pain: holistic care and nursing practice.* London: Baillière Tindall. This title is currently out of print, but you may be able to find library copies or second-hand copies.

Write brief notes for yourself on each theory and discuss your thoughts with your AL set.

Feedback

As Fordham and Dunn (1994) state, research into theories of pain has led to a greater understanding of the mechanisms of pain and of the therapeutic actions of various drugs. Furthermore, they suggest that the 'pragmatic, humanistic, physically non-invasive and psychosocial actions of patients in pain, nurses, doctors, psychologists and physiotherapists have regained a respectability and validity formerly submerged by the successful but partial view of scientific reductionism' (Fordham and Dunn, 1994: 32).

Fordham and Dunn (1994: 33) also identify the following 'puzzles of pain':

- Some rare individuals fail to feel pain at all.
- Some pathological conditions result in either the loss of the ability to feel pain or enhanced pain, or both, e.g. diabetes.
- Pain can be experienced without any apparent cause.
- Pain can be felt in absent parts of the body, i.e. following amputation.
- Pain can be excruciating when tissue damage is minimal, e.g. ureteric stones.
- Pain can be absent following massive injuries.
- Pain can be felt (in localised places only) at the site of tissue damage.
- Pain can be felt far away from the site of the tissue damage.
- Pain can be felt all over the body.
- Pain can move around the body.

Activity 3: Puzzles of pain

Have you encountered any of these puzzles, either through your own experience or through that of your patients?

Discuss these issues with your colleagues and the members of your AL set.

Feedback

We would suggest that these puzzling occurrences re-enforce the importance of listening to patients, of acknowledging each patient's experience as unique and of acknowledging the pain they tell you they experience, regardless of whether or not you can identify a cause.

Pain tolerance

A patient's pain threshold is the least experience of pain that the patient can recognise. A patient's pain tolerance is the greatest level of pain that the patient is prepared to tolerate. Pain tolerance varies considerably from person to person – what might be bearable to you may be severely painful for someone else. Furthermore, the sensory and emotional experiences will vary from person to person. When assessing and managing pain, it is important to consider both the physical pain and the distress caused by that pain, and to treat each separately where necessary. Pain tolerance is affected by a variety of factors, as illustrated in Figure 7.2.

For example, Tack (1990) suggested that there is a strong relationship between the symptoms of fatigue and pain, as respondents to her interview schedule frequently related fatigue to pain:

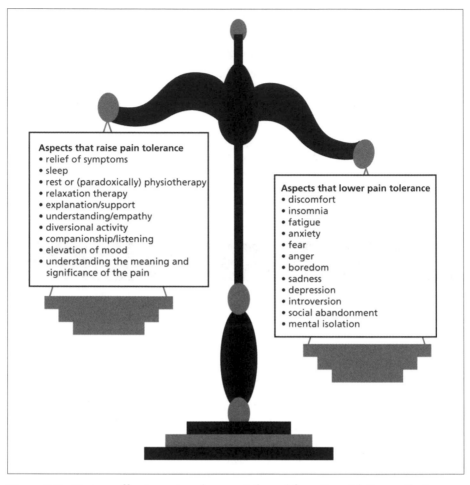

Figure 7.2 Factors affecting pain tolerance (adapted from Scottish Intercollegiate Guidelines Network (SIGN), 2000: 6)

Constant pain is very fatiguing. When I'm fatigued, I can't cope as well with the pain.

Patient, quoted in Tack (1990: 67)

This has been confirmed more recently in a study by Strong *et al.* (2006) looking at fatigue in myeloma patients.

Activity 4: Pain tolerance

Are there any strategies in place in your clinical area for increasing patients' pain tolerance? If so, make notes about them and compare them with our suggestions below. If not, discuss with the other members of your team how suitable strategies might be put into place.

Feedback

Many of the factors that decrease pain tolerance can be reduced if you establish a trusting, therapeutic relationship with the patient. You can provide explanation and support, companionship and a listening ear. By empathising with the patient, you can show that you understand the meaning and significance of the pain to them. We considered the importance of the therapeutic relationship in Chapter 5, 'Breathlessness', as well as the use of relaxation therapy.

Other factors may need particular forms of symptom relief, such as anxiety and depression (see Chapter 4), fatigue (see Chapter 6) and insomnia (see Chapter 4).

It may not be possible to distract patients who are experiencing severe pain, but it is worth at least asking patients if they would be interested in tackling small, interesting tasks. (Some examples of simple craft activities are given in Chapter 4.) Concentrating on something other than the pain may provide temporary distraction. Much will depend, however, on how ill the patients are, on how severe the pain is and on how each patient views the pain – what its meaning and significance is for each individual.

There are many ways of describing pain and many different types of pain. We will look at physical pain next and then go on to look at the concept of 'total pain'.

Physical pain

Physical pain can be divided into two major categories, acute and chronic, and we will start by looking at the differences between acute and chronic pain. We will then go on to consider the three types of physical pain: neuropathic, nociceptive (or somatic) and visceral pain. We will end our look at physical pain with a discussion of breakthrough pain – severe pain that breaks through routine analgesia.

Acute and chronic pain

Table 7.1 illustrates the differences between chronic and acute pain.

Acute pain can usually be resolved by treating the underlying cause or by using analgesics. Chronic pain is more difficult to manage as, often, the underlying cause cannot be treated, as in the cases of incurable cancer and osteoarthritis (in which the pain is referred to as chronic non-cancer pain, CNCP). CNCP is generally defined as pain lasting at least six months or of a duration longer than the expected time for tissue healing or resolution of the underlying disease process, or due to a condition where there is ongoing nociception. Even if the underlying cause cannot be

	Acute	Chronic
Onset	Sudden.	Slow.
Duration	Temporary, may last a few days.	Persists for an indefinite period.
Descriptors used by patients	Sharp, stabbing.	Aching, burning.
Signs of autonomic nervous system stimulation	Yes – patient may sweat and have tachycardia.	No.
Patient becomes	Anxious, afraid.	Withdrawn, depressed.
Examples	Traumatic injury, post-operative pain.	Lower back pain, cancer, arthritis.

Table 7.1 The differences between chronic and acute pain

treated, the pain itself can often be relieved by the use of analgesia. A further complication of chronic pain is that studies have suggested that between 30 per cent and 40 per cent of patients attending pain relief clinics for the treatment of chronic pain are depressed (Kramlinger *et al.*, 1983; Tyrer *et al.*, 1989). (We looked at the management of depression in Chapter 4.) However, more recent evidence still suggests that chronic pain is widely associated with psychological impairment, although training in this area is still variable (Weiner *et al.*, 2005).

However, remember that patients may be suffering more than one pain at a time and more than one type of pain at a time. A further complication is that some doctors make no distinction between acute and chronic pain, categorising both forms simply as 'pain'. However, in the palliative management of pain, it has been found helpful to make this distinction.

Activity 5: Acute or chronic pain?

Quickly look back to Activity 1. Was the pain you described an acute pain or chronic pain?

Review the notes of the patients in your clinical area who are experiencing pain. Is their pain described as acute or chronic? Do you agree with the description in each case? If not, why not?

Feedback

Acute and chronic pain are very different, as shown in Table 7.1, and it should be easy to identify whether a pain is acute or chronic, even where a patient is suffering more than one pain and/or more than one type of pain. The major difference is that chronic pain is not going to go away quickly. This can be a major problem for the patient and for health care professionals. If you believe that a patient's pain has been identified incorrectly, discuss the situation with your manager.

The attitudes of health care professionals, patients and their families towards chronic pain can be a major problem. Treating chronic pain as though it were acute and assuming that it will quickly get better leads to frustration for all involved, as exemplified in these quotes from patients taken from Seers and Friedli's report (1996: 1162–3)

> Can't understand how you can have so much pain and there is nothing they can do. Surely they must be able to find something. Every pain has a foundation. If it is not in my bones, it must be somewhere else. I get angry if they say they don't know. Have they tried everything – must have some idea of what it is.

> The hospital does the operation [laminectomy] and that is that. They don't want to know about the pain: it's not their problem. If they don't know, they don't want to know.

> I hate going to the GP – it's not nice feeling you're the one who got away. They feel useless and it's totally depressing.

Seers and Friedli (1996) suggest that the problem of treating chronic pain as though it were acute was at least partly caused by a lack of ongoing or even basic education of some health professionals in the area of pain management. They go on to cite Illich (1976: 141): 'only pain perceived as curable is intolerable'. So if a patient with chronic pain asks you when they can expect to be cured, it is best to tell them the truth.

Isolation is a crucial factor for patients with chronic pain. Chronic pain is experienced only by the patient, makes normal activities difficult and patients become further isolated due to low self-esteem (Rose, 1992). Morris (1991) describes a lack of cultural understanding of chronic pain – we believe that pain will go away or can be treated (i.e. we want chronic pain to behave like acute pain).

> Friends are amazed I'm no better. They think I should be able to have an operation and be cured from the pain.

> Friends stop phoning and don't come around to see me.
>
> Patients, quoted in Seers and Friedli (1996: 1165)

Social abandonment and isolation are likely to cause a patient's pain tolerance to decrease.

It may be possible to relieve both acute and chronic pain with analgesics but, as we have mentioned, pain is not just a sensory experience, it has an emotional impact too. We will look at this in more detail in 'Total pain'.

Types of physical pain

Neuropathic pain

Neuropathic pain is caused by an injury to the peripheral and/or central nervous system. Pain messages are generated either spontaneously or inappropriately in response to mild stimuli. The pain can be very sudden, intense and short-lived or lingering. Patients feel pain in the periphery of the body and describe the pain as burning, stabbing, shock-like or electrical. Examples include phantom limb pain after amputation, trigeminal neuralgia, pain following nerve trauma, post-herpetic neuralgia and pain due to the invasion of nerve plexuses by cancer. Unrelieved neuropathic pain is severe, unremitting and demoralising and accounts for 34 per cent of cancer-related pains (Ahmedzai, 2000). These conditions pose a major therapeutic challenge as they are unusually resistant to conventional analgesic drugs or neurosurgical measures.

Nociceptive pain

Nociceptive, or somatic, pain is due to the stimulation of the nociceptors in skin, bones, joints and viscera. Examples of nociceptive pain include bone pain and pain in soft-tissue masses, phantom limb pain after amputation, arthritis, fracture and cellulitis. The pain is usually described by patients as aching or throbbing and is generally well localised. Bone tumours and metastases are the most common cause of nociceptive pain in patients with cancer.

Visceral pain

Visceral pain is also due to the stimulation of the nociceptors in skin, bones, joints and viscera. Visceral pain is described by patients as deep and aching, and is often not well localised. Back pain caused by pancreatic cancer, peptic ulcers and mycocardial infarction are examples of visceral pain.

Activity 6: Physical pain

If you are interested in the pathophysiology of pain, read Section 9.2.1 'Pathophysiology of pain in cancer and other terminal diseases' in the following:

Doyle, D., Hanks, G. and MacDonald, N. (editors) (1998) *Oxford textbook of palliative medicine* (2nd Ed.). Oxford: Oxford University Press.

Make notes on what you read and compare them with the notes you made while doing Activity 2.

Feedback

Discuss your findings with members of your AL set.

Breakthrough pain

Breakthrough pain is a severe pain fluctuation that breaks through the analgesia administered for persistent pain. In the case of cancer patients it is defined as 'transient increases in pain in a cancer patient who has stable, persistent pain treated with opioids' (Portenoy and Hagen, 1990). It is experienced by 51–90 per cent of patients with cancer (World Health Organization, 1990 and Portenoy *et al.*, 1999, cited in Anderson, 2000).

Breakthrough pain should not be confused with 'end-of-dose failure', which is the pain a patient experiences when the effects of a regularly scheduled opioid come to an end. This may be because the regularly scheduled opioid analgesics are prescribed in inadequate quantities or because the intervals between administrations are too long. There is ongoing discussion as to whether movement-related pain (or incident pain) is a form of breakthrough pain (Colleau, 1999). There is agreement, however, that breakthrough pain may occur without any apparent cause. Rhiner and Kedziera (1999) state that episodes of breakthrough pain reach a maximum within three minutes and last an average of 30 minutes, and that a patient is unlikely to have more than four episodes a day.

Anderson (2000) describes breakthrough cancer pain as often incapacitating and debilitating, with a significant impact on quality of life. He suggests that patients who experience breakthrough pain are significantly more impaired in ability to function, mood and overall enjoyment of life, are more depressed and have more anxiety and social interference levels than those without it. Anderson cites Mercadante *et al.* (1992) and Bruera *et al.* (1995) in suggesting that patients who experience break-through pain are also more likely to have an overall poor response to opioid therapy.

Total pain

So far we have been considering mostly *physical* pain, but it is important to take a holistic approach when working with patients who are experiencing pain. The concept of total pain was based on observations that an individual's psychological, social, cultural and spiritual situations will affect their responses to physical pain (Figure 7.3). The concept of total pain has developed over many years and has been mainly attributed to the pioneering work of Dame Cicely Saunders, the founder of the modern hospice movement.

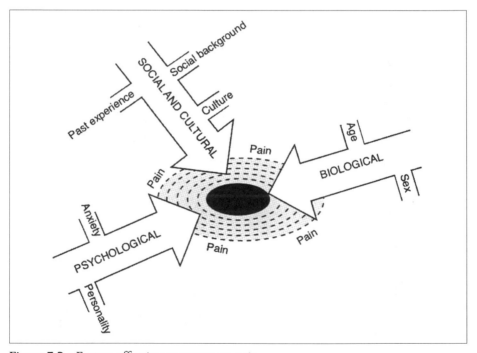

Figure 7.3 Factors affecting responses to pain

Physical pain is only one of the aspects of total pain. Physical pain can be exacerbated by social pain, psychological (or emotional) pain and spiritual pain, and can in turn exacerbate these forms of pain. (List and definitions adapted from Saunders and Baines (1989: 4), quotations from patients from Seers and Friedli (1996: 1164–6).)

Total pain includes:

- physical pain – the primary condition, adverse effects of treatment, other symptoms such as insomnia and chronic fatigue;

  . . . would never have believed you could have so much pain.

- social pain – loss of social position, job prestige and income, loss of role in family, sense of helplessness, disfigurement;

  All this brings loss of mobility, earnings, friends and loss of life.

- psychological pain – anger, caused by delays in diagnosis, unavailable or uncommunicative health care workers, failure of therapy, friends who do not visit; fear of hospital or nursing home; worry over family and finances; damaged body image, self-image, self-esteem, leading to anxiety and depression;

  Pain is warping my mind, it wipes out self-confidence, makes me feel miserable – I'm not me any more.

- spiritual pain – fear of pain and/or death, uncertainty about the future [to which we would add lack of meaning and hopelessness].

  Life is at a standstill and I feel it is finished. Sometimes I wonder if it is worth going on.

Patients may also experience cultural pain if, for example, their pain prevents them from taking part in events that are culturally important to them.

The patient's pain will inevitably affect their relationships with their families and so you need to be aware of the needs of other family members as well as the patient's needs. If relationships within the family are suffering, the anxiety about the situation will affect the patient's pain tolerance.

  Husband too drained to be sympathetic. Children affected by it – don't do things physically with them. They treat me as fragile. I have cheated him of a normal life.
  Patient, quoted in Seers and Friedli (1996: 1164)

Patients may feel guilt because of their pain and its effects on their family and carers. They may be unsympathetic when pain is experienced by other family members. They may feel unable to discuss their pain with their family or carers, because 'we've said it all' or because they feel that family members or carers don't understand their pain.

Note too that the psychological impact of life-threatening pain is greater than for non-malignant chronic pain, because the pain is perceived as a threat. Consequently patients experiencing cancer pain or angina suffer increased levels of anxiety and depression, as well as other psychological problems such as hypochondriasis, somatic focusing and neurotic symptoms.

Your aim is to relieve the patient's pain – their *total pain*, not just their physical pain. Drugs alone cannot control a person's pain. Empathy, understanding, diversion and elevation of mood are among the factors essential to relieve a patient's total pain. Figure 7.4 illustrates factors affecting the individual's responses to pain.

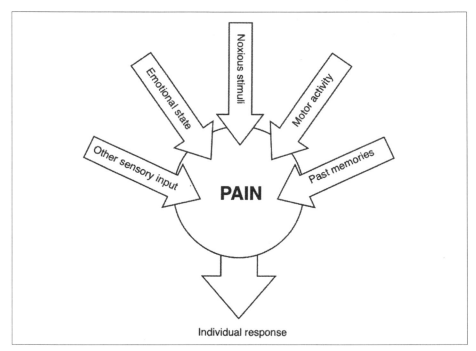

Figure 7.4   Factors affecting the individual's response to pain

Activity 7: Total pain

How do you currently help patients to relieve their total pain? Make brief notes on the strategies you use to help patients with:

• psychological pain;
• social pain;

- cultural pain;
- spiritual pain;
- their families' needs.

Feedback

Psychological pain – you may be able to help patients who are experiencing anger, fear, worry, anxiety or depression by talking to them, and allowing them to talk about how they feel. If you feel you cannot help, you may need to discuss with your team whether the patient should be referred on to a counsellor, psychologist or psychiatrist. This should also be discussed with the patient. If the psychological pain manifests itself as anxiety or depression, you will find Chapter 4 helpful.

Social pain – you may not be able to help with loss of social position, job prestige and income, or the loss of their role in the family. You may, however, be able to help them get over a sense of helplessness by involving them in their pain assessment and management, as we shall discuss later. There are also counselling and behavioural strategies for helping patients to get over the negative emotional impact of disfigurement. Bredin (1999), for example, suggests that a combination of listening to patients and providing therapeutic massage can be valuable in a multidisciplinary approach to preventing and treating distress in women who have had mastectomies. If the patient is having financial or work-related difficulties, assessment by a social worker can be very helpful. If the social pain manifests itself as anxiety or depression, you will find Chapter 4 helpful.

Cultural pain – ask the patient what you can do to help them and do your best to implement any changes they request. You may also find it helpful to discuss the situation with the patient's family, as they may be able to make suggestions of ways in which the patient's situation could be improved.

Spiritual pain – similarly, you may be able to support patients by discussing their fear of pain and/or death, their uncertainty about the future and by helping them find meaning in their experience. Patients with strong religious convictions may find it helpful to talk to another member of their faith. If you work in a hospital, you may be able to arrange for the chaplain to see the patient, if you don't feel confident about dealing with these issues on your own.

Families' needs – you can help by discussing these with the family and the patient, and ensuring that there are frank and open communications between them (while bearing in mind issues of confidentiality). You may be able to suggest other members of the health care team outside your clinical area who may be able to help the family more directly.

The relief of the patient's physical pain may also help with the other forms of pain; reducing these other forms of pain may help reduce the patient's need for drugs to relieve the physical pain.

The causes of physical pain

Patients may experience pain due to a variety of causes, including:

- pain due to the patient's condition or illness (e.g. cancer, rheumatoid or osteo-arthritis, post-herpetic neuralgia, etc.);
- pain due to treatment – surgery, radiotherapy, chemotherapy;
- associated conditions/complications – constipation, infection, pathological fractures, stomatitis;
- unrelated pre-existing conditions.

Activity 8: Causes of pain

What is the most common cause of pain in the patients that you look after? How well is this pain managed? If you think this pain could be managed better, make a list of suggestions for improving pain control.

Feedback

If patients are still complaining of pain, then pain control is clearly ineffective. You may feel that improved staffing and more time for each patient could help. Certain members of staff may believe that pain is inevitable and therefore fail to treat it. You may feel that the cause of the pain has been inadequately assessed. You may believe that not enough is known about the variety of pharmacological and non-pharmacological methods of managing pain. We will look at barriers to effective pain relief in greater depth in 'The management of pain' in Section 2 of this chapter.

The nurse's role

When you did some of the activities in Chapter 2 about what team members think other team members do, you may have found that people think that a nurse's role in pain management is simply to carry out assessments of pain and implement pain relief strategies. While nurses undoubtedly perform these tasks, they perform them in partnership with the patient – an important point that may be missed by others – and they also perform other tasks, many of which are not so easily identifiable (either by others or by nurses themselves).

An important part of working with patients receiving palliative care is the act of 'being with' the patient – the therapeutic relationship – which we looked at in some depth in Chapter 6. Fordham and Dunn (1994: 17) call this sort of relationship 'skilled companionship' and suggest that it is important when caring for those experiencing pain because of the isolation and abandonment that may be part of the experience of pain.

They identify three tasks that make up skilled companionship. The first is entering into the experience and establishing a presence. The goal is to share the same perception of pain, if possible, or at least to reduce the gap between the different perceptions of the patient and the nurse. The second task of skilled companionship is to sustain the connection and this may be easier for nurses than for other members of the team because of the nurse's more sustained contact with the patient. The third task is to help the patient make other connections, by helping the patient connect to (communicate with) other people on the multidisciplinary team who may be helpful.

Activity 9: The nurse's tasks

So far we have mentioned pain assessment and pain management as being part of the nurse's role, as well as the therapeutic relationship (or skilled companionship). What other tasks do you perform in your interactions with patients and other members of the care team in relation to managing pain?

Feedback

As well as assessing and implementing pain management strategies with the patient, you probably also monitor the effects of those strategies and regularly re-assess the patient's condition. You may identify the need for changes to the strategies employed or identify the need for additional strategies. You may therefore influence prescribing decisions and discuss the efficacy and side effects of the pain management strategies with other members of the team, with the aim of implementing the changes or additions to the strategies that you have identified as being necessary. Once you have ensured the implementation of new strategies, you would continue to monitor their effects on the patient's wellbeing, with a view to optimising the patient's quality of life.

In the next activity we will move away from the tasks that nurses perform to look at the roles nurses play in relation to patients, other carers and the environment.

Activity 10: The nurse's role

For this activity you will need the following book:

Fordham, M. and Dunn, V. (1994) *Alongside the person in pain: holistic care and nursing practice.* London: Baillière Tindall. This title is currently out of print, but you may be able to find library copies or second-hand copies.

Read Chapter 8: Role relationships in pain management (pp.125–35).

Discuss the role relationships identified by Fordham and Dunn with the other members of your AL set. Do you agree with their definitions? Are there other nursing roles that you can identify from your own experience? For example, if you or other members of your AL set work with patients living in their own homes, do you feel the roles are much the same as those described by Fordham and Dunn?

Feedback

The role relationships identified by Fordham and Dunn describe those involved in general nursing and, by the environment, they refer mainly to institutional environments such as hospitals and hospices. Specialist nurses and nurses in other environments may take on different roles, which you may have discussed with your AL set, perhaps expanding upon Fordham and Dunn's notes on roles in the community.

During your discussions with your AL set, there was probably general agreement that assessment and management of pain are a large part of the nurse's role. We will look at the assessment of pain in the next section and at the management of pain in the second section of this chapter.

The assessment of pain

The effective treatment of pain is not possible until an accurate assessment has been made. However, pain is extremely difficult to measure objectively as each person perceives, describes and reacts to pain differently. Assessment therefore requires in-depth history taking, accurate measurement and continuous observation (see Chapter 3 for further details). The initial assessment should be used as a baseline for comparison with further assessments, measurements and observations. Furthermore, as a patient may suffer from pain in several different places, due to several different causes, it is essential to accurately assess each pain as the treatment for each may also be different.

As we mentioned at the beginning of this chapter, research found that nurses greatly underestimated the pain that patients experienced after surgery (Seers and Goodman, 1987). In another study, Teske *et al.* (1983) found that, in the majority of cases, even skilled nurses erred in their assessment of pain when assessments were based solely on the nurse's observations. Hawthorn and Redmond (1998) acknowledge that there are many barriers to effective pain management and that poor assessment by the nurse is only one aspect of this – family members, for example, tend to overestimate the pain the patient is in (Elliott *et al.*, 1996). Therefore we would suggest that the person best placed to tell you about the patient's pain is *the patient*.

Ask the patient, not the doctor, where the pain is.

Hindu proverb

Furthermore, Cartmell and Coles (2000) state that a key element of successful pain control is patient empowerment through participation in the decision-making process, which includes ongoing assessment with the involvement of the patient.

As a nurse, you are in a unique position to assess the physical and psychological wellbeing of your patients. However, you must also communicate your findings to others, and assume responsibility for pain relief.

If we develop our skills in assessment and help the patient to communicate, we can fulfil our role as advocate to other team members, be they nursing colleagues or members of other professions. Three conditions are necessary for successful advocacy – firstly, a belief in the patient's communication of his/her pain experience, secondly the sensitivity to recognise pain provoking situations, especially for those who cannot communicate verbally, and thirdly, the fostering of a multi-disciplinary approach which includes the patient.

Fordham (1988)

Although written many years ago, we firmly believe Fordham's suggestions are still applicable to nursing practice in the twenty-first century. In fact, a recent study investigating palliative care in care homes found that the advocacy role was of the utmost importance to professional carers, as it allowed care to be provided in the way the resident wished (Phillips *et al.*, 2006).

By choosing to always believe the patient, you will be able to establish trust and build a therapeutic relationship with the patient. You can then build on your relationship with the patient to proceed with assessment and pain management strategies. This approach will encourage patients to share their experience of pain with you.

You may find this next activity quite emotionally demanding, so make sure you make full use of the support offered by your AL set and facilitator. Read through the activity – it is a role-play – and then discuss any issues that it raises for you with the members of your AL set. Some participants may choose not to do the role-play or may not be able to maintain it for long. When you have completed the role-play, discuss what happened, how you felt and why, with the members of your AL set, or, if you prefer to discuss it on a one-to-one basis, discuss it with your facilitator.

Activity 11: The importance of belief

Think about the pain you described in Activity 1. Imagine telling a colleague about the pain and having them refuse to believe you. You could perhaps show them the bruise or the x-ray – but what if there is no readily apparent cause for your pain, or your pain has been 'cured' – but still remains? How would you feel if people refused to believe that you were in pain?

Set up a series of role-plays (or a role-play with one other colleague, depending on people's availability and interest). Role-plays should consist of a pair of people – one explaining or attempting to prove their pain and the other refusing to accept its existence.

The 'patients' should then discuss among themselves how it makes them feel when the 'nurses' refuse to believe them and then share their feelings with the 'nurses'.

Run the role-play again, but this time the 'nurses' (they need not be the same 'nurses' as before) will be prepared to accept the patient's description of the pain and explain how they intend to help the patient manage the pain.

The 'patients' should then discuss among themselves how it makes them feel when the 'nurses' believe them and then share their feelings with the 'nurses'.

Feedback

You will probably find that having people refuse to believe your description of your pain is incredibly frustrating and makes you angry. Meeting this response continually and for long periods could make you withdrawn and depressed. These factors would reduce your pain tolerance and make your allegedly imaginary pain even greater.

On the other hand, having someone believe you and explain what steps they intend to take to help you is a relief – a huge relief if they are the first person to take you at your word. The consequent lifting of the anxiety and worry related to your pain experience would increase your pain tolerance, and could mean that you would need fewer drugs for pain relief.

Many tools for assessing pain have been devised but Dymock and MacConnachie (2000) suggest that some are complex, extensive and demanding of patient and staff time and therefore unworkable. Furthermore, they point out that pain is very subjective and pain tolerance varies widely between individuals so that it is difficult to uniformly apply good objective criteria in its assessment. Dymock and MacConnachie (2000: 12) recommend that you bear the following important points in mind when assessing pain.

- Believe the patient's reporting of pain. Objective parameters of acute pain such as tachycardia, sweating, pallor or facial grimacing are helpful when present, but are often absent in chronic pain.
- Sit, listen and reassure the patient that their pain can be controlled. Ask and observe. Do not wait for the patient to complain. Remember: patients with chronic pain do not always look as though they are 'in pain'.
- Take a careful pain history, including duration, location and quality. Assess the effect of pain on the patient's mood and how it affects day-to-day activities. Does the pain interfere with sleeping, eating or movement?
- Take a careful analgesic history, including present and past medication, response to analgesic therapy and the occurrence of side effects.

Note, however, that some patients, especially those with advanced cancer, experience pain that cannot be controlled. In this situation you cannot reassure patients that their pain can be controlled but you can assure them that you and your team will do everything possible to help control their pain.

Dymock and MacConnachie (2000: 12) also suggest that the doctor should 'accurately diagnose the cause of pain by (a) complete physical examination, and (b) relevant laboratory and radiological investigations'. You should discuss with the doctor his or her findings as to the cause of the pain, what he or she found on physical examination and what tests have been ordered to help pinpoint the cause.

Activity 12: Assessing pain

Note down how often you assess (and re-assess) patients' pain. (This need only be an estimate.)

Now look back over your patient records or care plans and make notes from them on how often you assess patients' pain.

Now compare your estimated number with the recorded number. If there is a difference, make notes on how you explain it.

What reasons can you think of for assessments not being routinely performed?

What could be done to encourage routine assessment in your workplace?

Feedback

Often there simply isn't time to perform assessments. Sometimes it is seen as being less important than all the other jobs that need to be done or people just forget to do it. People may assume that if the patient isn't complaining there's no problem. (Conversely, if patients frequently request medication, their responses are likely to be recorded more often.) Perhaps a patient is unconscious or semi-comatose, or unable to communicate verbally. Sometimes you may believe that because of the type of medication used, or the patient's diagnosis, it isn't necessary to assess their pain. Studies have also shown that pain assessment is often poor for children, the elderly and the dying (Hawthorn and Redmond, 1998). Discuss with your colleagues the link between infrequent assessment and poorly managed pain. We will look at the introduction of pain assessment procedures in the next activity.

Activity 13: Pain assessment procedures

How is pain assessed in your workplace? Make brief notes of how often pain is assessed, how it is assessed and by whom.

Is there a pain assessment procedure, which outlines how pain should be assessed, how often and by whom?

If not, discuss this with your colleagues. Discuss how such a procedure could be introduced.

Feedback

All members of the health care team (including the patient's family) should be encouraged to record details of the patient's pain management so that the overall picture is recorded.

de Rond *et al.* (2000) recommend that the most effective way of implementing an assessment process is to introduce the regular use of a standard assessment tool together with an education programme. In their pain monitoring programme, de Rond and colleagues introduced a simple tool, the numeric rating scale (which we will look at later), and educated nurses about pain, pain assessment and pain management. They found that the pain monitoring programme focused attention on patients' pain complaints and created a common language between patients and nurses.

One of the most important parts of assessment is communicating your findings to others. For instance, we recommend that when passing information on to the doctor you avoid saying. 'I believe . . .', or 'I feel

. . .', or 'I think . . .'. Give the doctor a detailed description so that he or she has something specific to work with, for example: 'Mrs Scott had her analgesia two hours ago, but she still has hot, burning pain in her left hip, radiating down to the back of her knee. It is more painful on movement and so is affecting her mobility.'

What should be included within assessment?

The first screening assessment of the patient (see Chapter 3) should have supplied you with details of the patient's history, as well as a full holistic assessment of the patient's situation, including physical, social, psychological, spiritual and cultural aspects of the patient's experience and the needs of the patient's family. In your focused assessment, however, you will need more information about the patient's pain than will be covered in the screening assessment. Detailed history taking should elicit the following details (adapted from Scottish Intercollegiate Guidelines Network, 2000: 7):

- site and number of pains;
- intensity/severity of pains;
- radiation of pain;
- timing of pain;
- quality of pain;
- aggravating and relieving factors;
- aetiology of pain;
  - pain caused by underlying disease,
  - pain caused by treatment,
  - pain associated with debility related to the underlying disease,
  - pain unrelated to the underlying disease or its treatment,
- type of pain;
  - somatic [nociceptive],
  - visceral,
  - neuropathic,
  - sympathetically mediated,
  - mixed,
  - anguish,
- analgesic drug history;
- presence of clinically significant psychological disorder, e.g. anxiety and/or depression.

See also *The management of pain in cancer patients: best practice statement* (NHS QIS, 2004) for excellent advice on the components of a pain assessment.

Activity 14: Pain descriptions

Think back to our descriptions of visceral, neuropathic and somatic pain. If you were assessing a patient for the presence of these types of pain, what sorts of words might they use to describe each type of pain?

- Visceral.
- Neuropathic.
- Somatic.

Feedback

Patients often use the following words to describe these types of pain:

- visceral: deep and aching;
- neuropathic: burning, stabbing, shock-like or electrical;
- somatic: aching or throbbing.

Fordham and Dunn (1994) suggest that as well as using specific words to describe pain, patients may gasp, sigh or make other vocalisations. They may speak in a different tone of voice from normal or in a different style from normal – curt or rambling. Some patients may be unable to describe their pain in words but be able to act it out. Others may be able to tell you what they would have to do to you that would make you feel the pain they are experiencing.

Physiological indications of acute pain include increases in heart rate, stroke volume and blood pressure (or decreases in some visceral pains). Other indications include pupil dilation and the patient sweating from the palms of the hands and soles of the feet. Note, however, that people in chronic pain do not have dramatic changes in physiology. Abbey *et al.* (2004: 9) also identify a variety of behavioural expressions of pain, given in Table 7.2.

These indications (verbal, physiological and behavioural) cover mainly the physical effects of pain but it is also important to consider the distress caused by pain. The Scottish Intercollegiate Guidelines Network (2000) states that failure to differentiate between the severity of the pain and the distress caused to the patient may lead to over-sedation of the patient.

Furthermore, it is important that your assessment should be holistic, as we discussed in Chapter 3, to enhance the effectiveness of prescribed analgesics. SIGN suggests that you should assess:

Vocalisation.	Whimpering, groaning, crying.
Body language.	Holding or protecting the part of the body that hurts, fidgeting, rocking.
Behavioural change.	Increased confusion, refusal to eat, alteration to usual patterns.
Physiological change.	Temperature, pulse or blood pressure outside normal limits, perspiring, flushing, pallor.
Physical change.	Skin tears, pressure areas, contractures, previous injury.

Table 7.2 Behavioural expressions of pain (Abbey *et al.*, 2004: 9)

- the physical effects or manifestations of pain;
- the functional effects: interference with the activities of daily living;
- psychosocial factors: level of anxiety, mood, cultural influences, fears, effects on inter-personal relationships, factors affecting pain thresholds (see 'Pain tolerance', earlier in this chapter);
- spiritual aspects: the effects of pain on the patient's sense of the meaning or purpose of life and death; it need not include a religious component.

We suggest that you also assess any cultural pain that the patient may be experiencing and the needs of the patient's family. The holistic aspects should already be covered to some extent in the notes from the screening assessment, but they may not focus on the effects of pain.

Activity 15: Initial assessment

Look through the notes of a couple of patients who are in pain or being treated for pain. Compare the details of their initial focused assessment with the items that we suggest should be included (listed above).

Are the assessments thorough? If not, how can they be made so?

Feedback

We would suggest that the introduction of a pain assessment procedure (see Activity 13) and a standardised assessment tool (see below) will help to make all pain assessments carried out in your clinical area more thorough.

Pain assessment tools

Assessment tools can be invaluable in aiding accurate pain assessment. Because of the subjective nature of pain, only the patient can measure their pain accurately. By providing them with an assessment tool, you are helping them to assess their pain and communicate it to others.

The tools should be simple, efficient and valid assessment instruments that can provide rapid evaluation in clinical settings of the major aspects of pain experienced by patients. They should measure:

- the intensity of the pain;
- relief of pain;
- psychological distress;
- functional impairment.

Pain assessment tools give patients a more active role in dealing with their pain and may also improve your relationship with the patient. Such formal, written documentation has the further advantage of providing proof or evidence of the patient's pain. As we have emphasised, being believed about their pain is essential for patients, who are not always taken at their word. The tools record the patterns of pain and the direction of change of pain (if any).

When used appropriately, assessment tools should also ensure the implementation of the most effective pain management measures and a resultant improvement in the patient's quality of life.

Activity 16: Why assess pain?

Read the following article:

Livneh, J., Garber, A. and Shaevich, E. (1998) 'Assessment and documentation of pain in oncology patients'. *International Journal of Palliative Nursing*, 4(4), pp.169–75.

Make notes on the article, identifying what you feel to be the most important points in the argument for implementing pain assessment procedures and using standard pain assessment tools in your clinical area. Discuss the points you have identified and the points listed below (if not included in your list) with your colleagues.

- Patients who do not report pain are assumed to be pain free.
- The presence of a palliative care trained nurse, responsible for managing the patient's pain and additional symptoms, resulted in patients receiving much better pain relief than those in other areas.
- Where the recording of treatment and relief of pain is inadequate, it is necessary to increase the dosage of pain-relieving medication.

- If medical staff do not continue to prescribe the opioids that the patient was receiving at home, patients will not receive analgesics unless their families bring them in from their home supply.
- In situations where oral opioids are not routinely administered, there may be no tablets available for patients.
- An inaccurate/incorrect pain assessment results in difficulty adapting the treatment to the patient's condition.
- Health professionals rely more on their own expectations and judgement than on what the patient reports; this leads to invalid assessment and a problematic adversarial relationship between the patient and the nurse.
- Even skilled nurses erred in their assessment of pain when assessments were based solely on the nurse's observations.
- The very act of making systematic notes improves the treatment of pain and the treatment of pain bears no relation to the type of tool used in the documentation.
- Documentation is the link between patients and staff, between pain and its treatment, and between various members of staff; it promotes communication between professionals and helps to ensure high-quality care and treatment.

Feedback

These issues, as well as any that are specific to your own workplace, should be enough to convince your colleagues of the need for pain assessment procedures and standard pain assessment tools.

Note, however, that in some instances pain assessment tools may make things worse for the patient by making them focus on their problems. Some specialists in palliative care prefer not to routinely use tools where patients have unresolved or intractable pain, as they serve only as a reminder of the problem to both patients *and* staff. Remember also that patients may be too tired or too ill to complete questionnaires.

However, don't simply start or stop using assessment tools without consulting the patient. Patients may think that you have started the use of tools because their situation is getting worse, or that you have stopped using the tools with them because their situation is hopeless. Good palliative nursing care should allow the patient to assess their problem in such a way as not to cause distress or anxiety. Conversely, no patient should be forced to use a tool against their wishes. You should therefore consider, for each patient, whether the use of assessment tools is of value, rather than use the tools routinely for all patients.

Activity 17: Pain assessment tools

Perform a literature review to identify the available types of pain assessment tool. Include simple tools that measure only pain intensity as well as more complex tools.

Collect copies of any pain assessment tools, e.g. forms, charts, etc. that are used in your workplace. You will need these for Activity 18.

Feedback

We review a selection of pain assessment tools below. We introduced several of these in Chapter 3 and you may find it helpful to look back at that chapter now.

Pain assessment tools which include simple measures of *pain intensity* only include:

- **Visual Analogue Scale (VAS)**
  The patient marks intensity of pain on a horizontal line with 'no pain' at one end and 'severe pain' at the other.
- **Numerical Rating Scale (NRS)**
  The patient rates pain on a vertical scale from 1 to 10. However, some patients are unable to use a numerical scale to rate their pain. The numbers may not make sense to them or they may not be able to apply numbers to their pain experience. In this case, you should use one of the other forms of scale.
- **Likert Scale**
  Subjects are asked to express agreement or disagreement with a set of attitude statements.
- **Verbal Rating Scale (VRS)**
  The patient rates pain verbally, e.g. 'none', 'mild', 'moderate' or 'severe'.

Some versions of these scales have faces drawn on them, which become increasingly unhappy as the pain level increases. This is sometimes referred to as the Wong Baker faces scale (Wong and Baker, 1988) and can be used very successfully with children, people with dementia and those whose literacy is poor.

It can be difficult to assess pain in patients with cognitive impairment. Often these people are unable to verbalise their pain and you would need to assess their pain using the observations given in Table 7.2. Many patients with cognitive impairment can use simple scales such as VAS. Where this is not possible, one of two tools specifically designed to assess pain in people with cognitive impairment should be used:

- the DOLOPLUS 2 scale named after the group who designed it (**www.doloplus.com** site accessed 30/6/08)
- the Abbey pain tool (Abbey *et al.*, 2004).

The Bourbonnais pain ruler is a specialised tool for pain assessment (Figure 7.5). The patient marks intensity of pain on a line with 'no pain' at one end and 'excruciating pain (no control)' at the other, and selects words that describe the pain, such as tender, crushing, squeezing, stabbing, etc. (Bourbonnais, 1981).

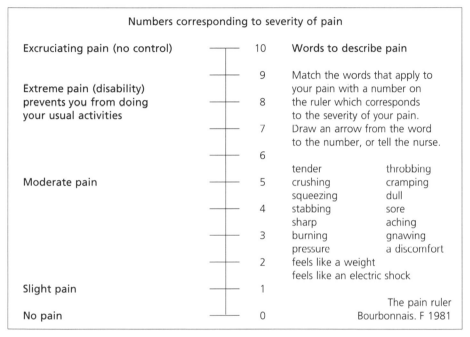

Figure 7.5 The Bourbonnais pain ruler (Bourbonnais, 1981: 279). Reprinted from Bourbonnais, F. (1981) 'Pain assessment: development of a tool for the nurse and the patient'. *Journal of Advanced Nursing*, 6(4), pp.277–82, with permission from Blackwell Publishing Ltd **www.blackwell-synergy. com/loi/JAN** (site accessed 30/6/08).

These simpler tools are used to record the answers when the patient is asked:

- How would you describe your pain now?
- How would you describe your pain at its worst intensity?
- How would you describe your pain at its least intensity?
- How would you describe your pain when it is at an acceptable level?

These scales can be easily completed by patients or by others under the patient's instructions. They provide clear, observable evidence of pain intensity, which can be shared with others. Their repeated use will demonstrate the direction of change of pain, which is crucial for monitoring the effectiveness of analgesia and other interventions.

It doesn't matter which scale is used, as long as it makes sense to the patient, the same scale is used every time and the parameters are specified so that the meaning of the pain rating is clear. For example, 5 on a scale of 0–10 is very different from 5 on a scale of 0–5.

More sophisticated tools include:

- **Memorial Pain Assessment Card** (Fishman *et al.*, 1987)
  A simple, rapidly completed questionnaire that measures intensity, relief of pain and psychological distress. Developed for use in hospitals.
- **Wisconsin Brief Pain Inventory** (Daut *et al.*, 1983)
  Measures intensity and relief of pain, psychological distress and functional impairment. A valid and reliably tested tool used in research studies. An example of the Brief Pain Inventory (short form), which is based on the Wisconsin Brief Pain Inventory, is shown in Figures 7.6 and 7.7.
- **McGill Pain Questionnaire** (Melzack, 1983) and **McGill Home Recording Chart**
  Very detailed and time-consuming to complete but a short form is available. Used in research.

These more complex tools may also assess:

- The location of the pain – by using a body chart on which the patient indicates the location of pain and, possibly, the severity, using different colours. This is also useful when pain exists in more than one place.
- The quality of the pain – by asking:
  'What words would you use to describe your pain?'
  'What would you do to me to have me feel the pain you have?'
  The patient's choice of descriptors is helpful in determining the origin of the pain and in implementing effective measures for its management.
- The onset, duration, variations and rhythms of pain – by asking:
  'How long have you had this pain?'
  'Has the intensity/quality changed since you first noticed it?'
  'Does anything change the nature of the pain, e.g. movement, hobbies, etc.?'
  'Is it better or worse at certain times of the day or night?'
- The patient's manner of expressing pain – by observing facial expressions and body posture. These may be the only indicators available in patients who cannot communicate verbally.
- What helps to relieve the pain and what makes it worse – by identifying all the coping mechanisms that the patient has found

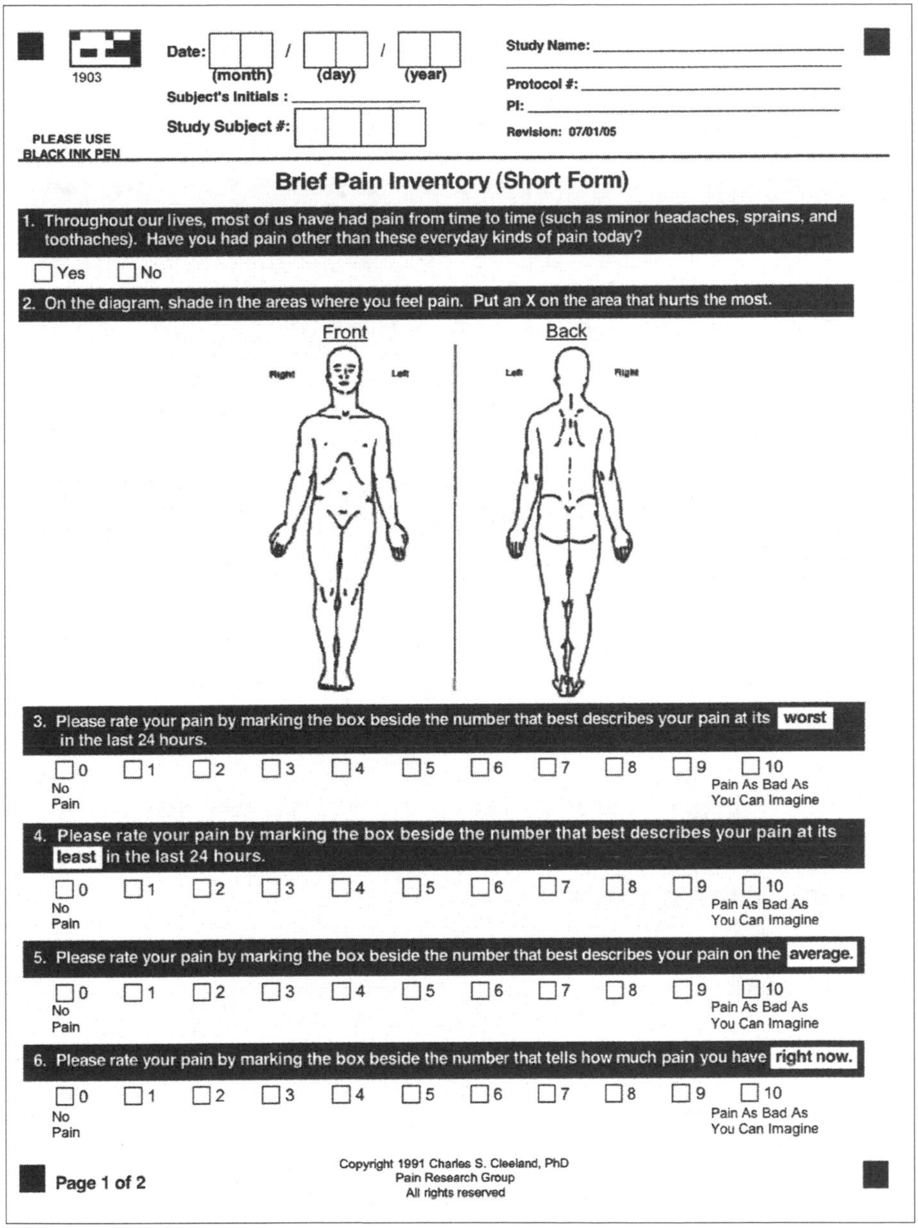

1903

Date: (month) / (day) / (year)

Subject's Initials :

Study Subject #:

PLEASE USE BLACK INK PEN

Study Name:

Protocol #:

PI:

Revision: 07/01/05

Brief Pain Inventory (Short Form)

1. Throughout our lives, most of us have had pain from time to time (such as minor headaches, sprains, and toothaches). Have you had pain other than these everyday kinds of pain today?

☐ Yes ☐ No

2. On the diagram, shade in the areas where you feel pain. Put an X on the area that hurts the most.

3. Please rate your pain by marking the box beside the number that best describes your pain at its **worst** in the last 24 hours.

☐ 0 No Pain ☐ 1 ☐ 2 ☐ 3 ☐ 4 ☐ 5 ☐ 6 ☐ 7 ☐ 8 ☐ 9 ☐ 10 Pain As Bad As You Can Imagine

4. Please rate your pain by marking the box beside the number that best describes your pain at its **least** in the last 24 hours.

☐ 0 No Pain ☐ 1 ☐ 2 ☐ 3 ☐ 4 ☐ 5 ☐ 6 ☐ 7 ☐ 8 ☐ 9 ☐ 10 Pain As Bad As You Can Imagine

5. Please rate your pain by marking the box beside the number that best describes your pain on the **average.**

☐ 0 No Pain ☐ 1 ☐ 2 ☐ 3 ☐ 4 ☐ 5 ☐ 6 ☐ 7 ☐ 8 ☐ 9 ☐ 10 Pain As Bad As You Can Imagine

6. Please rate your pain by marking the box beside the number that tells how much pain you have **right now.**

☐ 0 No Pain ☐ 1 ☐ 2 ☐ 3 ☐ 4 ☐ 5 ☐ 6 ☐ 7 ☐ 8 ☐ 9 ☐ 10 Pain As Bad As You Can Imagine

Page 1 of 2

Figure 7.6 Brief Pain Inventory (Short Form) page 1 (Duat *et al.*, 1983: 202). Copyright Charles S. Cleeland, PhD, Pain Research Group. Used with permission

helpful with a view to adopting them where possible and by identifying factors that make the pain worse and avoiding them.

- The effects of pain on the patient's quality of life, by asking questions about:
  – accompanying symptoms, e.g. nausea;

Figure 7.7 Brief Pain Inventory (Short Form) page 2 (Duat *et al.*, 1983: 202). Copyright Charles S. Cleeland, PhD, Pain Research Group. Used with permission

- sleep: does the pain interfere with sleep, and if so, how? How many hours of sleep does the patient get? Are they woken up by the pain?
- appetite;
- physical activity: is it limited by pain, and if so, how?
- relationships with others: have they changed?
- emotions, e.g. anger, crying;

– concentration;
– any other changes identified by the patient.

For further information on pain assessment tools, see Caraceni *et al.* (2002) for the recommendations of the European Association of Palliative Care (EAPC).

Activity 18: Choosing assessment tools

Look through the tools or charts you collected in Activity 17. Compare your pain assessment tools with the list we have given you (remember that there is an example of a more complex form on the next two pages) and with those you identified in your literature search in Activity 17.

Discuss the pros and cons of the tools you currently use, and other available tools that might be more useful, with your colleagues and with any patients who are interested. Several of the tools can be used for self-reporting, so it's important to have the patient's feedback if possible.

Based on the outcomes of your discussions, choose a tool that can be used within your workplace, bearing in mind the following guidelines (Carroll and Bowsher, 1993):

- Choose a simple tool that is quick and easy to use.
- Use a tool that has been validated and shown to work.
- Adapt existing tools if necessary.
- Ensure that those who are to use the tool understand it.
- Try out a selection of different charts to find which is most suitable.
- Find out from other users what they think – pros and cons.

Feedback

Carroll and Bowsher (1993) also suggest that you make sure that assessment and evaluation are performed regularly and that you act promptly on the results of the assessment. Test your tools in practice to see how effective they are. You might find that you need a complex tool for the initial assessment and further major re-assessments, but that a simple tool like the VAS will provide enough information to maintain effective pain relief from day to day.

When the initial focused assessment is complete, you should agree pain management strategies with the patient. When these strategies are implemented, regular re-evaluation is necessary to check that the pain management strategies are working. The frequency of the re-evaluation will depend on the level of pain control identified by the patient. If the patient is still in pain, it will be necessary to re-evaluate the situation and alter the pain management strategies until the pain is successfully controlled. This may mean re-evaluating the situation every four hours or, perhaps, even every 10–30 minutes if the pain is barely controlled. You should assess the patient's pain before you give them any analgesia and again after having given them analgesia, to find out whether it appears to have been effective. The interval between giving analgesia and checking on its effectiveness will depend upon the type, route and strength of the analgesia given. Once the patient identifies the pain level as being stable and more acceptable, it may be possible to extend the periods between re-evaluations. We will look at pain management strategies in the next section of this chapter, 'The management of pain'.

SECTION 2: THE MANAGEMENT OF PAIN

> To leave a person in avoidable pain and suffering should be regarded as a serious breach of human rights.
>
> Somerville (1995)

Two of the most important aspects of pain management are communication and teamwork. You might like to look through your work on those sections in Chapter 2 before starting work on this section, if you have not already done so. Communicating openly and honestly with the patient and their family and involving the patient and their family in team decisions is vital, although you should always bear patient confidentiality in mind. A particularly important reason for encouraging patients to take an active role in their pain management is that patient involvement improves pain control. A study by de Wit *et al.* (1997) showed that giving cancer patients an active role in their pain management had a beneficial effect on their pain experience. Your patients will therefore need you to give them information and instruction about their pain and the management of their pain, so that they can make informed decisions. For example, if the treatment for the underlying cause of the pain, e.g. surgery, is likely to cause ongoing chronic pain, you should discuss this with the patient *before* the surgery.

The Scottish Intercollegiate Guidelines Network (2000: 48) recommends that patients and their families should have a full explanation of how to take their medication, including the indications for the drug, its name, how often to take it, how to deal with breakthrough and incident pain, and the possible side effects of the drug. Seers and Friedli (1996), however, found that there was sometimes a mismatch between the expectations or perspectives of the patient and those of the doctor:

Not sure what I had done – an epidural and 'something else'. Doctor said, 'I won't tell you since it would mean nothing to you anyway'.

I asked consultant why I had a pain in my leg when it's my back. He said, 'I've explained that to you time and time again'. So I kept my mouth shut. He hadn't told me though.

Patients, quoted in Seers and Friedli (1996: 1163–4)

Activity 19: Keeping patients informed

Before starting this activity, read through the instructions and discuss them with your manager and your team. Identify patients of whom it would be appropriate to ask these questions. Also identify which member of the team is best placed to give the patients any information they request.

How well informed are patients in your area about the medication they are receiving for their pain? Select one or two patients who are known to you who are receiving analgesia, and ask them if they would be prepared to help you with this activity. If they are happy to help you, ask them if they know:

- the indications for the drug(s), i.e. why they are taking it;
- the name(s) of the drug(s);
- how often to take it/them;
- how to deal with breakthrough and incident pain (you may need to explain what you mean by breakthrough and incident pain);
- the possible side effects of the drug(s).

If they don't know all of these things, ask them whether they would like to know and direct them to the person you identified as being the best source of information.

Feedback

The probability is that some patients may not know a great deal about their medication. There may be several reasons for this: they may not have been given adequate information; they may just have too much on their mind; they may be too fearful to ask, given the frequent misconceptions and misunderstandings surrounding analgesics, especially opioids such as morphine (see 'Side effects of analgesics' later in this chapter). They may just not want to know. Some patients who are receiving palliative treatments may be too ill to take in what is happening to them. When and if a given treatment improves a patient's condition, it may be important to go back and talk with them about the medications they are receiving and explain things to them again. If you work in a hospital, you should also make sure that patients who are about to be discharged see the pharmacist before they are discharged. Patients must always be *given the choice to be fully informed about their medication* on a regular basis and it is also important to involve the family, as long as patient confidentiality is not breached. The involvement of the family is especially important if the patient's condition is such that they are unable to make their own choices.

Dymock and MacConnachie (2000: 12–13) suggest that you bear the following important points in mind:

- Treat the pain appropriately *while* completing the diagnostic evaluation.
- Institute appropriate *diagnosis-specific* therapy.
- If analgesics are indicated, use regular and adequate dosage, i.e. titrate dose against individual's pain tolerance. The aim is to prevent recurrence of pain rather than to treat it after it arises and there is *no place* for 'prn' (pro re nata – as required) analgesia, except to cover occasional breakthrough pain. Should this be required often, it is a signal to increase regular analgesia. Refer to the WHO Analgesic Ladder for choice of therapy [see 'Pharmacological methods' later in this chapter].
- Set realistic goals. For example:
  - achieve a pain-free, full night's sleep initially;
  - then maintain pain relief during the following day;
  - lastly, obtain freedom from pain on movement. May be difficult to achieve if there is skeletal instability, soft tissue inflammation or infiltration by tumour.
- Re-evaluate frequently (e.g. daily). Remember that increasing use of 'prn' or breakthrough analgesia indicates a need to revise regular analgesic therapy.

In addition to these points, we recommend that you re-assess the patient *at least daily* and, before increasing the dose of any analgesic, you give serious consideration as to whether it is the most appropriate analgesic for that patient. Note that in Dymock and MacConnachie's realistic goals it may be too much to expect a pain-free, full night's sleep with patients receiving palliative care. It may be more realistic to aim for a better night's sleep and some pain relief. Furthermore, it is implied that you 'maintain pain relief during the following day' while the patient is *at rest*. These goals can only be set with the full involvement and agreement of the patient.

As we mentioned in the section on assessment, when pain management strategies are implemented, regular re-evaluation is necessary to check that they are working. The frequency of the re-evaluation will depend on the level of pain control identified by the patient and the type, strength and route of the analgesia. If the patient is still in pain, it will be necessary to re-evaluate the situation and alter the pain management strategies until the pain is successfully controlled. This may mean re-evaluating the situation every four hours or perhaps even every 10–30 minutes if the pain is barely controlled. Once the patient identifies the pain level as being stable and more acceptable, it may be possible to extend the periods between re-evaluations. Breakthrough or 'prn' analgesia should be available to keep the patient comfortable but should not be relied upon as a way of managing pain. We will look at how you can decide what to do when a patient's pain is not responding to the current pain management strategy later, when we consider the WHO analgesia ladder.

Another way of evaluating pain management is for the patient to keep a diary of how well the pain is being controlled. If the pain management strategies are successful, a record of success may also boost the patient's mood, which will, in turn, increase their pain tolerance. If the patient agrees to share their diary with you, it will also show you whether the pain management strategies are working, so that you can identify whether the doses of any of the patient's drugs should be changed.

When managing pain, you should always try to avoid inflicting unnecessary pain and try to make painful procedures less painful where possible. For example, if patients find injections painful, you could apply EMLA® cream to the skin an hour or so before giving the injection. It numbs the skin so that the patient doesn't feel the needle. Alternatively, rubbing the skin with ice for 10 minutes produces local anaesthesia and can be used as a pre-procedural, short-term, superficial anaesthetic (Fordham and Dunn, 1994). However, before you use ice, you must check that there is no tissue damage to the patient's skin, especially with advancing disease. If there is tissue damage, do not use ice as an anaesthetic.

Activity 20: Making painful procedures less painful

Discuss with your team and members of your AL set what other procedures may be painful, and how those procedures may be made less painful.

Feedback

Other therapeutic activities that result in pain include lumbar puncture or procedures such as a dressing change or lying on a treatment couch for radiotherapy. Patients who are pain-free when at rest may find procedures such as bed baths and mobilisation painful. The pain associated with these activities can be minimised by the simple provision of pre-procedural analgesia (Fordham and Dunn, 1994), such as a subcutaneous injection of morphine 30 minutes before the procedure.

Furthermore, the Nursing and Midwifery Council (NMC) *Code of professional conduct* states that you should:

> ensure that no action or omission on your part, or within your sphere of responsibility, is detrimental to the interests, condition or safety of patients and clients.
>
> NMC (2004a)

This means that if you see someone else on your team causing a patient unnecessary pain, by action or omission, it is your responsibility to ensure that the pain the patient experiences is minimised. It is not enough for practitioners to simply *have* the knowledge and skills to control pain – they must *use* them.

Pain may be managed by pharmacological or non-pharmacological methods, or by a combination – analgesics used together with relaxation therapy, for example. We would suggest that empathy, understanding, diversion and elevation of mood are essential supplements to analgesics. We will go on to look at a range of pharmacological and non-pharmacological methods but we will start this section by looking at barriers to effective pain relief, and asking why, if almost all pain can be controlled, are so many patients still suffering unrelieved pain?

Barriers to effective pain relief

The Scottish Intercollegiate Guidelines Network (2000) identifies the following barriers to effective pain relief:

- the multidimensional, subjective nature of pain;
- lack of clearly defined language of pain;
- anxiety or depression;
- poor communication between patient and health care professional;
  - under-reporting by patient – some patients are reluctant to talk about their pain, or to ask for pain medication,
  - under-assessing by health professionals/carers,
  - language/ethnicity,
  - impaired hearing,
  - reduced cognitive ability,
  - reduced level of consciousness,
- lack of education of health care professionals regarding the mechanisms of pain, pain assessment and pain management;
- inadequate knowledge and inappropriate attitudes among health care professionals, patients and lay carers.

Activity 21: Barriers to pain relief

Discuss with your colleagues the effects on pain relief of the items on the following list:

- a belief that pain is inevitable;
- inaccurate diagnosis of cause;
- lack of understanding of analgesics, e.g. misconceptions and fears regarding opioids such as morphine;
- inadequate use of adjuvant analgesics;
- lack of knowledge of non-oral routes for the administration of analgesics;
- non-use of non-drug measures (i.e. failing to use non-pharmacological interventions);
- chronic pain in elderly people;
- unrealistic goals;
- infrequent review;
- insufficient attention to mood and morale;
- poor communication between professional carers and patients;
- lack of teamwork.

You may find it helpful to read the feedback to this activity during your discussion or to resume your discussion after reading the feedback. The feedback to this activity is quite lengthy because it considers each point in turn. It may help to expand your discussion as it may raise issues that have not been brought up previously.

Feedback

A belief that pain is inevitable leads to failure to treat the patient's pain properly or, in some cases, a failure to treat it at all and this is not acceptable in health care professionals. It should also be refuted if suggested by patients. Almost all pain can be controlled, except for a small but significant population for whom pain cannot be controlled.

Inaccurate diagnosis of cause leads to inappropriate treatment, especially if the patient is suffering from more than one pain. Regular reassessments are vital to ensure that new or recurring causes of pain are not missed.

A lack of understanding of analgesics, e.g. misconceptions and fears regarding opioids such as morphine (addiction, etc.), leads to health care professionals prescribing inappropriately. Analgesics may be too weak, insufficient, infrequent or given too late. The use of opioids is often delayed until the patient is 'really terminal' because of unfounded fears about their use. We will look at the fears about the side effects of analgesics experienced by both patients and practitioners later on. A lack of effective continuous analgesia may lead to reliance on prn (which some nurses consider to mean 'pain relief nil', as it is such an ineffective method of pain control). Another common misunderstanding may occur when acute pain causes a patient's blood pressure to drop and analgesia is withheld for fear of further lowering the blood pressure. But the patient needs analgesia to relieve the pain and raise the blood pressure.

Inadequate use of adjuvant analgesics will prevent patients achieving optimum pain relief. They are particularly important for pains that are relatively unresponsive to opioids and can greatly help conventional analgesics to achieve pain relief. (See the WHO ladder, later in this section, for further information.)

A lack of knowledge of non-oral routes for the administration of analgesics may lead to patients suffering unnecessary discomfort due to the chosen route, i.e. trying to take tablets when it is too painful to swallow or having an unnecessary number of injections. It may lead to ineffective pain control because the route chosen is not the most suitable for the type or quantity of analgesia they need. (See 'Routes for administering analgesics', later in this section.)

Failing to use non-pharmacological interventions will leave those pains that are not responsive to analgesics uncontrolled. Non-drug interventions have an important role to play, particularly nerve blocks and palliative radiotherapy. (See 'Non-pharmacological methods', later in this section.)

There are widely held beliefs that the elderly are less sensitive to pain and that pain is a normal part of ageing and therefore need not be treated, but there is no evidence to support these beliefs. There is, however, evidence that the elderly are more like to develop adverse reactions to pharmacological treatments for pain and that these reactions occur at much lower dosages than those seen in younger patients. However, there are guidelines for the management of the elderly patient that are applicable to all forms of analgesic medication (British National Formulary, 2006; Portenoy and Farkash, 1988, cited in Gagliese and Melzack, 1997). Although practitioners may not think that the elderly will be willing to participate in such treatments, evidence shows that the elderly benefit substantially from psychological treatment methods, including biofeedback and cognitive-behavioural therapy (Gagliese and Melzack, 1997).

Setting unrealistic goals will lead to the patient, their family and the members of the health care team becoming dissatisfied with treatment, if it appears unable to help the patient reach those goals. This may lead to the patient becoming despondent and this lowering of mood will lower their pain tolerance. Setting achievable goals will give the patient something which appears to be possible to aim for and achieving those goals will boost their mood, decreasing their total pain. (Examples of possible goals suggested by Dymock and MacConnachie (2000) are given at the beginning of this section.)

Infrequent review may lead to rejection of treatment and increasing levels of analgesics.

Insufficient attention to mood and morale may lead to mental isolation, social and spiritual problems, anxiety, depression and boredom, which can lower a patient's pain tolerance. Relief from these stresses can raise pain tolerance and can reduce the need for analgesia.

Reasons for poor communication between professional carers and patients include:

- lack of clearly defined language of pain;
- under-reporting by the patient (we looked at reasons why patients might under-report symptoms in Chapter 6, 'Fatigue'. Patients with cancer, for example, tend to under-report pain because they are afraid it means their cancer is spreading);
- under-assessing by health professionals/carers;
- language/ethnicity;
- impaired hearing;
- reduced cognitive ability;
- reduced level of consciousness.

A lack of teamwork may lead to conflicting approaches, unnecessary repetition or gaps in assessment and treatment, an ineffective and unco-ordinated approach to the patient's care. Aspects of the patient's pain will inevitably be missed and pain relief will be inadequate. Teamwork and communication are vital for effective pain control.

Having considered some of the potential barriers to effective pain relief, we will now go on to look at the two main approaches to managing pain – pharmacological and non-pharmacological methods.

Pharmacological methods

Pharmacological approaches have always had a valued place in the history of pain management. The introduction of non-steroidal anti-inflammatory drugs (NSAIDs) and various adjuvant analgesics has expanded the range of available drugs beyond the standard opioids. Furthermore, each member of the health care team has specialised knowledge that, if shared, can enhance the effectiveness of any drug regimen. The nurse's role in pain management includes:

- communicating with/listening to the patient;
- individualising the drug regimen;
- enhancing the action of the drugs;
- minimising the complications;
- monitoring the effects;
- influencing prescribing decisions;
- communicating the monitoring of the therapeutic efficacy and side-effects to the relevant team member;
- ensuring that appropriate adjustments are made.

When managing pain, whether due to cancer or to a chronic non-malignant cause, it is important to know which of the three pharmacological categories it falls into:

- opioid-responsive pain (mainly visceral pain);
- opioid-poorly-responsive pain (mainly nociceptive pain);
- opioid-resistant pain (mainly neuropathic pain).

In this section we will look at topics related to opioid-responsive pain such as the SIGN guidelines for control of pain in patients with cancer, the WHO analgesic ladder and ways in which you can help patients to manage breakthrough pain. We will briefly consider opioid-poorly-responsive pains and opioid-resistant pains, and then we will go on to consider the side effects of analgesics and the various routes of administration for analgesics.

Opioid-responsive pains

These include visceral pain. Patients should be prescribed an opioid, such as morphine, fentanyl, hydromorphone, oxycodone, methadone or tramadol. (See Twycross *et al.*, 1998 or **www.palliativedrugs.com** for information on the relative merits of these opioids. Site accessed 30/6/08.) The basic principles for prescribing in opioid-responsive pains are:

- by the route most feasible and acceptable to the patient (we look at routes of administration later in this section);
- by the clock – not 'as required';
- by the ladder – see the WHO analgesic ladder, below;
- for the individual – accurate assessment of pain followed by regular evaluation of analgesia.

The first, second and fourth principles are equally applicable to prescribing for opioid-resistant and opioid-poorly-responsive pain.

Activity 22: Guidelines for the pharmacological management of pain

What guidelines exist at your workplace for the pharmacological management of pain? Obtain copies of all the relevant systems, processes, etc., or, if you cannot obtain copies, make notes on the contents. Make a list of the titles of all documents, policies, etc.

Feedback

The documents you have identified may range from a simple photocopied sheet with instructions like the four given above the activity, to weighty books full of complicated instructions and calculations. All of them are useful. It's helpful to have the little reminders, but pain control can be very complex and you may find that you often need help, for example when converting from one form of analgesia to another. See Figure 7.8 for an example of changing from fentanyl patches to diamorphine via a syringe driver or pump.

Replacing fentanyl patches with diamorphine via a syringe driver

Remove the patch.

- Calculate the diamorphine dose by dividing the patch strength by two.

- Round this dose up to the most convenient diamorphine ampoule size and infuse the diamorphine over the next 24 hours via a syringe driver.
  e.g. Fentanyl 50 mcg patch/2 = 25 mg diamorphine
  infuse 25 mg diamorphine, via a syringe driver, over the next 24 hours.

- After 24 hours, give the whole of the previous patch strength as mg of diamorphine/24 hours, rounded up to a convenient diamorphine ampoule size.
  e.g. Fentanyl 50 mcg patch/1 = 50 mg diamorphine
  infuse 50 mg diamorphine, via a syringe driver, over the next 24 hours.

Figure 7.8 Replacing fentanyl patches with diamorphine via a syringe driver (based on recommendations from Sir Michael Sobell House, Oxford)

SIGN *guidelines*

The SIGN guidelines for control of pain in patients with cancer (Scottish Intercollegiate Guidelines Network, 2000: 13–15) state:

- The principles of treatment outlined in the WHO Cancer Relief Programme should be followed when treating pain in patients with cancer.
- This treatment strategy should be the standard against which all other treatment for pain in patients with cancer are tested.
- For appropriate use of the WHO analgesic ladder, analgesics should be selected depending upon initial assessment and the dose titrated as a result of ongoing regular assessment of response.
- A patient's treatment should start at the step of the WHO analgesic ladder appropriate for the severity of the pain.
- Prescribing of primary analgesia should always be adjusted as the pain severity alters.
- If the pain severity increases and is not controlled on a given step, move upwards to the next step of the analgesic ladder – do not prescribe another analgesic of the same potency.
- All patients with moderate to severe cancer pain, regardless of aetiology, should receive a trial of opioid analgesia.
- Analgesia for continuous pain should be prescribed on a regular basis not 'as required'.

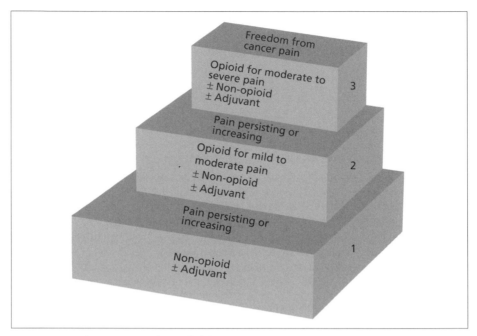

Figure 7.9 The WHO analgesic ladder **www.who.int/cancer/palliative/painladder/en/** (site accessed 7/7/08).

WHO analgesic ladder

The WHO analgesic ladder (Figure 7.9) was developed by the WHO programme for cancer pain relief as the general treatment strategy for cancer pain.

The WHO analgesic ladder is based upon the use of:

- paracetamol, aspirin, NSAIDs;
- weak opioids for moderate pain, e.g. coproxamol, dihydrocodeine;
- strong opioids for severe pain, e.g. morphine, fentanyl, diamorphine.

Step 1 – for persistent mild pain, the patient should be prescribed a non-opioid drug, such as paracetamol, aspirin or an NSAID. These drugs should be taken regularly ('by the clock'), not 'prn'/as required, up to the maximum dosage allowed. If necessary, an adjuvant drug should also be used. Adjuvant analgesics include several types of drugs, such as antidepressants, anticonvulsants and corticosteroids. If this treatment no longer relieves pain, move to Step 2.

Step 2 – for mild to moderate pain, a weak opioid drug should be prescribed. The patient may also take an adjuvant analgesic. Note that although the WHO ladder includes the option of '±non-opioid', there is no definitive information on the efficacy of NSAIDs as adjuvants to opioids (Jenkins and Bruera, 1999). If this treatment no longer relieves pain, or pain is not changed by moving to this step, there is no point in changing to another weak opioid – you should move to Step 3.

Step 3 – for moderate to severe pain, the patient should be prescribed a strong opioid such as morphine. The oral route is the recommended route of administration and should be used wherever possible. However, the route chosen should be that which is most feasible and most acceptable to the patient, e.g. oral, transdermal, subcutaneous, par rectum or spinal. A non-opioid may be given in addition to the strong opioid, if required. The patient may also take an adjuvant analgesic, if required. There is no upper limit to dosages of morphine and the dose should be titrated upwards until the pain is relieved. Where pain is not controlled with high doses of morphine, it may be necessary to try other opioids. One example is methadone, which is a synthetic opioid perhaps best known for its use as the maintenance drug in opioid addiction. It is also very effective at controlling cancer pain, but has a long and unpredictable half-life, which is associated with the risk of delayed toxicity (Manfredi *et al.*, 2001). The list of recommended reading includes three useful articles on managing chronic pain with methadone.

Note that although the WHO ladder refers to cancer pain, its recommendations on the use of opioids and adjuvant analgesics are commonly used for non-cancer chronic pain, including chronic neuropathic pain and osteoarthritis, and the use of opioids has been recommended for rheumatoid arthritis pain (Pal and Amlesh, no date).

Problems with the WHO ladder

If you compare the notes we have made about the steps with those outlined in the original WHO ladder published in 1986, you will find that they are not the same. This is because the steps cannot be set in stone, as new evidence and new drugs are constantly being introduced.

In fact, Ahmedzai (2000) has performed an analysis of the deficiencies of the original WHO ladder. His concerns include the fact that the division of opioids into 'strong' and 'weak' is arbitrary and tramadol, for example, crosses this boundary. The increasing availability of 'strong' opioids in formulations that allow very low dosing has led many experienced practitioners to restrict or even omit the second step, by going straight to a low dose of a 'strong' opioid. Another problem is the WHO emphasis on the oral route, which may not be possible, or may not be what the patient wants – there is no suggestion *of patient choice* in the ladder.

When implementing the WHO (1990) analgesic ladder . . . there are essential important issues for health professionals to take into consideration, which include patient choice, information and making time to allay fears and concerns.

Cartmell and Coles (2000: 37)

Ahmedzai (2000: 821) goes on to identify five further areas lacking in the WHO model.

- Radiotherapy for metastatic bone pain, chemotherapy in lung, colorectal and other solid tumours and hormone manipulation in breast and prostate cancers.
- Internal fixation or hip joint replacement is very effective for relieving pain from long bone metastases.
- Bisphosphonates are a new class of drugs, which are effective in controlling metastatic bone pain and may be further helpful on breast cancer by long-term prevention of bone fractures.
- The judicious use of local anaesthetic or neurolytic nerve blocks can give sufficient pain control to allow the reduction of oral medicine.
- Ketamine is very powerful against hard-to-manage pain (as we mention in 'Managing chronic neuropathic pain'). Methadone has a dual action on opioid and N-methyl-D-aspartate (NMDA) receptors.

All these treatments require consultation with or referral to specialists – surgeons, oncologists, palliative medicine teams or pain clinics.

Activity 23: The WHO ladder

What procedures do you follow when attempting to help a patient in pain? Create your own steps for the WHO ladder, outlining your procedures. You can just write out a list, if you prefer, or you may want to create a flowchart. If you are interested in creating a flowchart (or algorithm), you may find the following document useful:

Finlay, I.G., Bowdler, J.M. and Tebbit, P. (2000) *Are cancer pain guidelines good enough? Benchmarking review of locally derived guidelines on control of cancer pain.* London: National Council for Hospice and Specialist Palliative Care Services (now the National Council for Palliative Care). You can order it from the National Council's website: **www.ncpc.org.uk** (site accessed 30/6/08). It also includes position statements on the WHO ladder.

Feedback

Compare your notes with our notes above the activity. If you have any concerns, consult your manager or members of your AL set.

Managing breakthrough pain

The drugs currently used to manage breakthrough pain are morphine, hydromorphone and oxycodone. They are hydrophilic opioids often referred to as 'fast-acting' but their onset is about 30 minutes (unless given intravenously), by which time the breakthrough episode is likely to be almost over. Rhiner and Kedziera (1999) suggest that the medication used to relieve breakthrough pain should have the same profile as the pain; that is, it should have rapid onset, adequately cover the pain episode and be short in duration. They cite clinical research by the manufacturers of oral transmucosal fentanyl citrate (OTFC) that shows that OTFC produced faster pain relief and overall greater satisfaction than with previous breakthrough medications or placebos. We will look at the oral transmucosal route in more detail later in this section. Other possible methods include rectal preparations of liquid morphine, which can produce analgesia in 10 minutes, the intravenous administration of a bolus, which takes 2–5 minutes for methadone and 15–30 minutes for morphine and hydromorphone (Colleau, 1999), and the subcutaneous administration of opioids. The intravenous route, however, is rarely used in palliative care. The article 'Current thinking in the management of cancer breakthrough pain' (Davies, 2005) gives the most up-to-date advice on managing breakthrough pain.

Activity 24: Managing breakthrough pain

Perform a literature search for pharmacological methods of managing breakthrough pain.

Find out what the latest evidence-based recommendations are.

Feedback

It's likely that the results of your literature search will concur with the advice we have given but it is also possible that newer drugs have been identified.

Opioid-poorly-responsive pains

These include nerve compression pain and bone pain. For nerve compression pain patients should be prescribed a corticosteroid such as dexamethasone. Bone pain may be a new phase of the patient's illness – for example, bony metastases are a common cause of cancer pain. Find out whether there is a pathological fracture or any local tenderness over the affected bone. Investigate whether there is any involvement of the spine. Evidence of this includes back pain or signs of cord compression, such as urinary disturbance, weakness of the leg, leg pain or paraesthesia.

Any diagnosis should be confirmed by taking a plain radiograph of the whole bone involved and by taking a radioisotope scan of the whole skeleton. Any further hidden lesions will also show up on the scan.

For immediate control of pain, use an NSAID. There is a variability in the effectiveness of NSAIDs so if one does not help, it is worth trying another. Other analgesics that may be useful include corticosteroids, calcitonin, bisphosphonates and some radiopharmaceuticals (Doyle *et al.*, 1998).

If bone pain is very severe, consider the use of the parenteral form of the NSAID ketorolac. Because of the danger of gastrointestinal bleeding, this should be given subcutaneously via a syringe driver or infusion pump. Where there is impending spinal cord compression, dexamethasone should be prescribed pending consultation with a radiotherapist, orthopaedic surgeon or neurosurgeon. This consultation is a matter of urgency and should be sought at once. Paraplegia, even in a patient with only weeks to live, is a disaster and should be avoided at all costs. If there is a pathological fracture of a long bone or if there is vertebral involvement, contact the orthopaedic surgeon at once.

In the long term, palliative radiotherapy is the treatment of choice. However, patients should be made aware that the treatment is not expected to prolong life or to cure their illness. It is solely a pain relief measure, although it may improve the structural integrity of the bone in the medium term, with recalcification at the site of the metastases. External beam radiotherapy is the best treatment for localised metastatic bone pain, although radioactive isotopes such as strontium 192 can also be very effective for bone pain secondary to prostate cancer. A single dose seems to be as effective as fractionated treatment and is clearly more convenient for the patient.

Reassess the patient's situation approximately one week after irradiation, although bear in mind that pain relief resulting from the irradiation may not be experienced for up to two weeks after treatment. Consider whether the patient is taking the appropriate NSAIDs in the proper doses to control pain until such time as the palliative radiotherapy takes effect.

Opioid-resistant pains

These include nerve damage pain (burning or stabbing/shooting) and muscle spasm. For burning pains, patients should be prescribed a tricyclic antidepressant such as amitriptyline. For stabbing/shooting pains,

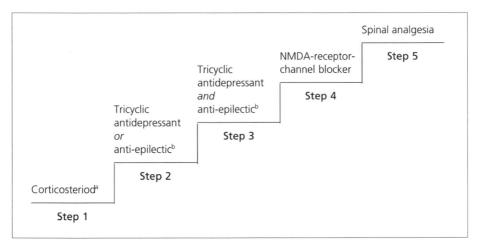

Figure 7.10 Adjuvant analgesics for neuropathic pain. If caused by cancer, use only if pain does not respond to the combined use of an NSAID and a strong opiod (Twycross and Wilcock, 2001: 55, Figure 2.14). Notes on Figure 7.10: [a]a trial of a corticosteriod is important when neuropathic pain is associated with limb weakness; [b]some centres use mexiletine, a local anaesthetic congener and cardiac anti-arrhythmic drug which blocks sodium channels, as an alternative to an anti-epileptic. Reproduced with the kind permission of Robert Twycross and Andrew Wilcock

patients should be prescribed an anticonvulsant such as carbamazapine. For muscle spasm, patients should be prescribed a muscle relaxant such as diazepam.

Twycross and Wilcock (2001) recommend a five-step analgesic ladder (Figure 7.10) as being useful for managing nerve injury pain. It may be used either alone or in conjunction with the WHO analgesic ladder (which we looked at in the section on opioid-responsive pains).

Managing chronic neuropathic pain

Neuropathic pain cannot be managed by conventional analgesics such as aspirin and NSAIDs. It is best managed by other pharmacological classes such as antidepressants, antiepileptics, local anaesthetics and derivatives, opioids, tramadol, capsaicin and NMDA antagonists (Attal, 2000).

In the last 10 years, particular attention has been paid to certain anti-epileptics, specifically gabapentin, lamotrigine and topiramate. Attal (2000) cites two studies by Rowbotham *et al.* (1998) and Backonja *et al.* (1998) as indicating significant, although moderate, overall efficiency for gabapentin. Quality of life and sleep impairment significantly improved and most side effects occurred during titration and were usually mild to moderate, consisting of dizziness and somnolence.

Attal (2000) describes lamotrigine and topiramate as seeming promising but states that their side effect profiles are generally less favourable than that of gabapentin.

Ketamine is an NMDA antagonist, which seems to have an analgesic role linked to an alteration in opioid sensitivity. Care should therefore be taken with opioid doses when ketamine is introduced – it may be necessary to decrease the opioid dosage (Fallon and Welsh, 1996). In specialist palliative care, ketamine infusions have been particularly useful for patients with intractable neuropathic pain, severe nerve pain on movement and those with painful cutaneous lesions (Makin, no date). Broadley *et al.* (1996) state that ketamine is a useful analgesic agent when given orally on a regular basis and that it may be of particular use in pain that is unresponsive to conventional treatments and/or when a syringe driver or pump is inappropriate. Side effects of the sub-anaesthetic use of ketamine include hypertension, hallucinations, confusion, delirium and vivid dreams (Fallon and Welsh, 1996; Mercadente, 1996). Before treating a patient with ketamine, we would recommend that you discuss your intentions with a palliative medicine consultant.

Chronic pain may also be treated by non-pharmacological methods. We will look at these in the next section, 'Non-pharmacological methods'.

Activity 25: Managing chronic neuropathic pain

Perform a literature search for pharmacological methods of managing chronic neuropathic pain. Find out what the latest evidence-based recommendations are.

Make notes on what the procedures for managing chronic neuropathic pain are in your workplace and compare them with the evidence-based guidelines you have found.

If you, or your patients, are interested in the use of cannabis (or cannabinoids) to manage chronic neuropathic pain, see if you can find any evidence supporting its use. Does your workplace have any guidelines covering the use of cannabis?

Feedback

It's likely that the results of your literature search will concur with the advice we have given, but it is also possible that newer drugs have been identified (or that older ones have been re-evaluated, as with ketamine). It is useful to have up-to-date knowledge on the medical advice regarding cannabis, as patients may express an interest in it and you need to know what current advice on its use is. Many organisations support the use of cannabis on a 'named patient' basis.

The following case study illustrates the complexity of pain, especially neuropathic pain, and its treatment.

Case study: The complexity of pain

Mrs Kerr, aged 48, currently has metastatic breast carcinoma with metastatic disease in the right side of her sacrum presenting with local bony pain at the right joint and sacral radicular pain with features of central hyper-excitability.

In 1998 she was diagnosed as having infiltrating ductal carcinoma of her left breast and had a mastectomy, axillary sampling, postoperative radiotherapy and adjuvant chemotherapy. In February 2000 she developed metastatic disease in her right pelvis, which was treated with radiotherapy with complete resolution of her pain. In December 2000 she developed further pain and a biopsy of her sacrum confirmed the presence of metastatic disease. She is currently waiting for further radiotherapy. She has a history of two types of pain:

1. Right sacral iliac pain that is constant and dull, maximally scoring 7 out of 10. It is exacerbated by walking and eased with Oramorph 10mg prn;

2. Right leg pain that radiates from hip to foot posteriorly. It is sharp and severe, maximally scoring 10 out of 10. It is associated with pain/hypersensitivity in her calf when it is touched lightly and her clothes irritate her skin in this area. She also complains of occasional lancinating pain in the right leg. There are no precipitating features and the pain is not improved by the current dose of Oramorph. She finds that the pain is more severe towards early evening. The neuropathic pain has improved since she started using a TENS machine.

She is currently taking Gabapentin 600 mg three times a day, Ibuprofen 400 mg three times a day, MST 30 mg twice a day, Nitrazepam 10 mg at night, and Oramorph 10 mg on average 3–4 times a day.

On examination Mrs Kerr was clearly uncomfortable, particularly when trying to stand up and walk. She is able to walk with no support and there are no focal neurological signs in her lower limbs. There is allodynia of the right calf and foot (S1 distribution). She is markedly tender over the right S1 joint.

Following radiotherapy, the lancinating pain that radiated down her thigh has been much improved. However, the allodynia affecting her lower right leg continues to be a major problem.

Her current drugs have helped her sacral pain, as has her radiotherapy, although they have had no impact on the allodynia affecting her foot. The team discussed various treatment options, including a trial of dexamethasone, a trial of ketamine

> and discussion with anaesthetist colleagues, who felt that a local nerve block may be of benefit. The pros and cons of each option were discussed with Mrs Kerr and it was decided to start with a trial of dexamethasone.

The side effects of analgesics

Health care professionals sometimes do not prescribe adequate analgesia for patients because they over-estimate the side effects of the drugs. There are many, largely unfounded, fears about the use of analgesics, particularly opioids, but we will start by looking at the side effects of non-opioids. Side effects of non-opioids include:

- Paracetamol has minimal toxicity at recommended doses but, at higher doses, can cause fatal hepatotoxicity and renal damage.
- Aspirin may be difficult to tolerate at analgesic doses due to the wide range of side effects, including bleeding and gastric ulceration.
- NSAIDs may cause serious and potentially fatal problems, including renal dysfunction, fluid retention and an increase in blood pressure and death from gastric bleeding. Groups shown to be at most risk of serious gastrointestinal side effects from NSAIDs are those over 60 years old, smokers, those with a previous history of peptic ulcer, those also receiving oral steroids or anticoagulants and those with existing renal disease, cardiac failure or hepatic impairment (Garcia Rodriguez and Jick, 1994). The British National Formulary (2006) also gives guidance on the side effects and contra-indications of NSAIDs.

Opioids have a variety of side effects:

- The majority of patients who take opioids become constipated and a suitable laxative should always be prescribed. Note that fentanyl causes less constipation than morphine (Twycross et al., 1998).
- Patients who haven't taken opioids before may develop nausea and vomiting, which will usually pass within 5–10 days.
- There may also be sedative effects, which will be exacerbated if the patient is taking other sedative drugs or drugs with sedative side effects. These pass in a few days.
- Patients may develop a dry mouth and should be encouraged to take sips of cool water.
- Less common side effects include hypotension, confusion, poor concentration, gastroparesis, urinary hesitancy or retention, itch, respiratory depression and hallucinations.

Patients on opioids for moderate to severe pain should be monitored closely for signs of opioid toxicity. If you realise that a patient is exhibiting opioid toxicity, seek advice from the palliative care team or local specialist palliative care unit. Although opioid toxicity is relatively uncommon, it's important to monitor for the subtle signs of its occurrence, so that you can stop it becoming more serious.

> Opioid toxicity can present as subtle agitation, seeing shadows at the periphery of the visual field, vivid dreams, nightmares, visual and auditory hallucinations, confusion and myoclonic jerks. Agitated confusion may be misinterpreted as uncontrolled pain and further opioids given. The sedated patient may then become dehydrated with resultant renal impairment. . . . The presence of opioid toxicity is an indication that the opioid dose is too high for the patient at this particular time, and it may warn of developing renal dysfunction.
>
> Scottish Intercollegiate Guidelines Network (2000: 25)

Other indicators of opioid toxicity include pinpoint pupils and decreased respiration.

The most common fears about the use of opioids are presented in Table 7.3.

Professional's fears	Patient's fears
Addiction.	Addiction.
Respiratory depression.	Side effects.
Excess sedation.	Impending death.
Confusion.	Tolerance.
	Decreased options for future pain relief.

Table 7.3 Fears about opioid use (Forbes and Faull, 1998: 122)

You can allay the most common of the fears about opioid use by reassuring patients and your colleagues that addiction does not occur when opioids are used for the management of pain. Opioids may cause drowsiness but this usually passes within a few days. Being given opioids does not mean that death is imminent. Starting opioids early does not mean that the dose will steadily increase to a very large dose and that if pain increases there will be no suitable analgesic available. Opioid doses for cancer pain have no standard ceiling, and can always be titrated upwards to relieve the patient's pain.

Patients also often have queries about the effect of analgesics on sex, drinking and driving. Strong analgesics shouldn't affect a patient's sex life. Drinking small amounts of alcohol isn't usually a problem while taking analgesics, but it's worth suggesting that if patients want to drink, they should check with their doctor first. Similarly, patients should check with their doctor whether they are fit to drive. You should point out, however, that should they drive against their doctor's advice, they are not covered by their motor insurance.

Respiratory depression is unusual. Patients who have not used opioids before may develop it if given a large dose for an acute pain. In chronic use, patients rapidly develop a tolerance to it. Patients starting opioids or increasing their dose may experience sedative effects, but these usually pass within 2–3 days. Patients will not become confused and unable to look after themselves. However, the elderly are more sensitive to the effects of morphine and those over 70 years old should be told that they may become muddled at times during the first few days, but they should persevere with the drugs as the effect will pass.

Drug abusers who are given an inadequate dosage of opioids may exhibit 'pseudoaddiction' – drug-seeking behaviour for pain relief – but this can be handled by the prescription of adequate analgesia.

Activity 26: Side effects

Create a side effect fact sheet for display in your workplace.

Identify the non-opioid and opioid drugs that are most commonly used in your workplace. Discuss side effects with the patients and with your colleagues. Make notes of the side effects they ascribe to each drug (regardless of whether they are correct). Perform a literature search for each drug to identify its acknowledged side effects and the means of countering those side effects.

There will probably also be patient information booklets or leaflets, often produced by the pharmaceutical companies, in your workplace. Collect a selection of these and read through their advice to patients. If there don't seem to be any booklets or leaflets in your clinical area, contact the pharmaceutical companies and find out what they can supply. These publications often present information about feared/potential adverse side effects very simply and clearly. The Internet incorporates a great wealth of information but always make sure that it comes from a reliable source.

Draw up a sheet with the following headings:

- drug;
- side effect;
- true/false;
- comment.

For each of the drugs you have selected, give its name; the side effects acknowledged in the literature, any others that have occurred in your experience, and those suggested by the patients and your colleagues. For each side effect, indicate whether the suggestion is true or false; cite (briefly) the evidence that supports that claim, and give brief details of the steps that can be taken to counter the side effects.

It is possible that you may have to have a sheet for each drug and you will certainly have to have more than one sheet in total!

If you have any queries, discuss them with your pharmacist. It may be a good idea to show them your work before you put it on public display.

Place your sheets somewhere where they can easily be consulted by patients and staff. If possible, it would help to laminate them or put them in plastic pockets.

Feedback

This activity will help with some of the points discussed in Activity 19 about the importance of keeping patients informed. It may also allay some of the fears that your colleagues have about the use of opioids. However, it's not enough just to put some sheets of paper up on a noticeboard somewhere. You need to tell patients and your colleagues about it, so that they know where they can consult it. It might be useful to have a smaller version that can be shown to patients who are less mobile.

Opioid rotation

Fallon (1997) defines opioid rotation as a switch from one opioid to another, with the aim of achieving a better balance between analgesia and side effects. To be beneficial, analgesia must be better (or the same) on the 'new' opioid and adverse effects the same (or less).

Fallon (1997) recommends the following approach to deciding whether it is necessary to change from the original opioid (commonly morphine):

- Review the clinical situation and pain syndrome.
- Review the adjuvant analgesics.
- Decrease the opioid dose avoiding sustained release preparations.
- Deal with the altered sensorium secondary to opioid toxicity using haloperidol.
- Correct any contributing abnormal biochemistry (opioid toxic patients simply do not drink enough).

If side effects are severe or pain is still uncontrolled, it may be worth considering an alternative opioid. Fallon (1997) identifies the major disadvantage of opioid rotation as being the fact that the clinician cannot know in advance whether an opioid switch will increase analgesia more than adverse effects. Furthermore, it may be difficult to judge the required dose of the 'new' analgesic. This is particularly problematic when patients are on very high doses. The right dose may be several times less than the clinician might expect.

Activity 27: Opioid rotation

Perform a literature search on the topic of opioid rotation and find out what the latest evidence-based recommendations are.

Feedback

You may find that opioid rotation is a rather controversial topic. Discuss your findings with the members of your AL set.

Routes for administering analgesics

In the normal course of life, most people take analgesics such as paracetamol, aspirin, etc. in tablet form, i.e. using the oral route of administration. However, at least 20 per cent of cancer patients need non-oral analgesia at some time in the course of their disease (Davis, 2000). In the terminal stage of palliative care, many patients may require non-oral administration. We list situations in which the oral route is not feasible below, but remember that patients may *choose* to take analgesics by a route other than the oral route, even when the oral route is feasible. Don't assume that all patients are happy with the oral route – explain that there are other options and find out which each individual patient prefers. Situations when the oral route may not be feasible include:

- decreased consciousness – patients are drowsy, comatose or semi-comatose;
- persistent nausea and vomiting;
- severe dysphagia;
- poor drug absorption when administered orally;
- where patients experience adverse effects after dosing and also experience breakthrough pain before the next dose;
- the requirement for an excessive number of tablets;
- the patient has an intestinal obstruction.

Non-oral routes of administering analgesics include transdermal, subcutaneous, oral transmucosal, par rectal and spinal.

The oral route

This is the most common route for administering opioids, with the exception of fentanyl, which is administered as sustained-release fentanyl patches. The oral route is recommended by WHO (1996, cited in Davies and McVicar, 2000) on the basis of cost and drug availability. It is non-invasive and is also the route that is most familiar to patients.

There are a variety of ways in which drugs that are administered orally can be taken, including:

- in tablet form;
- in liquid form;
- in soluble form;
- short-acting four hourly (e.g. morphine as a syrup);
- controlled-release – every 12 hours or every 24 hours;
- mixed into a drink, jelly or cold custard, with the patient's agreement.

If the oral route is the most feasible, or has been chosen by the patient, consult the patient on which form of oral administration is preferable.

The transdermal route

The principle of transdermal delivery is to apply an adhesive patch containing a concentration of drug sufficient to promote its diffusion into and across the skin (Davies and McVicar, 2000). It is therefore similar to subcutaneous infusion but without the need for an access point, syringe driver or infusion pump. Transdermal fentanyl and buprenorphine are the only opioids currently available for use in patches.

Both drugs are strong opioids delivered via a patch, although buprenorphine doesn't have as wide a therapeutic range as fentanyl. This can be seen in Table 7.4, showing the conversion from oral morphine to buprenorphine. It is recommended that no more than two buprenorphine patches are used at a time. Note also that buprenorphine is only

Buprenorphine (µg/h)	Oral morphine mg/24 hrs
35	30–60
52.5	90
70	120
2 × 70	240

Table 7.4 The conversion from oral morphine to buprenorphine (Cambridge and Huntingdon Palliative Care Group, 2005)

effective up to 240 mg of morphine per day – many patients may need more morphine than this.

Fentanyl may cause less constipation than morphine (Ahmedzai and Brooks, 1997), as may buprenorphine (**www.grunenthal.com**, 2006, site accessed 30/6/08). Both drugs are suitable for long-term use for patients with stable chronic pain. They are not licensed or recommended for acute pain. If you are unfamiliar with these drugs, before you transfer a patient onto the transdermal route, you should refer to the manufacturer's leaflets or seek advice from a pain relief specialist.

When the patch is first applied, the drug is absorbed across the skin's surface. Patients should have regular analgesia for the first 6–12 hours as the onset of action is 6–12 hours. The steady state is reached between 17 and 33 hours. Patients will then need the patch replaced every 72 hours, although some advice suggests that buprenorphine can remain on for 96 hours, so the patch can be changed twice weekly (NAPP, 2006). Check with your pharmacist for the local recommended practice. Always ensure that short-acting morphine is available prn for breakthrough pain in the correct dose.

Patches should be applied to a flat, clean, dry area of hairless skin, on the trunk, back or upper outer arm. Men may need to cut – not shave – body hair. Skin integrity must be preserved. The patches should not be cut. Although patches may be used by patients who have lymphoedema, they should not be used on oedematous limbs.

If it is decided to change to another opioid, the patch should be removed. Note that the drug in the skin will still remain active, delivering a decreasing dose for 24–48 hours. You should re-assess the patient regularly to ensure adequate pain control, bearing in mind the ongoing effect of the patch.

The patches still contain some medication when you remove them. Fold them with the adhesive sides inwards and dispose of them by placing them in a sharps bin (hospital) or dustbin (home). Wash your hands after handling them. Any unused patches should be returned to a pharmacy.

Patients who are in the final phase of a terminal illness may be comatose or semi-comatose and therefore unable to take oral breakthrough medication. You should continue to change the patch every 72 hours (unless there are toxic side effects), but you can also give additional analgesia if the patient is in pain. Table 7.5 gives the recommended doses of subcutaneous diamorphine depending on the strength of the fentanyl patch. No information is currently available (May 2008) on the conver-

Fentanyl patch strength (µg/h)	Four-hourly dose of subcutaneous diamorphine (mg)
12.5	2.5
25	5
50	10
75	15
100	20
150	30
200	40
300	60

Table 7.5 Recommended dose of additional analgesia depending on patch strength (Mersey Palliative Care Audit Group, January 2000)

sion of buprenorphine to diamorphine. If you have any concerns or queries, ask a pharmacist for advice.

If regular subcutaneous diamorphine is required over a 24-hour period, then you can give the equivalent diamorphine dose by a syringe driver or pump over the next 24-hour period. This is given in addition to the fentanyl patch.

The subcutaneous route

Patients who are unable to use the oral route, and who have unstable pain, may require frequent injections. In these situations it is often more convenient to use a syringe driver or infusion pump to administer continuous subcutaneous infusion (CSCI). The syringe driver or pump is a cost-effective method of delivering CSCI. A CSCI provides a safe and effective way of drug administration and can be used to maintain symptom control in patients who are no longer able to take oral medicine (Dickman *et al.*, 2005: v).

Diamorphine is the drug of choice in the UK as it can be dissolved in much smaller volumes than morphine, its onset is faster, its action more intense (if slightly briefer). It is also possible to administer two or more compatible drugs simultaneously and in well-controlled doses, although you will need to check your organisation's guidelines regarding the number and combinations of drugs that can be administered.

Risk management is clearly an issue with these devices, especially as errors (occasionally fatal) are still reported. It is recommended that only one type of driver or pump is used within a health authority/board area. There should also be a clear programme of staff training and education. The syringe and its contents should be checked regularly and these checks should be documented. Dickman *et al.* (2005) provide excellent guidance on the use of CSCI.

Staff should also be aware that certain drugs, although unlicensed for the subcutaneous route, have been used subcutaneously for many years, including:

- cyclizine;
- haloperidol;
- midazolam;
- metoclopramide.

Refer to your organisation's guidelines on the subcutaneous administration of these drugs.

If you are concerned about the use of a drug via an unlicensed route, refer to the NMC's *Guidelines for the administration of medicines* (NMC, 2004b), which state that:

> ... medication which is licensed but used outside its licensed indications may be administered under a patient group direction if such use is exceptional, justified by best practice and the status of the product is clearly described. In addition, you should be satisfied that you have sufficient information to administer the drug safely, and, wherever possible, that there is acceptable evidence for the use of that product for the intended indication.
>
> NMC (2004b: 13)

Activity 28: The subcutaneous route

Are syringe drivers or infusion pumps in use at your workplace? If so, who is responsible for training staff in their use? Find out from your colleagues who use a syringe driver or infusion pump, what training they received and from whom.

Obtain a set of the manufacturer's instructions for the syringe driver or infusion pump at your workplace. There are several types in current use – make sure the instructions you have are the correct ones for the syringe driver or infusion pump you use. Make brief notes on the manufacturer's instructions, recording what you consider to be the key safety points (including, for example, the conversion from the oral to the subcutaneous route and the setting of the rate of drug delivery).

Ask a colleague who is familiar with the use of a syringe driver or infusion pump (or who trains others in their use, if possible) to act as your 'student'. Explain to them how to use the syringe driver or infusion pump, based on your knowledge and experience, and the notes you have made. Ask them for feedback on your performance – do they feel that someone would be able to use a syringe driver or infusion pump safely following training from you?

Feedback

Someone from outside may come in to provide training, e.g. a trainer from the manufacturer, your Macmillan nurse, or someone from a local hospice or local palliative care unit. Someone else on your team, e.g. the district nurse, may be able to provide training. Everyone who uses the syringe driver or infusion pump should have received full training in its use.

In order to prevent mistakes and avoid potential tragedies, it's vital that you know how to use a syringe driver or pump properly, and how to explain its use safely to others.

For details of converting from oral morphine to subcutaneous morphine and back again, see the SIGN Guidelines (Scottish Intercollegiate Guidelines Network, 2000: 27–8) or Dickman *et al.* (2005).

The oral transmucosal route

The oral transmucosal route allows analgesics to move quickly into the body. Oral transmucosal fentanyl citrate (OTFC), a synthetic opioid, has been manufactured as a sweetened lozenge on a handle. When placed against the cheek and allowed to dissolve, a portion of OTFC is rapidly absorbed through the oral mucosa so that it becomes effective in 5–10 minutes (Nugent, 2006).

Rhiner and Kedziera (1999) state that OTFC is indicated 'only for breakthrough cancer pain only in opioid-tolerant cancer patients: those taking, and tolerant to, strong opioids around the clock'. For further information on OTFC, see Rhiner and Kedziera's article and refer to the manufacturer's instructions.

The rectal route

Although the EAPC recommends both rectal and subcutaneous routes for patients unable to take opioids orally, suppositories are not commonly used in the UK. The effectiveness is so similar to that of oral morphine that the same dose can be used. However, conventional immediate-release suppositories must be administered four to six times daily and disintegrate after insertion. Consequently, they are rarely used for the treatment of chronic pain in the UK.

A 24-hour morphine sulphate hydrogel suppository (MSHS) – sometimes also referred to as a morphine hydrogel suppository (MHS) – has been developed (Davis, 2000). The morphine is contained in a ribbed, water-insoluble, hydrogel polymer rod, which in the dehydrated form is firm and rigid. When it is inserted into the rectum it absorbs water, swells and becomes soft and rubbery. It then releases morphine at a constant rate.

The suppository remains intact after insertion and can easily be removed if necessary – at the end of a dosing period or if something adverse occurs. Morphine release stops immediately on its removal. The suppository should be removed after 24 hours, either by natural bowel movement or through insertion of a suppository to aid defecation.

Use of a suppository is not suitable for patients with severe diarrhoea, constipation or anorectal disorders. It is also inappropriate if the patient's morphine requirement is outside the suppository's dosage range, or if frequent changes in the dose of analgesia are required.

Don't assume that patients will not want to use a suppository. Many cancer patients are used to using suppositories to manage constipation or haemorrhoids. In some European countries, suppositories are routinely used in preference to the oral route. A study by Colbert *et al.* (1998) looking at attitudes to suppositories suggested that patients are more tolerant to the idea of using a suppository than doctors. Davis (2000) reports that most patients in her study found the MSHS easy to insert and remove and were unaware of its presence. Further, Davis found that stable pain control was achieved in one day for 95 per cent of patients evaluated and pain control was considered successful in all 26 patients who completed three days of treatment.

The spinal route

This approach can be very useful for a small proportion of patients (Ahmedzai, 2000). It is associated with a reduction in side effects, by avoiding systemic administration, although physical hypotension, urinary retention and severe itching sometimes occur.

Activity 29: Routes for the administration of analgesia

Does your workplace have guidelines for what administration route should be used in a given situation? Is there an acknowledgement of the patient's right to choose the route of analgesia? Do they identify what types of non-oral routes can be used? Do they include patches, syringe drivers or infusion pumps, lozenges and suppositories? If they do not include a particular option, make notes about it, so that you can present a coherent argument for its inclusion.

Discuss the route(s) that is/are excluded with your colleagues, emphasising any important points about effectiveness, safety and any contraindications. Find out how the range of options might be increased to include all available routes.

Feedback

Maximising the number of available routes for analgesia is an important aspect of patient choice and should therefore be taken very seriously.

Activity 30: Patient choices

Before starting this activity, read through the instructions and discuss them with your manager. Together, identify patients of whom it would be appropriate to ask these questions.

How well informed are patients in your area about the routes via which they can take the medication they are receiving for their pain? Select one or two patients who are known to you who are receiving analgesia and ask them if they would be prepared to help you with this activity. If they are happy to help you, ask them what they know about the following:

- the oral route;
- the transdermal route;
- the subcutaneous route;
- the oral transmucosal route;
- the par rectal route;
- the spinal route.

Patients may find it easier to understand what you mean if you say tablets or syrups and liquids, patches, syringe drivers/infusion pumps, lozenges or suppositories.

Find out how they feel about each of the routes, and reflect upon how you would feel in their situation – for example, are you uncomfortable with the thought of suppositories? Find out if they want to change from the route that they are currently using.

Feedback

The probability is that some patients may not know a great deal about their medication routes. There may be several reasons for this: they may not have been given adequate information; they may just have too much on their mind; they may be too fearful to ask. Often patients who are receiving palliative treatments are too ill to take in what is happening to them. Patients must always be *given the choice to be fully informed about their medication* on a regular basis and it is also important to involve the family – especially if the patient's condition is such that they are unable to make their own choices.

Most patients will probably be fairly relaxed about oral, transdermal and oral trans-mucosal routes, although patients may start to dislike the oral route if they regularly have to take large numbers of pills. Patches may be seen as a form of freedom – the patient doesn't have to 'watch the clock' so much or remember to take their tablets everywhere they go. Patients' concerns about the subcutaneous route may include a needle phobia and with syringe drivers or pumps include a fear that the analgesic might run out before the nurse can change it for them. Patients may be embarrassed about the use of suppositories. Discuss with your AL set how you can help allay these concerns or any others raised by your patients.

If the patient or their family chooses to change the route of administration of analgesia, discuss this process with your manager. Ensure that any change of route is in the patient's best interest and not simply for the convenience of others.

Patient choice can have a positive impact upon the patient experience. Patient choice should include the appropriateness of route of administration and acceptability of side-effects, and therefore of the opioid selected. This relies upon patients being partners in their care and having the necessary information in order to make such decisions.

Davies and McVicar (2000: 477)

Non-pharmacological methods

Non-pharmacological methods include medical and complementary approaches, and take a holistic approach, considering the patient's physical, psychological, social, cultural and spiritual distress, and the needs of the patient's family.

Medical non-pharmacological methods

Medical non-pharmacological methods of pain management include radiotherapy, cordotomy and nerve blocks, which we will look at below. Other methods include skeletal stabilisation, surgical interruption of pain pathways, central nervous system stimulation procedures and intraventricular analgesic infusions.

Radiotherapy is a very effective way of controlling pain in the bones. It helps to relieve pain and enables the bone to grow strong again. The dose is usually quite low and often the main side effect is a slight tiredness, although this depends on the site at which the radiotherapy is directed.

If directed at the base of the spine, it can cause diarrhoea, which is unpleasant and exhausting for the patient. Oesophagitis may be a problem after radiotherapy to the lungs. If the patient is experiencing pain at a number of sites, e.g. throughout the pelvis, the use of 'hemibody irradiation' may be recommended. This involves treating the upper or lower half of the body in a single treatment or fraction. Acute side effects such as nausea or diarrhoea are common and the patient should be prescribed medication to prevent or alleviate these side effects.

Cordotomy (an operation on the spinal cord) can provide complete analgesia in about two-thirds of patients (Lahuerta *et al.*, 1994). If a patient has widespread pain, but one location where it is not controlled by simple measures, then cordotomy may be useful in controlling that pain. However, cordotomy affects only one side of the body and a bilateral cordotomy will still not relieve midline pain. Analgesia will still be needed for midline pain after the operation and the pain relief from the cordotomy will last no longer than a year in most patients.

Nerve blocks can be done at specialist pain clinics, which specialise in the treatment of all types of chronic pain. Pain specialists may also visit inpatients to perform nerve blocks. The nerves are blocked to stop them receiving pain messages. This can be done using a long-acting local anaesthetic, heat, cold or certain chemicals. Research suggests that nerve block prior to surgery may prevent the development of persistent pain.

Activity 31: Pain clinics

Find out whether there is a pain clinic in your area. Obtain contact details, opening hours, guidelines for referral and details of what interventions are available. Many pain clinics welcome professional visitors. Make contact with your local pain clinic and arrange to visit. You can find out much useful information from helpful specialists.

Feedback

If there is a central information source (perhaps a folder or a filing cabinet) in your clinical area containing details of external services offering pain relief, make sure that the details of the pain clinic are included in it and are correct.

Complementary therapies

Complementary approaches to pain management are becoming increasingly popular with patients and nurses. When used wisely, in conjunction with other medical treatments, they can be of benefit in coping with stress, promoting wellbeing and reducing symptoms. They appear to be popular because they are regarded as 'holistic', since they have the potential to address a number of differing dimensions of the patient's experience – body, mind and spirit. They also help decrease the sense of powerlessness patients and their families can feel when at the receiving end of medical treatments, by encouraging self-awareness, self-care and the chance to have a more active role in treatment. It would also seem that time spent by a nurse offering a simple massage or relaxation can enhance the therapeutic relationship (Bredin, 1999; Corner *et al.*, 1995) and encourage patients/families to articulate their fears and difficult emotions and find meaning in their suffering.

One of the problems with using complementary therapies is the lack of research studies demonstrating clear benefits to patients and the difficulties of regulating such a vast range of diverse therapies (Pan *et al.*, 2000). However, many forms of complementary medicine are gaining acceptability within the current health care system, and health care practitioners are seeking ways to integrate complementary medicine more fully and effectively (Foundation for Integrated Medicine, 1997). Within the speciality of palliative care, complementary therapies are now offered in many hospices and palliative care units, and most hospitals now have policies regarding their use. As with pharmacological interventions, the main issues to consider are patient safety, ease of use, cost effectiveness and efficacy of treatment. Some examples of complementary therapies are given in Table 7.6.

Complementary therapies for pain management

Acupressure	Meditation
Acupuncture	Music
Aromatherapy	Perfume
Biofeedback	Prayer
Copper	Reflexology
Hypnosis/hypnotherapy	Relaxation
Laying-on of hands	Story-telling
Magnets	Visualisation
Massage	

Table 7.6 Complementary therapies for pain management

The approaches listed in Table 7.6 are included because we know that they have been used and advocated by patients. Their inclusion does not denote general professional acceptance, but you should be aware of the types of therapies that patients may find helpful, or may turn to in desperation to relieve their pain. We discuss some of these therapies in more detail below.

Acupuncture is thought to work by causing the body to release endorphins to control pain. A number of specialist NHS pain clinics offer acupuncture. If you are interested in acupuncture, you may find Section 9.2.8 in Doyle *et al.* (1998) helpful and informative.

Aromatherapy and massage help to manage pain by interrupting the pain signals going to the brain and by helping the muscles to relax.

Biofeedback (Flor *et al.*, 1983, cited in Fordham and Dunn, 1994) is primarily an extension of relaxation, in which the person learns to gain a measure of control over normally unconscious functions, such as reducing muscle tension or increasing alpha brain activity. Visual feedback of physiological parameters is provided by an electronic monitoring machine (e.g. an electromyograph or electroencephalograph).

Hypnotherapy is unlikely to control pain by itself, but self-hypnosis can be a useful part of the relaxation process.

Learning to relax can help patients to forget their fears and anxieties, even if only for a few minutes a day. Relaxation can also reduce muscle tension. We looked at relaxation techniques in Chapter 5, 'Breathlessness'. However, do not assume that relaxation will be useful for every patient. Patients may feel their pain is too bad to be helped by relaxation and it is difficult to relax while you are in pain:

> . . . like putting your hand in the fire and relax at the same time is very difficult . . . your mind is subconsciously divided.
>
> Patient, quoted in Seers and Friedli (1996: 1165)

Visualisation is used in a number of ways, from visualising the pain away (Levine, 1986) to visualising a relaxed and calm situation/environment in order to help shut out the awareness of pain, reduce stress and promote relaxation and wellbeing. There is a useful section ('Distraction techniques') that includes a bit about visualisation in Chapter 5, 'Breathlessness'. Chapter 5 also has a section on complementary therapies in the recommended reading.

Activity 32: Complementary therapies

Make a list of the complementary therapies that you know about.

Contact the individuals, companies and organisations offering complementary therapies and ask for details and research evidence where available.

Look at the literature surrounding the use of complementary medicine and familiarise yourself with the debates regarding safety of treatment and cost effectiveness.

Identify colleagues/practitioners within or outside your place of work who may have training/expertise or an interest in complementary therapies and find out their views.

Talk to patients and find out about their experience – it is likely that some will already have sought out some form of complementary medicine.

Feedback

Many complementary therapies have not been adequately researched, which is unfortunate if it limits their use when they are in fact beneficial. Other therapies are on the fringe of medical respectability, use pseudo-scientific language and tend to be expensive. You should bear these things in mind when treating hard-to-manage pain and giving advice to patients and their families. Just because something is expensive does not mean it is effective. Similarly, just because something is under-researched or inexpensive does not mean that it is ineffective.

We have a responsibility to be as fully informed as possible about the various complementary therapies on offer to patients receiving palliative care. We need to know how these therapies work and what the benefits/side-effects are. In this way we can help patients make informed choices about their care and treatment and hopefully – alongside medical treatments – improve the patient's quality of life.

Other non-pharmacological approaches

Other ways of managing pain include:

- cold;
- cutaneous stimulation;
- diet;
- exercise;
- heat;
- ice (not the same as cold);
- keeping the patient comfortable;
- peer support groups/counselling;
- spiritual support;
- splints;
- transcutaneous electrical nerve stimulation (TENS);
- vibration, e.g. vibrating cushions.

We discuss some of these below.

Cold, although a more effective method of pain management than heat (LaFoy and Geden, 1989, cited in Fordham and Dunn, 1994), is not used as frequently as heat, nor does it have the same connotation of relaxation or comfort (Fordham and Dunn, 1994).

Exercise is an important strategy in the fight against chronic pain (Fordham and Dunn, 1994). As most chronic pain is not a sign of injury, exercise poses no greater risk of damage than to a fit, healthy person. There are such enormous benefits to be gained from exercise that unless movement is medically contraindicated (as in an acute flare-up of arthritis), the risk of experiencing pain because of the exercise is worth taking (Fordham and Dunn, 1994).

Heat has been used to relieve pain for centuries. In a survey of cancer patients to identify non-pharmacological methods of pain relief and their effectiveness, heat methods were used most frequently and helped control pain to some degree in 68 per cent of patients (Barbour *et al.*, 1986, cited in Fordham and Dunn, 1994).

The way a patient sits or lies down can affect their pain. Positions that were comfortable at first may become uncomfortable after 15–20 minutes. Encourage patients to change position frequently (unless they are in a special bed) as they may develop pressure sores, and help them as often as necessary. Find out from the physiotherapist or occupational therapist whether bed cradles are available. They can help keep the weight of the bedclothes off aching bodies and limbs.

Attending peer support groups or visiting a counsellor can help patients by enabling them to talk about worries and fears that they may not feel able to discuss with family and friends. Anxiety and depression can make pain worse and so treating these symptoms can help patients manage their pain better. (See also Chapter 4, 'Anxiety and depression'.)

Patients who know they are unlikely to recover from their illness may suffer considerable spiritual pain, regardless of any religious conviction. Spiritual support may help patients address issues that they feel no other form of support can address.

The aim of TENS is to stimulate the nerves reaching the brain, causing the body to release its own natural analgesics, endorphins. The nerve fibres involved are A-beta and A-delta (see 'Theories of pain' in Section 1 of this chapter). TENS is particularly useful if the pain is confined to specific parts of the body. If you are interested in TENS, you may find Section 9.2.8 in Doyle *et al.* (1998) helpful and informative.

People in pain and those who care for them are . . . rising up in revolt against their passive waiting until a cure appears. One reaction is to search the classical folk remedies abandoned by modern medicine. Another reaction is to demand better day-to-day care of the patient, which is another way of describing control of symptoms, principally pain.

Wall and Jones (1991: 20)

Activity 33: Review activity

Having completed this chapter, reflect on the new knowledge and skills you have gained. You may find it helpful to read through the summary on the next page.

What challenges can you identify in implementing your new knowledge and skills in your day-to-day work with people experiencing pain?

Feedback

Discuss the challenges you have identified with your AL set, your team and your manager. Identify ways of overcoming those challenges.

SUMMARY

In this chapter we have emphasised the importance of believing the patient in pain. We have looked at various different types of pain, including total pain, and investigated why pain should be accurately assessed and how this can be done. We have expressed the belief that almost all pain can be controlled and discussed a variety of pharmacological and non-pharmacological ways of managing pain. Having completed this chapter, you should be able to:

- describe the components and complexities of pain;
- outline the possible causes of pain;
- summarise the nurse's role in working with patients experiencing pain;
- list the aspects of the patient's pain experience that should be assessed;
- justify the introduction of a pain assessment process in your workplace;
- summarise the relative merits of the tools that can be used to assess pain in your patients;
- compare the different approaches that can be taken to the management of pain in your practice setting;
- discuss the following aspects of the pharmacological management of pain;

– the WHO analgesic ladder,
– the side effects of analgesics,
– oral and non-oral routes of drug administration
- outline non-pharmacological methods of managing pain, including medical and complementary approaches;
- critically evaluate how the management of pain can impact on the quality of life of patients receiving palliative care.

USEFUL WEBSITES

www.doloplus.com
Website of the DOLOPLUS study group, from which you can download the DOLOPLUS 2 scale. Site accessed 13/5/08.

www.iasp-pain.org
The International Association for the Study of Pain is an international, multidisciplinary, non-profit professional association dedicated to furthering research on pain and improving the care of patients with pain. Site accessed 13/5/08.

www.nhshealthquality.org
This site offers access to information on the work of the NHS QIS in Scotland, and aims to provide an informative and useful tool for healthcare professionals and the general public. Site accessed 13/5/08.

www.pain.com
This is a worldwide congress on pain. Site accessed 13/5/08.

www.palliativecarescotland.org.uk
Website of the Scottish Partnership for Palliative Care. Site accessed 13/5/08.

www.palliativedrugs.com
Provides 'essential, comprehensive and independent information for health professionals about the use of drugs in palliative care'. Site accessed 13/5/08.

www.pallcare.info
Includes a database of compatibility of drug mixtures used in syringe drivers. Site accessed 13/5/08.

www.sciencedirect.com/pain
This is an online pain journal which will give evidence for current good practice. Site accessed 13/5/08.

www.sign.ac.uk
Homepage of the Scottish Intercollegiate Guidelines Network. Site accessed 13/5/08.

www.stoppain.org
Department of Pain Medicine and Palliative Care at Beth Israel Medical
Center. Site accessed 13/5/08.

RECOMMENDED SOURCES OF INFORMATION

Titles followed by O/P are out of print – but you may be able to find
library copies.

On general pain management

Caraceni, A., Cherney, N., Fasinger, R., Kaasa, S., Poulain, P., Radbruch,
L. and DeConno, F. (2002) 'Pain measurement tools and methods in
clinical research in palliative care: recommendations of an expert
working group of the European Association of Palliative Care'. *Journal
of Pain and Symptom Management*, 23(3), pp.239–55.

Carroll, D. and Bowsher, D. (editors) (1993) *Pain management and
nursing care.* Oxford: Butterworth-Heinemann.

Doyle, D., Hanks, G. and MacDonald, N. (editors) (2005) *Oxford textbook
of palliative medicine* (3rd Ed.). Oxford: Oxford University Press.

Fallon, M., Hanks, G. and Cherny, N. (2006) 'ABC of palliative care:
principles of control of cancer pain'. *British Medical Journal*, 332,
pp.1022–4.

Fordham, M. and Dunn, V. (1994) *Alongside the person in pain: holistic
care and nursing practice.* London: Baillière Tindall. O/P

McCaffery, M. and Beebe, A. (1999) *Pain: clinical manual* (2nd Ed.). St
Louis: Mosby.

NHS Quality Improvement Scotland (2004) *The management of pain in
patients with cancer: best practice.* Edinburgh: NHS Quality Improvement Scotland.

Scottish Intercollegiate Guidelines Network (2000) *Control of pain in
patients with cancer: a national clinical guideline.* Edinburgh: SIGN.

Seymour, J., Clark, D. and Winslow, M. (2005) 'Pain and palliative care:
the emergence of new specialists'. *Journal of Pain and Symptom
Management*, 29(1), pp.2–13.

Simpson, K. and Budd, K. (2000) *Cancer pain management: a comprehensive approach.* Oxford: Oxford University Press.

Wootton, M. (2004) 'Morphine is not the only analgesic in palliative care:
literature review'. *Journal of Advanced Nursing*, 45(5), pp.527–32.

Twycross, R., Wilcock, A. and Thorp, S. (2002) *Palliative care formulary*
(2nd Ed.). Oxford: Radcliffe Medical.

On guidelines on pharmacological interventions

Dickman, A., Schneider, J. and Varga, J. (2005) *The syringe driver* (2nd
Ed.). Oxford: Oxford University Press.

Hanks, G.W., de Conno, F., Cherny, N., Hanna, M., Kalso, E., McQuay, H.J., Mercadente, S., Meynadler, J., Poulain, P., Ripamonti, C., Radbruch, L., Roca i Casas, J., Sawe, J., Twycross, R.G. and Ventafridda, V. (2001) 'Expert working group of the research network of the European Association of Palliative Care, Morphine and alternative opioids in cancer pain: the EAPC recommendations'. *British Journal of Cancer*, 84(5), pp.587–93

Finlay, I.G., Bowdler, J.M. and Tebbit, P. (2000) *Are cancer pain guidelines good enough? Benchmarking review of locally derived guidelines on control of cancer pain.* London: National Council for Hospice and Specialist Palliative Care Services (now the National Council for Palliative Care). You can order it from the National Council's website: **www.ncpc.org.uk/publications/pubs_list2.html** Site accessed 30/6/08.

On the use of methadone in managing pain

Jamison, R.N., Kauffman, J. and Katz, N.P. (2000) 'Characteristics of methadone maintenance patients with chronic pain'. *Journal of Pain and Symptom Management*, 19(1), pp.53–62.

Makin, M.K. and Morley, J.S. (2000) 'Subcutaneous methadone in terminally-ill patients (letter by Mathew, P., and authors' response)'. *Journal of Pain and Symptom Management*, 19(4), pp.237–8

Manfredi, P.L., Gonzales, G.R., Cheville, A.L., Kornick, C. and Payne, R. (2001) 'Methadone analgesia in cancer pain patients on chronic methadone maintenance therapy'. *Journal of Pain and Symptom Management*, 21(2), pp.169–74.

REFERENCES

Abbey, J., Piller, N., De Bellis, A., Esterman, A., Parkes, D., Giles, L. and Lowcay, B. (2004) 'The Abbey pain scale: a 1 minute numerical indicator for people with end stage dementia'. *International Journal of Palliative Nursing*, 10(1), pp.6–13.

Addington-Hall, J. and McCarthy, M. (1995) 'Dying from cancer: results of a national population-based investigation'. *Palliative Medicine*, 9(4), pp.295–305.

Ahmedzai, S. (2000) 'Can we finally get it right with cancer pain control?' *Hospital Medicine*, 61(12), pp.820–1.

Ahmedzai, S. and Brooks, D. (1997) 'Transdermal fentanyl versus sustained-release oral morphine in cancer pain: preference, efficacy and quality of life'. *Journal of Pain Symptom Management*, 13(5), pp.254–61.

Anderson, S. (2000) 'Breakthrough cancer pain: definition and characteristics', in *A breakthrough in breakthrough pain?* Symposium at the 11th International Conference on Cancer Nursing, Oslo, Norway, 1 August (unpublished work).

Attal, N. (2000) 'Chronic neuropathic pain: mechanisms and treatment'. *Clinical Journal of Pain*, 16(3 Supplement), pp.S118–S130.

Backonja, M., Beydoun, A., Edwards, K.R., Schwartz, S.L., Fonseco, V., Hes, M., LaMoreaux, L. and Garofolo, E. (1998) 'Gabapentin for the symptomatic treatment of painful neuropathy in patients with diabetes mellitus: a randomized controlled trial'. *Journal of the American Medical Association*, 280(21), pp.1831–6.

Barbour, L.A., McGuire, D.A. and Kirchhoff, K.T. (1986) 'Nonanalgesic methods of pain control used by cancer outpatients'. *Oncology Nursing Forum*, 13(6), pp.56–60.

Bourbonnais, F. (1981) 'Pain assessment: development of a tool for the nurse and the patient'. *Journal of Advanced Nursing*, 6(4), pp.277–82.

Bredin, M. (1999) 'Mastectomy, body image and therapeutic massage; a qualitative study of women's experience'. *Journal of Advanced Nursing*, 29(5), pp.1113–20.

British National Formulary (2006) BNF No 51, BMJ Publishing. **www.bnf.org** (site accessed 13/5/08).

Broadley, K.E., Kurowska, A. and Tookman, A. (1996) 'Ketamine injection used orally'. *Palliative Medicine*, 10(3), pp.247–50.

Bruera, E., Schoeller, T., Wenk, R., MacEachern, T., Marcelino, S., Hanson, J. and Suarez-Almazor, M. (1995) 'A prospective multicenter assessment of the Edmonton staging system for cancer pain'. *Journal of Pain Symptom Management*, 10(5), pp.348–55.

Cambridge and Huntingdon Palliative Care Group (2005) 'Factsheet 5: guidelines for the use of transdermal opioids – fentanyl and buprenorphine "patches"'. **www.arthurrankhouse.nhs.uk** (site accessed 13/5/08).

Caraceni, A., Cherny, N., Fainsinger, R., Kaasa, S., Poulain, P., Radbruch, L. and de Conno, F. (2002) 'Pain measurement tools and methods in clinical research in palliative care – recommendations of an Expert Working Group of the European Association of Palliative Care'. *Journal of Pain and Symptom Management*, 23(3), pp.239–55.

Carroll, D. and Bowsher, D. (editors) (1993) *Pain management and nursing care*. Oxford: Butterworth-Heinemann.

Cartmell, R. and Coles, A. (2000) 'Informed choice in cancer pain: empowering the patient'. *British Journal of Community Nursing*, 5(11), pp.560–4.

Colbert, S.A., O'Hanlon, D., McAnena, O. and Flynn, N. (1998) 'The attitudes of patients and health care personnel to rectal drug administration following day case surgery'. *European Journal of Anaesthesiology*, 15(4), pp.422–6.

Colleau, S.M. (1999) 'The significance of breakthrough pain in cancer'. *Cancer Pain Release*, 12(4), pp.1–4.

Corner, J., Cawley, N. and Hildebrand, S. (1995) 'An evaluation of the use of massage with addition of essential oils on the well-being of cancer patients'. London: Centre for Cancer and Palliative Care Studies, Institute of Cancer Research (unpublished work).

Daut, R.L., Cleeland, C.S. and Flanery, R.C. (1983) 'Development of the Wisconsin Brief Pain Questionnaire to assess pain in cancer and other diseases'. *Pain*, 17(2), pp.197–210.

Davies, A. (2005) 'Current thinking in the management of breakthrough cancer pain'. *European Journal of Palliative Care*, Supplement 4–6.

Davies, J. and McVicar, A. (2000) 'Balancing efficiency, cost-effectiveness and patient choice in opioid selection'. *International Journal of Palliative Nursing*, 6(10), pp.470–8.

Davis, C. (2000) 'A new 24-hour morphine hydrogel suppository'. *European Journal of Palliative Care*, 7(5), pp.165–7.

de Rond, M.E., de Wit, R., van Dam, F.S. and Muller, M.J. (2000) 'A pain monitoring programme for nurses: effects on communication, assessment and documentation of patients' pain'. *Journal of Pain and Symptom Management*, 20(6), pp.424–39.

de Wit, R., van Dam, F., Zandbelt, L., van Buuren, A., van der Heijden, K., Leenhouts, G. and Loonstra, S. (1997) 'A pain education program for chronic cancer pain patients: follow-up results from a randomized controlled trial'. *Pain*, 73(1), pp.55–69.

Dickman, A., Schneider, J. and Varga, J. (2005) *The syringe driver* (2nd Ed.). Oxford: Oxford University Press.

Doyle, D., Hanks, G. and MacDonald, N. (editors) (1998) *Oxford textbook of palliative medicine* (2nd Ed.). Oxford: Oxford University Press.

Dymock, B. and MacConnachie, A. (2000) *Relief of pain and related symptoms: the role of drug therapy* (3rd Ed.). Edinburgh: Scottish Partnership for Palliative Care. (Available from SPPC, 1A Cambridge Street, Edinburgh EH1 2DY.)

Elliott, B.A., Elliott, T.E., Murray, D.M., Braun, B.L. and Johnson, K.M. (1996) 'Patients and family members: the role of knowledge and attitudes in cancer pain'. *Journal of Pain Symptom Management*, 12(4), pp.209–20.

Fallon, M. (1997) 'Opioid rotation: does it have a role?' *Palliative Medicine*, 11(3), pp.177–8.

Fallon, M.T. and Welsh, J. (1996) 'The role of ketamine in pain control'. *European Journal of Palliative Care*, 3(4), pp.143–6.

Finlay, I.G., Bowdler, J.M. and Tebbit, P. (2000) *Are cancer pain guidelines good enough? Benchmarking review of locally derived guidelines on control of cancer pain*. London: National Council for Hospice and Specialist Palliative Care Services (now the National Council for Palliative Care). You can order it from the National Council's website: **www.ncpc.org.uk/publications/pubs_list2.html** (site accessed 13/5/08).

Fishman, B., Pasternak, S., Wallenstein, S.L., Houde, R.W., Holland, J.C. and Foley, K.M. (1987) 'The Memorial Pain Assessment Card: a valid instrument for the evaluation of cancer pain'. *Cancer*, 60(5), pp.1151–8.

Flor, H., Haag, G., Turk, D.C. and Koehler, H. (1983) 'Efficacy of EMG biofeedback, pseudotherapy, and conventional medical treatment for chronic rheumatic back pain'. *Pain*, 17(1), pp.21–31.

Forbes, K. and Faull, C. (1998) 'The principles of pain management', in Faull, C., Carter, Y. and Woof, R. (editors) *Handbook of palliative care*. Oxford: Blackwell Science, pp.99–133.

Fordham, M. (1988) 'Pain', in Wilson-Barnett, J. (editor) *Patient problems: a research base for nursing care*. London: Scutari, pp.119–47.

Fordham, M. and Dunn, V. (1994) *Alongside the person in pain: holistic care and nursing practice*. London: Baillière Tindall.

Foundation for Integrated Medicine (1997) *Integrated health care: a way forward for the next five years?* London: Royal Society of Medicine.

Gagliese, L. and Melzack, R. (1997) 'Chronic pain in elderly people'. *Pain*, 70(1), pp.3–14.

Garcia Rodriguez, L.A. and Jick, H. (1994) 'Risk of upper gastrointestinal bleeding and perforation associated with individual non-steroidal anti-inflammatory drugs'. *Lancet*, 343, 26 March, pp.769–72.

Hawthorn, J. and Redmond, K. (1998) *Pain: causes and management*. Malden, MA: Blackwell Science.

Illich, I. (1976) *Limits to medicine*. London: Boyars.

Jenkins, C.A. and Bruera, E. (1999) 'Nonsteroidal anti-inflammatory drugs as adjuvant analgesics in cancer patients'. *Palliative Medicine*, 13(3), pp.183–96.

Kramlinger, K.G., Swanson, D.W. and Maruta, T. (1983) 'Are patients with chronic pain depressed?' *American Journal of Psychiatry*, 140(6), pp.747–9.

LaFoy, J. and Geden, E.A. (1989) 'Postepisiotomy pain: warm versus cold sitz bath'. *Journal of Obstetrics, Gynaecological and Neonatal Nursing*, 18(5), pp.399–403.

Lahuerta, J., Bowsher, D., Lipton, S. and Buxton, P.H. (1994) 'Percutaneous cervical cordotomy: a review of 181 operations on 146 patients with a study on the location of "pain fibers" in the C-2 spinal cord segment of 29 cases'. *Journal of Neurosurgery*, 80(6), pp.975–85.

Levine, S. (1986) *Who dies?* Bath: Gateway.

Livneh, J., Garber, A. and Shaevich, E. (1998) 'Assessment and documentation of pain in oncology patients'. *International Journal of Palliative Nursing*, 4(4), pp.169–75.

Makin, W. (no date) 'Christie Hospital NHS Trust: Information on the use of ketamine infusions in intractable cancer pain'. Manchester: Christie Hospital Specialist Palliative Care Support Team (unpublished work).

Manfredi, P.L., Gonzales, G.R., Cheville, A.L., Kornick, C. and Payne, R. (2001) 'Methadone analgesia in cancer pain patients on chronic methadone maintenance therapy'. *Journal of Pain and Symptom Management*, 21(2), pp.169–74.

McCaffery, M. (1972) *Nursing management of the patient in pain*. Philadelphia: Lippincott.

McCaffery, M. (1980) *Nursing management of the patient with pain* (2nd Ed.). Philadelphia: Lippincott.

Melzack, R. (1983) 'The McGill Pain Questionnaire', in Melzack, R. (editor) *Pain measurement and assessment*. New York: Raven Press, pp.41–7.

Mercadente, S. (1996) 'Ketamine in cancer pain: an update'. *Palliative medicine*, 10, pp.225–30.

Mercadante, S., Maddaloni, S., Roccella, S. and Salvaggio, L. (1992) 'Predictive factors in advanced cancer pain treated only by analgesics'. *Pain*, 50(2), pp.151–2.

Mersey Palliative Care Audit Group (2000) 'Guidelines for the use of fentanyl in dying patients'. Merseyside: Mersey Palliative Care Audit Group (unpublished work).

Merskey, H. and Bogduk, N. (editors) (1994) *Classification of chronic pain* (2nd Ed.) prepared by the International Association for the Study of Pain Task Force on Taxonomy. Seattle: IASP Press.

Morris, D.B. (1991) *The culture of pain*. Berkeley: University of California Press.

NAPP Pharmaceuticals (2006) *Transtec 35, 52.5 and 70 micrograms transdermal patch*. Go to: **www.emc.medicines.org.uk** and do a quick search (using the search box at the top right-hand corner) for 'transtec'. Site accessed 13/5/08.

NHS QIS (2004) *The management of pain in patients with cancer: best practice*. Edinburgh: NHS Quality Improvement Scotland.

NMC – see Nursing and Midwifery Council.

Nugent, M. (2006) 'The management of breakthrough cancer pain: is current practice best practice?' *European Journal of Palliative Care*, 13(1), pp.10–12.

Nursing and Midwifery Council (2004a) *Code of professional conduct*. London: NMC.

Nursing and Midwifery Council (2004b) *Guidelines for the administration of medicines*. London: NMC.

Pal, B. and Amlesh, H. (no date) 'Opioids and other analgesic use in rheumatoid arthritis patients: a review and recommendations'. Manchester: South Manchester University Hospitals NHS Trust (unpublished work).

Pan, C.X., Morrison, R.S., Ness, J., Fugh-Berman, A. and Leipzeig, R.M. (2000) 'Complementary and alternative medicine in the management of pain, dyspnea and nausea and vomiting near the end of life – a systematic review'. *Journal of Pain and Symptom Management*, 20(5), pp.374–87.

Phillips, J., Davidson, P., Jackson, D., Kristjanson, L. and Daly, J. (2006) 'Residential aged care: the last frontier for palliative care'. *Journal of Advanced Nursing*, 55(4), pp.416–24.

Portenoy, R.K. and Farkash, A. (1988) 'Practical management of non-malignant pain in the elderly'. *Geriatrics*, 43(5), pp.29–47.

Portenoy, R.K. and Hagen, N.A. (1990) 'Breakthrough pain: definition, prevalence and characteristics'. *Pain*, 41(3), pp.273–81.

Portenoy, R.K., Payne, D. and Jacobsen, P. (1999) 'Breakthrough pain: characteristics and impact in patients with cancer pain'. *Pain*, 81(1/2), pp.129–34.

Rhiner, M. and Kedziera, P. (1999) 'Managing breakthrough cancer pain: a new approach'. *American Journal of Nursing*, 99(3), supplement pp.3–12.

Rose, K.E. (1992) *The experience of chronic pain: an anthropological interpretation*. MSc dissertation, Medical Social Anthropology, Keele University.

Rowbotham, M., Harden, N., Stacey, B., Bernstein, P. and Magnus-Miller, L. (1998) 'Gabapentin in the treatment of postherpetic neuralgia: a randomized controlled trial'. *Journal of the American Medical Association*, 280(21), pp.1837–42.

Saunders, C. and Baines, M. (1989) *Living with dying: the management of terminal disease* (2nd Ed.). Oxford: Oxford University Press.

Scottish Intercollegiate Guidelines Network (2000) *Control of pain in patients with cancer: a national clinical guideline*. Edinburgh: SIGN.

Seers, K. and Friedli, K. (1996) 'The patients' experiences of their chronic non-malignant pain'. *Journal of Advanced Nursing*, 24(6), pp.1160–8.

Seers, K. and Goodman, C. (1987) *Anything for pain?* Julian Aston for North West Thames Regional Health Authority, (Nursing Research video no. 1).

Somerville, M.A. (1995) 'Opioids for chronic pain of non-malignant origin: coercion or consent?' *Health Care Analysis*, 3(1), pp.12–14.

Strong, A., Karavartas, S. and Reicherter, E.A. (2006) 'Recommended exercise protocol to decrease cancer-related fatigue and muscle wasting in patients with multiple myeloma: an evidence-based systematic review'. *Topics in Geriatric Rehabilitation*, 22(2), pp.172–86.

Tack, B. (1990) 'Fatigue in rheumatoid arthritis: conditions, strategies, and consequences'. *Arthritis Care and Research*, 3(2), pp.65–70.

Teske, K., Daut, R. and Cleeland, C.S. (1983) 'Relationships between nurses' observations and patients' self-reports of pain'. *Pain*, 16(3), pp.289–96.

Twycross, R. and Wilcock, A. (2001) *Symptom management in advanced cancer* (3rd Ed.). Oxford: Radcliffe Medical.

Twycross, R., Wilcock, A. and Thorp, S. (editors) (1998) *Palliative care formulary*. Oxford: Radcliffe Medical.

Tyrer, S.P., Capon, M., Peterson, D.M., Charlton, J.E. and Thompson, J.W. (1989) 'The detection of psychiatric illness and psychological handicaps in a British pain clinic population'. *Pain*, 36(1), pp.63–74.

Wall, P. and Jones, M. (1991) *Defeating pain: the war against a silent epidemic*. New York: Plenum Press.

Weiner, D., Turner, G.H., Hennon, J.G., Perera, S. and Hartman, S. (2005) 'The state of chronic pain education in geriatric medicine fellowship training programs'. *Journal of American Geriatrics Society*, 53(10), pp.1798–805.

Wong, D. and Baker, C. (1988) 'Pain in children: a comparison of assessment scales'. *Pediatric Nursing*, 14(1), pp.9–17.

World Health Organization (1990) *Cancer pain relief and palliative care*. Geneva: WHO (Technical report no. 804).

World Health Organization (1996) *Cancer pain relief* (2nd Ed.). Geneva: WHO.

www.grunenthal.com (2006) Key Products 1: pain therapy. Site accessed 30/6/08.

Chapter 8

Quality Improvement

Elaine Stevens and Linda Kerr

INTRODUCTION

Quality improvement is an ongoing process aimed at improving the quality of care experienced by patients and their families. It makes you think about *what* you are doing, *why* you are doing it, and *how* you could do it better (Kitson, 1990: 32). You can use it to identify problems in practice and improve care. It can help you to focus time and resources on effective aspects of care, rather than ineffective (or even harmful) aspects. It also allows organisations to meet national standards, e.g. the *National Service Framework for older people* (DOH, 2001a), *National care standards: hospice care* (Care Commission Scotland, 2002; DOH, 2002) and standards for the care of adults with cancer (NICE, 2004).

Bruera (1996) suggests that quality assurance may also enable palliative care to gain the acceptance of academic health care institutions and health care planners, with the following benefits:

- access to palliative care for increasing numbers of patients and families;
- increased education of medical students, residents, staff physicians [i.e. house officers and specialist registrars] and other disciplines;
- the provision of the protected time and infrastructure necessary for palliative care workers to perform research;
- future funding for palliative care in times of a worldwide crisis on the funding of health care.

In this chapter we will start off by considering clinical governance – the source of quality improvement in terms of good practice and evidence-based practice. We will investigate the way in which the policies, protocols and standards that are set at national and local level impact upon those working in palliative care. We will introduce the audit cycle as a means of ensuring that your practice meets the requirements of national and local standards and clinical guidelines, through the development, implementation and evaluation of policies, protocols and standards about and for your work.

LEARNING OUTCOMES

When you have completed this chapter you will be able to:
- discuss the impact of clinical governance on the provision of palliative care within your care setting;
- explain how evidence-based practice can improve the standard of palliative care provided to patients;
- explain the process of clinical audit;
- perform a clinical audit in your workplace by:
  - defining best practice,
  - implementing best practice,
  - monitoring and comparing against best practice,
  - taking action to improve
- evaluate the process of clinical audit.

Preparation

We recommend that you read the following before you start this chapter.

- Lugton, J. and McIntyre, R. (editors) (2005) *Palliative care: the nursing role* (2nd Ed.). Edinburgh: Churchill Livingstone. Chapter 11 'Research and audit: demonstrating quality' is a useful and interesting introduction to quality, audit and research in palliative care.
- Robbins, M. (1998) *Evaluating palliative care.* Oxford: Oxford University Press.

For Activity 1 you will need the following document:

A first class service: quality in the new NHS. Health Service Circular 113/98. Available from: **www.dh.gov.uk/en/Publicationsandstatistics/Publications/PublicationsPolicy AndGuidance/DH_4006902** (site accessed 13/5/08).

For Activity 6, you might find the following article helpful:

Higginson, I.J. (1999) 'Evidence-based palliative care?' *European Journal of Palliative Care*, 6(6), pp.188–93.

For Activity 10 you will find it useful to have the criteria for appraising research papers and systematic reviews available from CASP (Critical Appraisal Skills Programme), Oxford Institute of Health Sciences, PO Box 777, Oxford OX3 7LF. Available from: **www.phru. nhs.uk/Pages/PHD/resources.htm** (site accessed 13/5/08).

In Activity 11, we ask you to obtain copies of the DOH (2004) *Standards for better health* or the Trent palliative care standards. Your local nursing or hospice library may have copies. Alternatively, they are available from:

- Department of Health. **www.dh.gov.uk/en/Publicationsandstatistics/Publications/ PublicationsPolicyAndGuidance/DH_4086665** (site accessed 13/5/08).
- Ahmedzai, S.H., Hunt, J. and Keeley, V. (1998) *Palliative care core standards. A multidisciplinary approach.* From Trent Hospice Audit Group, Sheffield: The University of Sheffield. Available from: Sheffield Palliative Care Studies Group, Academic Unit of Supportive Care, Division of Clinical Sciences (South), Section of Surgical and Anaesthetic Sciences, University of Sheffield, K Floor, Royal Hallamshire Hospital, Glossop Road, Sheffield, S10 2JF. Tel. +44 (0)114 271 2950 e-mail: **pallmed@ sheffield.ac.uk**

You will need copies of at least one of the following items when preparing to perform a clinical audit:

- Morrell, C. and Harvey, G. (1999) *The clinical audit handbook: improving the quality of health care.* London: Baillière Tindall/RCN. This chapter uses the model of clinical audit described in this book. The book includes interesting examples from clinical audit in practice, and some useful sample audit forms.
- Glickman, M. (1997) *Making palliative care better: quality improvement, multiprofessional audit and standards.* Occasional Paper 12. National Council for Palliative Care Services. You can find order details for this publication here: **www.ncpc.org.uk/ publications/pubs_list2.html** (site accessed 13/5/08).
- Higginson, I. (editor) (1993) *Clinical audit in palliative care.* Oxford: Radcliffe Medical Press.

In Activity 14, and other later activities, you will be asking patients and their families about the quality of care they have received. It is advisable to check with your manager before you do these activities.

Other useful documents include:

- Gold Standards Framework. **www.goldstandardsframework.nhs.uk** (site accessed 13/5/08).
- NHS QIS (2002) *Standards for specialist palliative care.* Edinburgh: NHS QIS. Available from: **www.nhshealthquality.org/nhsqis/files/SPC.pdf** (site accessed 13/5/08).
- SPPC (2003a) *Beyond the randomised trial: evidence and effectiveness in palliative care.* Edinburgh: SPPC. Available from: **www.palliativecarescotland.org.uk/publications/ Beyond the randomised trial.pdf** (site accessed 13/5/08).
- *Cancer in Scotland: action for change*, available on the Scottish Executive website at **www.scotland.gov.uk/library3/health/csac-00.asp** (site accessed 13/5/08).
- *The NHS cancer plan*, available at **www.dh.gov.uk/en/Publicationsandstatistics/ Publications/PublicationsPolicyAndGuidance/Browsable/DH_4098139** (site accessed 13/5/08).

Preparatory activity

In this chapter you will be performing an audit of practice in your workplace. Before you do this, it will be helpful if you have done some preparatory work on the skills and experience needed.

In *Clinical governance: how nurses can get involved*, the RCN (2000) identifies the following skills and experience as being essential for the competent setting of standards, monitoring and improvement of practice:

- literature searching – for example, knowing how to search databases and the internet, identifying which journals are covered by which databases;
- critical appraisal of evidence;
- constructing standards;
- establishing user views by methods such as interviewing, producing and interpreting questionnaires;
- consensus building;
- working in a multiprofessional team;
- designing audit tools and collecting appropriate data;
- evaluating data;
- influencing the team to change practice;
- understanding the role of other professionals involved in care;
- communication (written and oral);
- facilitating;
- disseminating results;
- presentation.

Review your own skills and experience in these areas. Identify the areas where you need the most help, training or practice, and create an action plan for improving your skills/experience in those areas.

Feedback

Your manager and other members of the care team may be able to help you with sources of relevant information and training. You could also consult your local audit facilitator or Trust audit facilitator, your clinical effectiveness co-ordinator or the person responsible for audit in your local specialist palliative care team.

CLINICAL GOVERNANCE

In *A first class service: quality in the new NHS* (DoH, 1998), clinical governance is defined as:

a framework through which NHS organisations are accountable for continuously improving the quality of their services and safeguarding high standards of care by creating an environment in which excellence in clinical care will flourish.

The RCN explains:

Put simply, it means putting doctors and nurses in charge of the way things are done – and making both clinicians and managers account-able for the quality of patient care. It is about helping health care services make decisions based on clinical judgement – not just on how much things cost.

RCN (1998: 9)

Clinical governance was proposed by the Government to ensure high-quality health care, and makes health care providers, including NHS Boards and Trusts and individual health care practitioners, responsible for:

- giving care which is based on the best possible evidence;
- monitoring and evaluating care;
- demonstrating quality care;
- giving a public account of their practice to patients, health care providers and purchasers and professionals.

The RCN has produced a couple of useful guides to clinical governance – *Guidance for nurses on clinical governance* (RCN, 1998) and *Clinical governance: how nurses can get involved* (RCN, 2000; RCN, 2003).

Clinical governance is part of a framework for setting, delivering and monitoring standards. The proposed framework for England is shown in Figure 8.1 as an example.

Three of the key initiatives shown in Figure 8.1 are:

- National Institute of Clinical Excellence (NICE) – will promote clinical effectiveness and cost effectiveness, and the production and dissemina-tion of clinical guidelines. It is a nationwide appraisal body established to determine the best approach for treating the patient.
- National Service Frameworks – will bring together the best evidence of clinical effectiveness and cost effectiveness with the views of service users, to determine the best ways of providing particular services.
- The Commission for Health Improvement, whose functions were taken over in 2004 by the Healthcare Commission. The Healthcare Commission supports and oversees the quality of clinical governance

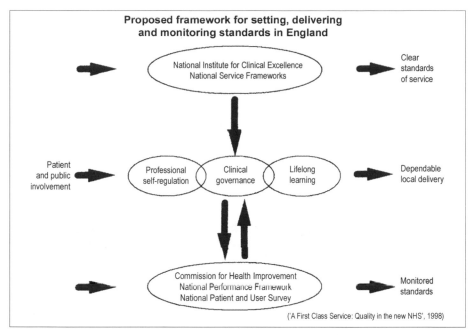

Figure 8.1 Delivering improved quality (DOH, 1998: Introduction: 5). Reproduced under the terms of the Click-Use Licence.

and clinical services. The Healthcare Commission is playing a crucial role in modernising the NHS in England and Wales. By raising standards in clinical care through regular reviews of NHS organisations, the Healthcare Commission aims to improve the quality of patient care. The Healthcare Commission also investigates serious service failures in the NHS and monitors the implementation of National Service Frameworks and National Institute for Clinical Excellence guidance. It also plays a role in advising the NHS on best practice.

Wales will link with England on NICE and the Healthcare Commission. Scotland has its own structures for quality improvement including SIGN (Scottish Intercollegiate Guidelines Network), CRAG (Clinical Resource and Audit Group) and the Clinical Standards Board, which together form part of NHS Quality Improvement Scotland, **www.nhshealthquality.org** (site accessed 13/5/08).

Under clinical governance, Chief Executives have statutory accountability on behalf of the organisation for assuring the quality of services. Individual practitioners are also accountable for demonstrating high-quality, clinically effective care. Arrangements for clinical governance have also been made for primary care groups (England) and community health partnerships (Scotland). The principles for clinical governance apply to all those who provide or manage patient care services in the

NHS and are the same for large and small organisations. (They also apply to those in the independent sector, in principle but not in regulation.) Key elements of the clinical governance framework include:

- clear lines of responsibility and accountability;
- quality improvement programmes, including clinical audit, evidence-based practice, standard setting and monitoring;
- risk management programmes, including learning from complaints, learning from incidents, helping staff to reflect on and develop their practice. (RCN, 2000: 5)

Activity 1: Clinical governance

Obtain a copy of the government document *A first class service: quality in the new NHS* (DoH, 1998). Available from: **www.dh.gov.uk/en/Publicationsandstatistics/ Publications/PublicationsPolicyAndGuidance/DH_4006902** (site accessed 13/5/08). Skim through it quickly to get a general idea of its contents. Then read through it more slowly, and make notes on how this quality system affects:

- your own professional practice;
- the care provided to palliative care patients in your clinical area.

If your Trust or Health Authority has a clinical governance strategy, obtain a copy of any documentation for it. Work through the documents identifying how the strategy affects:

- your own professional practice;
- the care provided to palliative care patients in your clinical area.

Discuss your findings with the members of your AL set.

Feedback

Your discussion of the effects of clinical governance may have included the following points:

- the development of a culture that promotes and supports improvements in practice and patient care; is open and blame-free rather than revolving around disciplinary procedures; is truly multiprofessional; develops partnership with patients;
- the encouragement of practitioners to share information and to develop communication skills and presentation skills;
- the development of patient-centred leaders through: the management of self, building, developing and managing effective relationships with team members, focusing on the patient, networking and increasing political awareness;

- the implementation of continuing professional development programmes, to encourage lifelong learning;
- the enforcement of professional self-regulation, making nurses responsible for the quality of their clinical practice and for their professional conduct;
- a commitment to quality improvement, involving nurses in standard setting, monitoring and making improvements and re-auditing;
- the implementation of risk management programmes, involving nurses in reporting incidents, the implementation of risk assessment and prevention strategies, handling complaints, clinical supervision, dealing with poor performance and continuing professional development.

RCN (2000: 8–19)

Activity 2: Keeping up to date

Keeping your professional knowledge up to date meets many of the criteria of clinical governance.

If you have a few colleagues who are interested in reading new articles, you may be able to set up a journal club, to review new evidence that might have an impact on your practice. Each member could agree to read articles on a particular topic and to report back to the club at regularly scheduled meetings.

It may be easier if you all agree to create and maintain a resource file on current issues in palliative care.

Feedback

The provision of current literature will enable the care team to form educated opinions about issues in palliative care.

A nurse's experience of quality improvement

All nurses want to improve the quality of care they provide, yet many feel frustrated and weary because they've not been listened to in the past. Sometimes the way things are organised just doesn't make sense – despite the fact that nurses often put forward ideas about how to make things run more smoothly. Clinical governance will provide nurses at every level with a framework through which they can channel their concerns about the quality of patient care.

This quote is from the following article – an interesting illustration of how nurses can use clinical governance to improve practice. It's only a couple of pages long and is well worth a read: Harvey, G.

> (1998) 'Improving patient care: getting to grips with clinical governance'. *RCN Magazine*, Autumn 1998, pp.8–9.

Evidence-based practice

> Evidence-based practice is the conscious, explicit and judicious use of current evidence in making decisions about the care of individual patients.
>
> Sackett *et al.* (1996)

Health care professionals often base their decisions about how to meet patients' needs on past practice, perhaps not asking how effective their chosen strategy is or whether other approaches exist that might be more successful. Evidence-based practice, which is a tenet of clinical governance, requires the evaluation of the effectiveness of medical and nursing interventions, the dissemination of the results of the evaluation and the application of the findings to practice. In this section, we will consider what we mean by 'evidence', ask you whether your own practice is evidence-based and investigate how evidence-based practice can improve the standard of care provided to the patient with palliative care needs.

What is evidence?

> Evidence is the combination of research, clinical expertise and patient choice.
>
> Sackett *et al.* (1996: 71–2)

Often, however, the term 'evidence-based practice' is used in the health service to refer to getting *research* evidence into practice. This doesn't mean that your experience or the wishes of the patient and family don't count – just that you also need to integrate the best available external evidence from systematic research into your practice. Problems arise when there is no evidence in a particular area or where the evidence that exists is unclear.

Research evidence will be either quantitative or qualitative. Morgan (1997: 44) defines these types of evidence.

- **Quantitative evidence.** Some clinical areas have been the subject of randomised-controlled trials (RCTs), seen as the 'gold standard' for determining the effectiveness of an intervention. These are large-scale, scientifically constructed research projects that are conducted in a way which ensures the results are valid and unbiased. RCTs can measure and display the impact of an intervention, proving whether it is as effective as – or more effective than – other options. This type of evidence is relatively easy to obtain in some fields of care where there are ways of quantifying the health outcome for the patient.

- **Qualitative evidence.** Nursing care concerns the wellbeing or quality of life of the patient and it is not always possible to assign numerical values for this. Instead, research designs and methods are used to gain an understanding of patients' and their families' perceptions of interventions or care. Alternatively patients and their families may be asked to describe their experiences and/or satisfaction with the care given. Researchers look for recurring themes and patterns in the data/information and look for similarities and differences both within a case and across cases.

The major drawback with quantitative research is that it tends mainly to focus on areas such as drug trials and wound care, where the results are easily quantified. Aspects that are more useful in palliative care, such as quality of life, altered bereavement outcomes or quality of care, are more difficult to measure, and may therefore be excluded. Furthermore, the RCT is not an appropriate way to study these areas.

> Palliative care is characterised by care that is delivered with sensitive attention to the diverse reactions and needs of people coming to terms with life-threatening illnesses and the personal suffering that this often entails. It aims to address the physical, psychological, social and spiritual needs of the dying and their families. The danger of concentrating on areas that are amenable to measurement, such as patients' physical symptoms, is that the areas less easily measured are given less attention in the quest for improving and demonstrating quality of care. . . . palliative care is complex and, in its totality, beyond measurement.
>
> Lugton and Kindlen (1999: 279)

Qualitative research is also appropriate in nursing situations because it accesses people's perceptions and experiences of care and caring.

Increasingly, researchers who are concerned with demonstrating effectiveness will seek both types of evidence, seeing them as complementary. However, you will notice that many guideline documents do not rate qualitative research as highly as quantitative research in terms of the level of evidence it provides. You can find details of research evidence in:

- systematic reviews;
- clinical guidelines;
- National Service Frameworks.

We look at each of these briefly below and also at some other sources of evidence, including databases such as MEDLINE and CINAHL.

Systematic reviews

A systematic review is a process whereby a group of specialists investigate research evidence and that which is deemed acceptable is then brought into one place – often a CD-ROM or internet database. Systematic reviews therefore contain only rigorous, well-conducted studies and are a major source of synthesised evidence. Three key sources are the Cochrane Collaboration, the NHS Centre for Reviews and Dissemination, and Health Technology Assessments.

The Cochrane Collaboration – within the Cochrane Collaboration, an international group of clinicians, methodologists and consumers produce systematic reviews of randomised trials of health care interventions. The systematic reviews are updated each time an important new trial is reported, providing the highest levels of evidence ever achieved on the efficacy of preventive, therapeutic and rehabilitative regimes.

The Cochrane Library is published on computer disk and CD-ROM, on the internet and in a variety of other forms. It includes:

- CDSR (the Cochrane Database of Systematic Reviews);
- DARE (Database of Abstracts of Reviews of Effectiveness), a related database of published systematic reviews abstracted by the NHS Centre for Reviews and Dissemination at the University of York;
- the Cochrane Controlled Trials Register (CCTR), a bibliography of over 100,000 controlled trials including many not included in MEDLINE or other bibliographic databases;
- the Cochrane Review Methodology Database (CRMD), an invaluable source of information on RCTs and the strengths and weaknesses of systematic reviews.

There is a separate database specifically dedicated to midwifery and childbirth issues.

There is also a Cochrane Review Group – the Pain, Palliative Care and Supportive Care Group (PaPaS) – that prepares, maintains and disseminates systematic reviews of RCTs of interventions concerned with:

- the prevention and treatment of pain, both acute and chronic;
- the relief of symptoms resulting from both the disease process, and interventions used in the management of disease and symptom control (this involves palliative care in its widest sense);

- supporting patients and carers through the disease process.

You can find more details about the PaPaS Group at **www.jr2.ox.ac.uk/ cochrane** (site accessed 13/5/08).

The NHS Centre for Reviews and Dissemination – The NHS Centre for Reviews and Dissemination (CRD) was established in January 1994 to provide the NHS with important information on the effectiveness of treatments and the delivery and organisation of health care. CRD, by offering rigorous and systematic reviews on selected topics, a database of good-quality reviews, a dissemination service and an information service, helps to promote research-based practice in the NHS.

CRD collaborates with a number of health research and information organisations across the world and is a UK member of the International Network of Agencies for Health Technology Assessment (INAHTA). CRD produces a database of HTA projects and publications. You can find out more about CRD at **www.york.ac.uk/inst/crd** (site accessed 13/5/08).

Health Technology Assessment – the HTA programme is a national programme of research established and funded by the Department of Health's Research and Development programme. The purpose of the programme is to ensure that high-quality research information on the costs, effectiveness and broader impact of health technologies is produced in the most effective way for those who use, manage and provide care in the NHS. You can find out more about HTA at **www.ncchta.org** (site accessed 13/5/08).

Clinical guidelines

National clinical guidelines or clinical practice guidelines are:

> Systematically developed statements to assist practitioner and client decisions about appropriate health care for specific clinical circumstances.
>
> Institute of Medicine, 1992, cited in Duff *et al.* (1996: 889)

These provide information about the care for a particular condition, including options, and make recommendations, based on research evidence, which can be adapted locally to suit a particular situation and patient. The NHS library holds the national database for approved evidence-based guidelines at **www.library.nhs.uk/guidelinesfinder** (site accessed 13/5/08). In Scotland, the Scottish Intercollegiate Guidelines

Network (SIGN) holds guidelines and in Northern Ireland they can be found at the DHSS. The RCN has a leaflet (*Common questions about guidelines*) on clinical guidelines. In addition, the RCN Information Service will be able to give you more information about guidelines, where to find them and how to evaluate them. Local guidelines, or protocols, are based on national clinical guidelines, but take into account local issues like resource levels and individual patient information and needs. Clinical audit, which we look at later in this chapter, can be used as a framework for the implementation of clinical guidelines.

The National Service Frameworks

These set national standards and define service models for a specific service or care group. NICE has put in place programmes to support their implementation. The NSFs will also establish performance measures against which progress within an agreed timescale will be measured. *The NSF for older people* (DOH, 2001a) is one example. Further information on NSFs can be found at **www.library.nhs.uk** (site accessed 13/5/08).

The National Institute for Clinical Evidence (NICE) is an independent organisation responsible for providing national guidance on promoting good health and preventing and treating ill health. NICE helps health professionals implement their guidance by providing tools such as cost templates, audit criteria and slide sets. More information on NICE can be found at **www.nice.org.uk** (site accessed 13/5/08).

Other sources of evidence

Other sources include general and specialised bibliographic databases, both in print and in electronic form. For the most part, electronic media, whether on computer disk, CD-ROM, or the internet, are making paper sources obsolete. Electronic media are generally much more accessible, much more thoroughly indexed and, most importantly, have the potential to be much more up to date.

> If you are computerless, make friends with a librarian; if you are computer-phobic, sign up for desensitisation right away!
>
> Sackett *et al.* (1997)

The main databases that have information on research evidence relevant to health care are:

- CINAHL (Cumulative Index of Nursing and Allied Health Literature). CINAHL covers virtually every nursing journal published. The allied health areas covered are physical therapy, occupational therapy and emergency services. Website: **www.cinahl.com** (site accessed 13/5/08).

- BNI (British Nursing Index). BNI contains references to over 220 nursing and allied health journals from 1994 onwards. It is a collation of NMI and Nursing Bibliography and RCN Nurse ROM. Websites: **www.bournemouth.ac.uk/library/resources/nursing.html** and **www.ovid.com/site/catalog/DataBase/28.jsp** (site accessed 14/7/08).

- MEDLINE (a computerised version of the *Index Medicus*) and EM-BASE (a computerised version of the *Excerpta Medica*). The US National Library's MEDLINE, and EMBASE, its European and more commercial counterpart, are general purpose databases, covering all of biomedical research and many other areas. Their major drawbacks are that they cover only about 6,000 of the 20,000 (primarily English language) journals published worldwide. They find only those trials which are electronically indexed (about half the total) and they find only those trials which are actually published (which are usually biased towards the positive). MEDLINE website: **www.medscape.com**. EM-BASE website: **www.embase.com** – however, you can access most of this information through the NHS e-libraries. Sites accessed 13/5/08.

These are available in most teaching hospitals' libraries and on the Internet. The NHS e-libraries are also good resources which allow access to these databases. Furthermore, there are journals that are dedicated to conducting and publishing systematic reviews, e.g. *Evidence-based Medicine*, *Evidence-Based Nursing* and the *Journal of Clinical Effectiveness*.

> [*Evidence-Based Nursing*] has evolved as a direct response to the dilemma of practitioners who want to use research, but are thwarted by overwhelming clinical demands, an ever burgeoning research literature, and for many, a lack of skills in critical appraisal.
>
> Mulhall (1998: 4)

Finally, some textbooks are still good sources of evidence. *Evaluating palliative care: establishing the evidence base* (Robbins, 1998) examines the methodological issues in the evaluation of palliative cancer care and encapsulates the (pre-1998) state of palliative care research.

Activity 3: Evidence-based practice within your clinical area

Is evidence-based practice a priority within your clinical area? Discuss this with your manager and colleagues, including those in other disciplines. Find out whether people are in favour of integrating evidence into practice and what they think the issues and challenges might be.

Feedback

Evidence-based practice aims to provide patients with an improved quality of care and to prevent staff from implementing ineffective interventions. However, given the complexities of providing care for patients and of health care systems generally, applying research is not straightforward. There are many considerations:

- Those responsible for budgets may point out that it may save money by identifying the most cost-effective measures. However, the best treatments may also be expensive.
- Taking time out to search for and appraise the evidence may be difficult for practitioners.
- Many clinical staff have not had the opportunity to attend training in using research and how to know if research studies have been well conducted.
- There may be limited research evidence in some clinical areas or the research that exists may not clearly indicate which treatment is best for which patient.
- Even if the evidence is clear, colleagues who have been practising in a certain way for many years may not be willing to change their practice. Implementing change is one of the biggest challenges of introducing evidence into practice.
- There may also be resource considerations, such as getting hold of the right equipment and acquiring the training to use certain equipment.
- Balancing the research evidence, clinical expertise and the preferences of the patient may also be a challenge.

Your own practice

In the next two activities we will ask you to consider whether your own practice is evidence-based, what evidence you have to support your answer (if 'yes') and what you can do to make your practice evidence-based (if you answer 'no').

Remember that research evidence isn't the only form of evidence. The term 'evidence' also includes your own clinical expertise and patient choice. In fact one of the simpler definitions of evidence-based practice avoids mentioning evidence at all, but defines it as:

> doing the right thing in the right way for the right patients at the right time.
>
> Duff *et al.*, 1997

Activity 4: Doing the right thing

Think about an intervention that you use frequently in your everyday practice. How do you know that you are doing:

- the right thing;
- in the right way;

- for the right patients;
- at the right time?

Make notes of the evidence, knowledge or experience upon which you base your actions.

Feedback

Your answer may be that it was what you were taught to do in your basic education. If this was some time ago, there may be new evidence supporting different interventions and it will be worthwhile investigating the current evidence for the best intervention. You may have come across recent evidence supporting the intervention while reading around your subject or doing work for your continuing professional development. You may not have any *research* evidence to support your use of this particular intervention, but remember the importance of counting your own practice knowledge and experience as evidence.

We recommend that you integrate the use of evidence through reflective practice. By regularly refreshing your knowledge of the best available evidence through reflection, you will be able in practice to make the best decision as quickly as possible. The model of reflective practice we introduced in Chapter 2 allows you to look back on an incident in a structured way, investigating:

- what actually happened;
- what you thought and how you felt about the experience;
- the appropriateness of the actions you took during the incident, the effectiveness of the care you provided and whether it was based on the evidence that underpins good practice;
- what you learned from the incident and how you can improve your future practice.

We recommend that in the third stage of this reflective cycle (or a suitable stage of a reflective model that you are already familiar with) you use the sources we have suggested to identify relevant evidence with which to compare your actions and the effectiveness of the care you provide. Where there is good, relevant evidence, you will also discover ways of improving your future practice.

Activity 5: Is your practice evidence-based?

The checklist below (Greenhalgh, 1996, cited in Higginson, 1999) comprises a series of questions based on good practice and evidence-based practice. (If you quickly skim through the list, you will realise that the anticipated answer to each question is 'yes'.)

Reflect upon your recent work with a palliative care patient, then work through the list, ticking the appropriate box.

If you tick 'yes', make a note on a separate sheet of paper of what evidence you have to support your assertion. For example, you may be able to get 'testimony' evidence from the patient, their family or your colleagues, or you may have notes or other materials documenting what decisions you have made and how you made them.

If you tick 'no', make notes on what you could do now (or what you could do in the future) so that in, say, a few days' time, or a week, you could tick 'yes'.

	Yes	No
1. Have I identified and prioritised the clinical, psychological, social and other problems, taking into account the patient's and family's perspective?	☐	☐
2. Have I performed a sufficiently competent and complete assessment (including examination) to establish the likelihood of completing the diagnosis?	☐	☐
3. Have I considered additional problems and risk factors that may need opportunistic attention?	☐	☐
4. Have I, where necessary, sought evidence from systematic reviews, guidelines, clinical trials and other sources pertaining to the problem?	☐	☐
5. Have I assessed and taken into the account the completeness, quality and strength of the evidence?	☐	☐
6. Have I applied valid and relevant evidence to the particular set of problems in a way that is both scientifically justified and intuitively sensible?	☐	☐
7. Have I presented the pros and cons of different options to the patient and family in a way they can understand, and incorporated the patient's and family's wishes into the final recommendation?	☐	☐
8. Have I arranged review, recall, referral or further care as necessary?	☐	☐

Feedback

Even where your answers are 'yes', you may still need to do further work to ensure that your practice really is evidence-based. For example, if you are making decisions informed by data you looked up, say, five years ago, you cannot be sure that your practice is still evidence-based. In the intervening five years, research may have identified more efficient or cost-effective ways of doing what you are doing. We recommend the use of reflective practice as a way of integrating research evidence and issues of patient choice into your practice.

Activity 6: Improving the standard of care

Create an information sheet to win over those people who are not in favour of the integration of evidence into practice. Ask yourself the question:

'How can evidence-based practice improve the standard of care provided to the palliative care patient?'

You could use headings similar to the ones below:

- identification of most effective intervention;
- efficient use of staff time and other resources;
- cost effectiveness;
- using your own expertise;
- giving the patient a voice.

Support your argument, where possible, by the inclusion of practice evidence from your own practice or that of your colleagues – give examples of situations in which the integration of evidence into practice has improved the standard of palliative care provided to a patient.

You may find the following article helpful:

Higginson, I.J. (1999) 'Evidence-based palliative care?' *European Journal of Palliative Care*, 6(6), pp.188–93.

Feedback

You can find useful and interesting examples of the impact of evidence-based practice on patient care in the journal *Evidence-based Nursing*.

CLINICAL AUDIT

> Clinical audit is a systematic and critical analysis of the quality of clinical care. This includes procedures used for diagnosis, treatment and care of patients, the associated use of resources and the effect of care on the outcome and quality of life of the patient.
>
> Clinical Outcomes Group (1993)

Clinical audit may also be viewed as an internally applied mechanism for quality improvement, as the control and ownership of clinical audit projects rest with the staff involved (Morrell and Harvey, 1999: 12).

Clinical audit is a way of reviewing clinical practice through multiprofessional, patient-centred audit. A multiprofessional approach is vital in palliative care, because care teams often include professionals such as social workers and chaplains in addition to clinical staff. Glickman (1997) states that it is important for all those providing care, including administrative staff supporting the clinical team, and volunteers where appropriate, to be involved in evaluating and improving the service. He also asserts that patients and their families/carers should also be involved wherever possible. Glickman (1997) suggests that it may be helpful to think of this broad-based approach as multiprofessional audit.

Put simply, clinical audit is about looking at practice and changing practice to improve the quality of care experienced by patients. Morrell and Harvey (1999) suggest that the audit cycle has four phases, as shown in Figure 8.2.

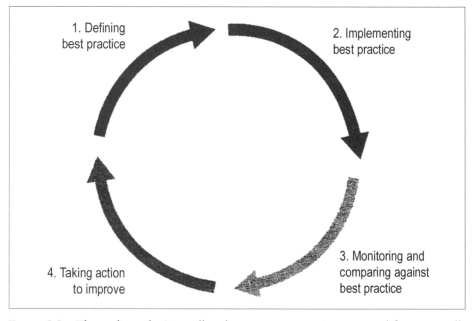

Figure 8.2 The audit cycle (Morrell and Harvey, 1999: 10). Reprinted from Morrell, C. and Harvey, G. (1999) The clinical audit handbook: improving the quality of health care, with permission from Elsevier. **www.elsevier.com** (site accessed 13/5/08)

Morrell and Harvey (1999) then go on to break each phase down into smaller, more detailed steps:

- Defining best practice:
  - choose a topic for audit;
  - describe current practice;
  - enlist the support of all staff involved;
  - critically review the available evidence;
  - develop a standard, i.e. objective and criteria.

- Implementing best practice:
  - disseminate the standard;
  - develop a monitoring tool [or use an existing one, such as the Palliative Care Outcome Scale (Higginson, 1998) or the Edmonton Symptom Assessment System (Bruera *et al.*, 1991)]
  - implement the criteria.
- Monitoring and comparing against best practice:
  - identify sources of data and methods for sampling;
  - collect valid and reliable data;
  - compare the results to the objective.
- Taking action to improve:
  - feedback to participants;
  - generate a team action plan and implement;
  - re-audit and evaluate.

An important thing to bear in mind about the audit cycle is that you don't just do one cycle and then stop. It is an ongoing process, a continuous effort to improve the quality of care you provide. Furthermore, bear in mind that:

> If through the process of audit or research patients are disturbed beyond what would be normally required for clinical management, ethics approval should be sought.
>
> Lugton and Kindlen (1999: 281)

The approach to clinical audit described by Morrell and Harvey (1999) is criterion-based audit. Other approaches to audit that Morrell and Harvey (1999) suggest you may encounter include:

- **Benchmarking** – involves the same process of definition, implementing, measuring and action planning as criterion-based audit, but the audit results are shared across clinical units and organisations with a view to learning from those who do it best. The Department of Health has produced a resource pack called *Essence of care: patient-focused benchmarking for health care practitioners* (DoH, 2001b), which provides benchmarking tools for improving the quality of care in eight fundamental aspects of care.
- **National clinical audit** – co-ordinated by Medical Royal Colleges and professional bodies – you may have been involved in collecting data for a national or regional audit project.
- **Care pathways** – similar to standards but follow the patient through a number of clinical interventions rather than focusing on one, which clinical audit more commonly does. The Liverpool Care Pathway (**www.mcpcil.org.uk/liverpool_care_pathway** site accessed 13/5/08), for example, provides guidance on best practice in the patient's last 48 hours of life.

- **TELER system** – a method for making and using clinical notes, requiring staff to use a scale to describe the achievement of treatment or care objectives.
- **Peer review** – including case review, critical incident analysis and clinical supervision.

Four of the following five sections take you through Morrell and Harvey's four stages of clinical audit. The section that follows 'Defining best practice', which is called 'Outcomes in palliative care', looks at outcomes (and outcome measures) in palliative care, which have an impact on the formulation of standards in palliative care.

Note that we are not expecting you to perform a huge, all-encompassing audit of the quality of care provided to palliative care patients. You may simply be looking at one small area of your own practice – a sort of mini-audit. In fact, Higginson (1993) suggests that 'small audits with frequent feedback may be more successful'. Furthermore, she recommends that you use the mnemonic ARISE to help you remember some important points about feedback, review and repeating the audit cycle:

- A – Analyse often so that the results are considered early, not when a large amount of data has been collected.
- R – Review the results, the progress of the audit and the positive and negative effects on staff and patients to plan the future developments.
- I – Instigate change both in working practice and in the audit method used, even if the changes are relatively small, before the audit cycle is repeated.
- S – Set new standards – to be monitored in a new audit cycle.
- E – Effect new cycle, building on the results of the previous audit.

If you are particularly interested in auditing spiritual care, you will find the following article useful. It includes a standard for spiritual care and an audit form for capturing patients'/carers' views.

Catterall, R.A., Cox, M., Greet, B., Sankey, J. and Griffiths, G. (1998) 'The assessment and audit of spiritual care'. *International Journal of Palliative Nursing*, 4(4), pp.162–8.

Clinical audit: Phase 1 – Defining best practice

Morrell and Harvey (1999) define the steps to be taken in this part of the audit cycle as:

- choose a topic for audit;
- describe current practice;

- enlist the support of all staff involved;
- critically review the available evidence;
- develop a standard, i.e. objective and criteria.

We will look at each step in turn.

1. Choose a topic

The choice of topic is crucial in clinical audit because the often significant resources involved in the project must be seen to have been used wisely. Topics chosen therefore often include areas of care or interventions that patients experience frequently, that are costly in terms of human or financial resources, where problems are apparent or where great risk is involved in the procedure.

Activity 7: Choosing a topic

Discuss with your colleagues possible topics for audit. Identify:

- the area of palliative care that is most common or intervention that is most frequent in your clinical area;
- the most expensive area of care or intervention;
- any area that seems to be causing problems;
- interventions or procedures that involve a great deal of risk.

It is also vital to get patients involved in clinical audit but remember that if patients will be disturbed beyond what would normally be required for clinical management, you should obtain approval from your organisation's ethics committee.

Now that you have identified these four items, you need to narrow your choice to a single topic. You might like to investigate one of the problem areas identified by nurses in a *Nursing Times* survey on the provision of care for dying patients (Munro, 2001):

- a lack of training;
- a lack of support from medical colleagues;
- a lack of necessary equipment;
- nursing shortages;
- difficulties gaining access to specialist support.

For example, you might like to investigate the availability of clean bed-linen, appropriate food or necessary drugs, if these issues came up in your discussions with your colleagues or patients. Other questions you need to answer before making your choice include:

- Are systematic reviews of research in that area available?

- Are there existing national clinical guidelines in the area?
- Is it an area in which it is actually possible to promote sustainable improvement?

Feedback

Having identified the topic you wish to audit, the next step is to describe current practice.

2. Describe current practice

Morrell and Harvey (1999: 19) suggest that reasons for collecting data at this early stage include the identification of problems and areas for improvement, and a better chance of identifying improvements in practice when they occur. If you don't have a clear picture of what you're doing now, how can you be sure that the changes you implement actually improve the situation?

Activity 8: Describe current practice

Morrell and Harvey (1999) identify the following as useful sources of information:

- letters from patients, complaints or comments from external agencies;
- critical incident reports – where members of staff have described and analysed important concerns following one incident;
- summaries of team meetings where the issue has been discussed;
- information from routine data sources, including number of patients involved;
- variance data from care pathways;
- data collected from externally applied audits – educational audit, or national audit projects;
- patient stories or feedback from focus groups;
- direct observation of care.

Obtain access to as many as possible of these sources where they are relevant to the topic you have chosen. Make notes, or take copies of documents, and try to build up a clear picture of current practice.

Feedback

You should find evidence supporting your choice of topic in these documents. If you do not, you may need to reconsider your choice, to ensure that the resources invested in your audit project are being used on something worthwhile.

Once you have described current practice, and are sure that your choice of audit topic is appropriate, the next step is to enlist the support of all staff involved.

3. Enlist staff support

The most effective way to enlist support is by forming a clinical audit group (Morrell and Harvey, 1999: 19). The group should have six to eight members representing the following individuals/groups:

- managers;
- the clinical audit committee;
- the clinical director and any others for whom the project may have implications;
- patients upon whom the project may have an impact;
- the professional groups involved.

Your clinical audit group may therefore include one or more members of your local specialist palliative care team or a representative from a local palliative care provider, depending on your audit topic.

If you have chosen to do a mini-audit (i.e. just one small area of your own practice), you may not need to set up a formal group like the one described by Morrell and Harvey above. It may be enough to involve your manager and those of your colleagues and patients who will be affected by the change in your practice. Members of your AL set may also be able to provide support and advice. However, if your audit project may have far-reaching or serious consequences, or require a large investment of staff time, or other forms of organisational resources, we recommend that you follow the formal audit process as described by Morrell and Harvey.

Activity 9: Setting up a clinical audit group

Read pp.19–22 of Morrell and Harvey (1999). This is about enlisting support from staff and goes into more depth on setting up and running meetings of a clinical audit group.

Discuss with your manager and colleagues who should be in the clinical audit group and how to obtain the support of those groups and individuals. Contact those groups and individuals who express an interest in joining the clinical audit group and schedule a meeting to discuss the project. You can use examples from your description of current practice as illustrations of why you have chosen this topic for audit.

Feedback

It may take some considerable time to create a clinical audit group, get meetings scheduled and so on. But hopefully you will eventually achieve a group comprised of people who not only support the audit project but who do so enthusiastically. Enthusiastic support is more likely to make any project a success.

The first task of the group is to critically appraise the available evidence for the topic concerned (Morrell and Harvey, 1999: 22).

4. Critically review the available evidence

We defined what we mean by evidence earlier in this chapter and suggested a variety of sources of evidence. If no research evidence is available on the topic you have selected, you may decide to review your choice. Alternatively, you may choose to seek other types of evidence, such as professional consensus or patient preferences.

Activity 10: Reviewing available evidence

Identify what types of evidence are available regarding your audit topic, i.e.:

- systematic reviews (e.g. those performed by the Cochrane Collaboration);
- individual research projects (e.g. journal articles – databases such as MEDLINE and CINAHL are good sources of these);
- national clinical guidelines (it may be necessary to adapt these to local conditions);
- previous audit or quality projects.

Obtain copies of the documents detailing the available evidence.

Once you have obtained your evidence, you need to critically appraise it, unless – like information contained within systematic reviews, for example – it has already been appraised. To help with this task, we suggest you obtain the criteria for appraising research papers and systematic reviews available from CASP (Critical Appraisal Skills Programme), Oxford Institute of Health Sciences, PO Box 777, Oxford OX3 7LF. Available from: **www.phru.nhs.uk/Pages/PHD/resources.htm** (site accessed 13/5/08).

Several other useful publications are listed in the 'Recommended sources of information' at the end of this chapter, under the heading 'Critical appraisal'.

If research evidence is not available, find out whether professional consensus or patient preferences have been recorded for your audit topic.

If they have not, you may wish to review your choice of topic. Researching professional consensus and patient preferences is extremely time-consuming. Unless your audit topic is extremely important or problematic, it may be better to choose another topic.

Feedback

If you decide to adapt a clinical guideline, you will find it helpful to read the section on guidelines in Chapter 9 of Morrell and Harvey (1999). If you need to investigate patient preferences, you will find it helpful to read the section on consumer involvement in Chapter 7 of Morrell and Harvey (1999).

Now that you have collected and critically reviewed the available evidence, the next step is to develop a standard.

5. Develop a standard

This is the final step in the definition of best practice – a standard is a statement of best practice. It is expressed in terms of an objective and criteria. The criteria can be measured to evaluate compliance with the standard. An example of a palliative care standard (SPA, 1996) is shown in Figure 8.3. The standard statement is the objective. The criteria are listed in terms of structure (what you need), process (what you do) and outcome (what you expect) – we explain these in more detail below. When you look at Figure 8.3 you will see that questions to help you audit the implementation of the standard are supplied as part of the standard. Criteria may be defined for:

- **structure** – what must be provided in order to achieve the standard, e.g. physical environment, ancilliary services, equipment, staff, policies/procedures, organisational system, etc.
- **process** – what action must take place in order to achieve the standard, e.g. assessment techniques, methods of care delivery, intervention, education, giving information and documentation, how resources are used, evaluation, etc.
- **outcome** – the expected results or effect of the care/treatment provided, e.g. the pain is controlled to a level that is acceptable to the patient. Outcome measures need to be:
  – evidence-based;
  – valid;
  – reliable;
  – easy to use;
  – cost effective;
  – ethically sound (Marr and Giebing, 1994).

This focus on structure and process as well as outcomes is known as a systems approach. Glickman (1997: 10–11) identifies the following potential benefits of a systems approach to quality improvement:

CORE STANDARD:	STANDARD REFERENCE:	CARE GROUP:	STANDARD STATEMENT:
Specialist Palliative Care	Symptom Management	Palliative Care/Patients/Families	All patients have their symptoms managed to a degree that is acceptable to them, and achievable by multidisciplinary team intervention within current palliative care knowledge
STRUCTURE: • Availability of suitably qualified staff with demonstrable enhanced communication skills – to include: Nursing Medical Physiotherapy Occupational Therapy Social Work Chaplaincy • Clear concise documentation. • Clear policies/protocols. • Opportunities for inter-disciplinary discussions. • Opportunities for discussion between staff and patients/carers. • Appropriate specialist equipment.	PROCESS: • In-patients' symptoms are assessed on admission and reviewed at least daily by multidisciplinary team. • Out-patients are assessed on first contact, and reviewed at each subsequent contact. • Assessment takes into account all aspects of holistic care. • Patient/advocate/relatives are consulted about care options and plans for care. • Care is reviewed and monitored to achieve best possible symptom relief. • Close liaison within the multidisciplinary team takes place. • Care delivered is based on sound knowledge and current research.	OUTCOME: • Symptom management can be shown to be of a comparable standard to that delivered in other specialist units. • Physical symptoms are managed to an acceptable level. • There is evidence that emotional, spiritual, social and psychological needs have been addressed and given equal importance. • The wishes/desires of the patient/advocate were taken into account. • There is evidence of inter-disciplinary team work in the planning and delivery of care. • There is evidence that care plans are reviewed regularly and kept up to date.	AUDIT: Do personnel files identify the qualifications of each staff member and provide evidence of ongoing professional development? Do care plans indicate that needs are clearly identified and care evaluated? Are policies and protocols available and in use? Do regular multidisciplinary meetings take place and are decisions recorded? Is suitable equipment available, is it maintained, are staff proficient in its use? Can it be demonstrated that the patient's symptoms have been managed to an acceptable level? Is there evidence that the patient has been involved in the decision-making process?

Figure 8.3 Standard No 1: Symptom management (SPA, 1996: 5)

- concentration on the process of care as it affects the patient, across departmental and professional boundaries (patient-focused care);
- improvements in efficiency by revealing outdated practices, 'bottle-necks', duplication of effort and gaps in communication;
- clarification of complex procedures, resulting in better understanding by staff of each other's aims, roles and problems;
- production of flowcharts and process descriptions, which can be used in staff induction and training.

There are, however, problems with measuring outcomes in palliative care, which we will look at next, in 'Outcomes in palliative care'. You may find that when the members of your clinical audit group attempt to identify the criteria that are necessary for the success of the standard, they create impossibly long lists. We will look at how to refine your criteria in the section following 'Outcomes in palliative care'.

In 2001, the Nuffield Trust published a policy document, *Care of the dying in the NHS* (Nuffield Trust, 2001). The document identifies the key challenges facing those trying to deliver high-quality care for the dying within the NHS and recommends that leaders within the health professions produce an authoritative, evidence-based document on best practice to be made available nationally for use by health professionals wherever they practise. It furthermore recommends that central government should take a lead in setting national standards for provision and training in care of the dying, which should include requiring each NHS area to prepare a plan for driving forward a continuing commitment to improving care of the dying.

This policy document was published to coincide with a survey published in the *Nursing Times* that found that one in four nurses felt that the health service fails to provide decent care for dying patients (Munro, 2001). As we mentioned in Activity 7, the study found five key areas that caused nurses particular concern:

- a lack of training;
- a lack of support from medical colleagues;
- a lack of necessary equipment;
- nursing shortages;
- difficulties gaining access to specialist support.

We believe that in every hospital and health care setting there should be clear lines of responsibility for ensuring that basic equipment and the drugs needed to care for dying patients are available. And staff should be given enough time to perform their roles in listening to and helping patients.

John Wyn Owen, Secretary of the Nuffield Trust (quoted in Munro, 2001: 5)

Since the publication of *Care of the dying in the NHS* (Nuffield Trust, 2001), the Health Care Standards Unit (HCSU) has worked with the Department of Health to improve the use of standards within the NHS. One of the HCSU's key aims is to develop and maintain the *Standards for better health* (SfBH, DOH, 2004), which were published in July 2004. All NHS organisations are required to take the SfBH into account when developing, providing and commissioning health care and the Healthcare Commission will use the standards as a key component of its assessments. HCSU will be working with the NHS and the Department of Health to ensure the standards are useful to staff, patients and other stakeholders. (Website: **www.hcsu.org.uk** accessed 30/6/08.) The Association of Palliative Day Care Leaders has modified the SfBH for day hospices to adopt as standards of best practice. (Website: **www.apdcl.org.uk** accessed 13/5/08.)

Activity 11: Identifying relevant standards

Make a list of the following where they exist in your clinical area and are relevant to the topic you have selected for audit:

- goals;
- objectives;
- clinical guidelines;
- protocols;
- care packages;
- standard statements.

Obtain copies of the documentation for these, together with a copy of the *Standards for better health* (DOH, 2004) or the Trent standards (Ahmedzai *et al.*, 1998). (See 'Preparation' at the beginning of this chapter for details of how to obtain these standards.) They may not be exactly what you need so try contacting the audit department or talk to a member of the care team at the local specialist palliative care service about clinical audit and standard setting. What kinds of strategies and standards do they have? Are they locally devised or adapted from national ones? If adapted from national standards, find out which standards they came from. If devised locally, ask if you could have a copy.

Feedback

It is probable that standards exist that are relevant to your audit topic, but they may not reflect local conditions very closely. We will go on to look at how you can set standards, possibly by altering existing standards to suit your needs, later in this section. Keep your notes with this book as you will need them for Activity 14.

If you have obtained standards relevant to your audit topic, you may still have to do some work on them to make them worthwhile implementing. There are problems that may be encountered when attempting to implement standards and we will look at these next.

Problems with standards and their implementation

There are a number of principles on which standards should be based. We recommend that your standards:

- are owned and controlled by practitioners;
- include the participation and involvement of practitioners;
- are patient/client focused;
- are situation based;
- set achievable standards;
- are potentially multidisciplinary (adapted from RCN, 1990).

However, in practice, you may have encountered standards that appear to be:

- imposed on practitioners by management;
- set by others with little or no consultation, e.g. core or generic standards;
- nurse or organisationally focused;
- lacking in relevance to local issues or problems;
- sometimes unrealistic considering the available resources;
- lacking in input from other disciplines.

Some of these are problems with the standards themselves and some are problems due to the way in which the standards are implemented.

Activity 12: Problems with standards

Discuss the problems inherent in creating standards for palliative care with your clinical audit group. Make notes of any problems you identify over and above the ones we have listed above and, for each problem, identify a solution, if possible.

Feedback

The problems we have listed above this activity can be solved by ensuring that standards are defined from the bottom up and involve consultation with patients and with other disciplines, which may in turn ensure that they are realistic and achievable. Other problems you may have identified include the fact that nursing standards are often mechanistic and reductionist. They describe only a small part of nursing and very few address the caring, empathetic, compassionate side of nursing. They are written in the language of theory – remote, impersonal and unfeeling – which trivialises and dehumanises nursing. Furthermore, the setting of uniform standards goes against the tenets of individualised care.

Schroeder (1988) identifies three other problems with standards.

- Confusing terminology. This has made it difficult for nurses to talk clearly, caused significant duplication in effort and resulted in so much confusion that the practising nurse who is supposed to use them is put off by their complexity or by the seeming irrelevance of semantics.
- A plethora of standards from a variety of sources. How do standards fit together to form an organised framework of care? How can standards from different sources be pulled together? How can national and local standards be integrated?
- The constantly changing health care environment. How can the contents of standards reflect changes in the health care environment, such as changes in throughput (e.g. more acutely ill patients)?

Bear these issues in mind when creating your standards and you may be able to minimise any problems you might encounter during the implementation phase. A further problem specific to palliative care is the definition and measurement of outcomes.

Outcomes in palliative care

When auditing palliative care, one problem is the measuring of outcomes:

> Outcome and quality of life measures need to be sensitive to the wider aspects of palliative care, not merely mortality, function, or absence of symptoms.
>
> Higginson (1999: 188)

However, there are at least four good reasons for using outcomes measures (Jenkinson, cited in Hearn and Higginson, 1997: 193). They enable you to:

- obtain more detailed information about the patient for clinical monitoring to aid and improve patient care;
- audit the care provided, by determining whether standards are being met and identify potential areas for improvement;
- compare services/care before and after the introduction of a service, which can be of value in assessing the efficacy of a service and the cost-effectiveness;

- use the analysis of the data generated to inform purchasers and thereby secure resources for future services.

We will look briefly at tools for measuring outcomes in 'Outcome measures', next.

Outcome measures

Hearn and Higginson (1997) state that information generated using outcome measures to measure the effectiveness of palliative care interventions is potentially invaluable but that that information is only as good as the method used to obtain it. They performed a review of 41 outcome measures to identify the ones that seemed to be the most useful in palliative care for patients with advanced cancer. The 12 outcome measures that met their criteria are:

- An Initial Assessment of Suffering (MacAdam and Smith, 1987);
- Edmonton Symptom Assessment Schedule (Bruera *et al.*, 1991);
- European Organisation for Research of Treatment of Cancer – EORTC QLQ-C30 (Aaronson *et al.*, 1993);
- Hebrew Rehabilitation Centre for Aged Quality of Life Index – HRCA-QL (Morris *et al.*, 1986);
- The McGill Quality of Life Questionnaire – MQOL (Cohen *et al.*, 1995);
- The McMaster Quality of Life Scale – MQLS (Sterkenburg and Woodward, 1996);
- Palliative Care Assessment – PACA (Ellershaw *et al.*, 1995);
- Palliative Care Core Standards – PCCS (Ahmedzai *et al.*, 1998);
- Rotterdam Symptom Checklist – RSCL (de Haes *et al.*, 1990);
- Support Team Assessment Schedule – STAS (Higginson, 1993);
- Symptom Distress Scales – SDS (McCorkle and Young, 1978);
- The Schedule for the Evaluation of Individual Quality of life – SEIQoL (O'Boyle *et al.*, 1994).

You might find one or more of these tools relevant when evaluating palliative care outcomes. A brief description of each of these tools is given in Hearn and Higginson (1997).

Another tool that you may find useful is POS (Palliative Care Outcome Scale – Higginson, 1998). We looked at this in Chapter 3. POS was developed in 1998, after Hearn and Higginson's (1997) research was completed. For details of POS, see: **www.kcl.ac.uk/schools/medicine/ depts/palliative/qat/pos.html** (site accessed 13/5/08). You need to register to use POS but registration is free.

When selecting a tool, make sure it has been validated for the use to which you wish to put it. Ask your AL facilitator or your local audit/clinical governance team for advice on how to do this. Many of these tools are designed for use by patients but there are challenges in involving patients receiving palliative care in the measurement of outcomes.

Activity 13: Challenges in measuring outcomes

Discuss the challenges that may be encountered when measuring outcomes in palliative care with your clinical audit group. Consider in particular patient-focused outcomes, i.e. those which require patients to complete self-report tools such as VASs or other forms of questionnaire or checklist. Consider also the validity of making a link between a specific intervention and the resulting outcome.

Feedback

A major challenge is that patients may die early during care, so you may not get a chance to ask them their opinions about the outcomes of care. They may be too ill or too fatigued to complete a questionnaire or survey by themselves or they may find it too difficult to concentrate. They may not wish to take part in audit or research, although some may be willing to do so if they believe it will improve things for others. If patients do agree to take part, they may adjust their responses so as not to offend or upset professionals or relatives. If the patient cannot participate directly, but agrees that a health care professional or relative or carer may complete a questionnaire on their behalf, the results may not be valid. Surveys completed by the family or professionals after a patient's death may not be true reflections of the patient's experience and responses may be affected by the family's grief. It may be difficult to demonstrate that a particular outcome was produced by a particular intervention or to illustrate that the interventions carried out had any impact at all on the client. Outcomes may have everything to do with the care provided or they might have nothing to do with it. Outcomes are particularly difficult to measure when the outcome is something that does not happen.

In this section so far we have looked at what we mean by the term standard, examples of relevant standards, problems with standards and challenges in measuring outcomes in palliative care. Earlier we mentioned that when identifying the criteria for your standard, the members of your clinical audit group might create impossibly long lists – we will look at how to cut those lists down to a more sensible size next.

Refining criteria

Morrell and Harvey (1999) suggest that you use the acronym DREAM to help you to remember the necessary attributes for your criteria:

D **Distinct** – does it identify something new, rather than repeating other criteria?

R **Relevant** – is it crucial to the achievement of the objective?

E **Evidence-based** – is the source of information clear?

A **Achievable** – is it realistic within current resources?

M **Measurable** – most importantly, can it be measured?

If you set a standard with criteria that do not have the DREAM attributes, the probability is that practice will not live up to the standard. Unfortunately, when it is realised that the standard is the problem, rather than practice, and that this is because the criteria are irrelevant, for example, or unachievable, the standard will be discredited and, possibly, the entire clinical audit process.

When creating your own standards, or amending existing standards, try to refine your criteria so that the standard can be easily audited. Note that national or generic standards have very wide topic areas – this enables them to be refined at local level.

Activity 14: Developing standards

When developing your standards, you need to share information with everyone who will be affected by the implementation of the standard and set up a feedback system so that they can tell you what they think. We will look at ways of doing this in the next section, 'Implementing best practice', as this is when it is most important, but you should start doing it now, if you haven't already done so.

1. From the information you collected in Activity 11, identify four or five standard statements that are relevant to your audit topic. Discuss the standards with your clinical audit group and identify the one that best expresses the statement of best practice for your topic. If there does not seem to be one, you will have to write a standard statement of your own – see the second part of this activity.

If you are going to use or alter an existing standard, you may need to contact the people who created it to obtain their permission to use it. You will need to agree with your clinical audit group what changes need to be made to it to make it relevant to your audit topic (if any). Remember to involve patients, so that they can have a say in the setting of outcomes. Check that the standard is expressed in terms of structure, process and outcome, and check the criteria using the DREAM acronym.

Remember to refer to the information you gathered in Activity 8 (Describe current practice) and Activity 10 (Reviewing available evidence) when writing your standard.

2. If you are making a brand-new standard, you will need to identify the criteria in terms of:

- structure;
- process;
- outcome (bearing in mind the issues surrounding palliative care outcomes).

Refine your criteria using the DREAM acronym.

Remember to refer to the information you gathered in Activity 8 (Describe current practice) and Activity 10 (Reviewing available evidence) when writing your standard.

Feedback

You should now have a statement of best practice expressed as an objective and accompanying criteria.

When you consider, for example, whether the structure and process criteria can easily be fulfilled within current resources, consider ways of overcoming this obstacle before implementing the standard. Can your manager obtain more resources? Will local charities provide funding for equipment, etc.? Contact a palliative care provider and ask for advice on overcoming problems related to structure and process.

Now that we have identified best practice, we need to implement it.

Clinical audit: Phase 2 – Implementing best practice

We will look at the following stages of implementing best practice:

- disseminate the standard;
- develop a monitoring tool;
- implement the criteria.

1. Disseminate the standard and develop a monitoring tool

Morrell and Harvey (1999) suggest the following ways of informing those who will be affected by the implementation of the standard:

- circulation of draft documents;
- notice boards;
- newsletters;
- hand-over meetings;
- other regular meetings;
- ward rounds.

Meetings and ward rounds may also act as feedback systems, where people can comment on the information you give them. Involving people like this is very important. If people feel that they have not been told what is happening or why, or they feel that any concerns they may have expressed about the standard have not been listened to, they are unlikely to implement it.

Next you need to develop a monitoring tool, i.e. something that enables you to measure whether a criterion has been achieved. Structure criteria (what you need) either exist or they do not. Process criteria (what you do) can either be observed directly (when someone does something) or the result of the process can be checked. With patient-focused outcome criteria (what you expect), it is usually best to ask patients about their experience of care. As we mentioned earlier, this may be difficult when working with patients who are receiving palliative care.

Tools may include checklists, questionnaires, interviews and written records or video recordings of care. If you are basing your standard on a clinical guideline, you may find that it includes an audit tool. You may remember that the standard shown in Figure 8.3 includes audit questions. It may be possible to re-order the phrases of your standard to create audit questions. For example, if the standard is 'X must happen at regular intervals and at least twice a day', your questions could include: 'Has X happened?', 'At what intervals has X occurred?', 'How often has X occurred in a 24-hour period?'. There may be other existing relevant measurement tools, like those we listed in 'Outcomes in palliative care', such as the Palliative Outcome Scale (Higginson, 1998) or the Edmonton Symptom Assessment System (Bruera *et al.*, 1991).

Activity 15: Develop a monitoring tool

1. Before attempting this activity, you may find it helpful to look through the sources of information listed at the end of this chapter, specifically those on the following topics:

- evaluation;
- questionnaires;
- research instruments.

Developing a monitoring tool is a skilled task and it may be better to identify an existing tool that will enable you to measure your criteria. Discuss existing monitoring tools with your clinical audit group and select the most appropriate one, if there is such a tool.

If there is no existing tool relevant to your criteria, contact the clinical audit staff within your organisation and draw on their expertise to create a valid monitoring tool.

2. Use your monitoring tool to measure how well or otherwise the criteria of your standard are currently being met.

Feedback

1. If you are having problems finding or creating a tool to measure your criteria, it may be a good idea to reassess the criteria – perhaps they are not measurable after all.

2. Your findings should mirror your description of current practice. It's also a good way of testing how practical your monitoring tool is and how measurable your criteria are.

This process of measuring what is happening before the implementation of the standard is known as 'collecting baseline data'. It gives you a baseline with which to compare the situation once your standard has been implemented. Small improvements that may have gone unnoticed should be apparent when compared with the baseline data.

Now that you have your monitoring tool and are confident in its use and in your ability to measure your criteria, the next step is to implement your standard.

2. Implement the criteria

You should already have been disseminating information about the standard. Before implementing the standard you must obtain more formal recognition from the senior staff within your organisation who will be responsible for agreeing the resources you will need to implement the standard. (Although this may not be necessary if you are performing a mini-audit.) These senior staff may be members of the clinical audit committee or quality steering group, or the clinical director or manager. You also need to agree a schedule for the implementation of the criteria and the standard as a whole. Remember that the idea is to analyse often – not to wait until huge amounts of data have been gathered (see Higginson's (1993) ARISE criteria, on p.16).

Activity 16: Implementing the criteria

Find out who will be responsible for authorising the resources for your project and make sure you have their formal agreement to the implementation before you go any further.

Before implementing your standard, make sure that you explain the purpose of the standard to the care team and explain why the clinical audit group felt it was necessary to devise a standard for this area of care. The care team should already be aware of the standard if you have been disseminating the standard by circulating draft documents, etc. as we recommended. However, an education session on the standard immediately before its implementation would be a good way of spreading information about the standard and the ways in which you intend to monitor compliance. People are more likely to become involved if they understand what they are doing and why.

Agree an implementation date for the standard and a series of evaluation dates for the criteria (i.e. when you will use your monitoring tool). For a relatively simple criterion, the evaluation date may be fairly short term, e.g. less than six weeks. But bear in mind that it's worth allowing time for people to become used to working to a standard before you evaluate the situation.

Feedback

It may take some time for an innovation in practice to take root, but it's worthwhile having intermediate target dates to check that the process is going smoothly. You may set a series of short-term, medium-term (less than six months) and long-term (more than six months) dates for evaluating the various criteria for your standard. Your results may suggest changes to the standard or the criteria, or steps that you should consider when your prepare to take action to improve the situation or when you prepare to re-audit.

Next we will look at monitoring the implementation of the standard.

Clinical audit: Phase 3 – Monitoring and comparing against best practice

The stages in this part of the clinical audit process are:

- identify sources of data and methods for sampling;
- collect valid and reliable data;
- compare the results to the objective.

We will look at each point in turn.

1. Identify sources of data and methods for sampling

The monitoring tool you developed for your audit project should be an ideal source of data. As we mentioned in the section on developing a monitoring tool, it may be:

- a checklist;
- a questionnaire;
- an interview;

- written records or video recordings of care;
- audit tools supplied as part of the implementation procedure for a clinical guideline;
- audit questions incorporated in a standard (as in Figure 8.3);
- other existing relevant measurement tools, like those we listed in 'Outcomes in palliative care'.

You may also find the following sources of data useful:

- patient records;
- hospital and GP information systems;
- cancer registries;
- infection control data;
- discharge data;
- contracts monitoring.

When preparing to use your monitoring tool, you need to consider how many people to seek feedback from and who those people should be. For example, you may not be able to survey everyone who is affected by your project if it affects a large number of people. You may just want to select a representative sample and extrapolate the results from their responses. There are two main categories of sampling – probability and non-probability sampling. Each of these categories includes a number of sub-categories, described briefly in Morrell and Harvey (1999: 51–3).

Activity 17: Data sources and sampling methods

Discuss with the members of your audit group whether it would be appropriate to use data from any of the sources identified above in addition to the data collected when using your monitoring tool. If any of the data sources is identified as being useful, agree who will be responsible for obtaining the data.

Read pp.51–7 of Morrell and Harvey (1999) for a brief overview of sampling methods. We recommend that you do more in-depth reading on the topics of sampling, data collection and comparison and analysis. Ask your librarian, AL set facilitator or your organisation's clinical audit/clinical governance team for advice on sources of useful information on these topics. We recommend that you start reading about data collection and comparison and analysis now, as these are complex topic areas. They are time-consuming and crucial to the project. The data you collect must be valid and reliable, and the comparisons you draw and analyses you make must be correct, as you are going to base your actions for improvement on them.

When you're doing your reading on sampling methods, you may find it helpful to discuss the different approaches with other members of your AL set. If you have identified a method that seems appropriate for your audit project, discuss the reasons for your choice. Your AL set may confirm your choice – or cause you to re-assess it. In either case, you will be better prepared when you discuss sampling methods with your audit group.

Discuss the variety of sampling methods available with your audit group, and agree:

- the method you will use;
- the sample size;
- the timeframe for data collection.

Feedback

Whether existing generic data is useful to you will depend on your audit topic. For example, if your audit topic is in the area of cancer care, then cancer registries will contain useful data.

The background work you have done on sampling methods should have ensured that the members of your audit group have chosen the most appropriate method of sampling for your audit topic. If you are concerned that they have not, approach the subject again. There is no point in collecting data from the wrong people. The sample size should be neither too big nor too small. With too large a sample, data collectors (or auditors) may become discouraged, or the timeframe may turn out to be unrealistic. As sample size decreases, you cannot place as much confidence in your results. (Although here we are considering a quantitative approach, which we looked at in 'What is evidence?' Sample sizes in qualitative research are often small but the researchers may not be trying to extrapolate the results of their sample into the wider population.) When discussing the timeframe for data collection, remember to allow for expected absences such as annual leave, unexpected occurrences such as illness and seasonal variations in your audit sample – cold weather and flu viruses regularly increase the numbers of elderly people requiring care, for example.

2. Collect valid and reliable data

Before collecting your data, you need to agree with your audit group who will collect the data (the auditor). There may be one auditor or several and they need not belong to the audit group. Auditors may either be impartial observers of the area being audited, or they may be representatives from groups directly affected by the audit. If you are performing a mini-audit, you may consider doing the data collection yourself but bear in mind that it may be worth considering asking a colleague to do it for you. The people you survey may give you the answers they think you want to hear, but be more forthcoming with an impartial auditor.

It is also necessary to make contact with the people who make up your audit sample. Through letters, meetings and other forms of contact, you need to explain to the members of the audit sample what help you require in the data collection process and why. You should answer any questions about the audit project, make sure that it is clear that they are not under any obligation to take part and that they can drop out at any point in the process. Your ethics committee may require you to obtain written consent from everyone involved in providing data to your auditors. Depending on your sample and your audit tool, you may be able to (or have to) do this some time in advance of the data collection process. Alternatively, auditors may take these steps immediately before the interview or other form of data collection.

The decision on how to collect the data may already have been made – for example, a monitoring tool in the form of a questionnaire or checklist is also a data collection sheet. Otherwise, you may need to create data collection sheets, using word processing or spreadsheet software, or specialised audit software.

3. Compare the results to the objective

The way in which you compare and analyse your data will depend on whether it is quantitative or qualitative.

Quantitative data

Quantitative data can be analysed in a huge number of ways, from simple approaches such as pie charts, bar charts and histograms, through to the use of extremely complex statistical software packages. If you have already done some background reading on data collection and comparison and analysis, you may have been amazed by the number of approaches possible. Factors to consider when identifying the way in which you will perform comparison and analysis include the timeframe and your familiarity with the various approaches.

Will you be able to perform the analysis in time? If you have any doubt, consider choosing a method that is simple and therefore quick to learn and apply or with which you are already familiar. These should also be your criteria from the point of view of accuracy. You don't want to waste all the effort people have already put into the project by making mistakes at this point. If you feel that you cannot perform the comparison and analysis to a suitably high standard, there may be someone in the clinical audit group who may be able to perform this task or your organisation's clinical audit staff may be able to help you.

Your aim is to show the differences between current practice and best practice as identified in your standard. However, it is probable that practice has been improving during the implementation phase. You may therefore find it useful to compare and analyse your baseline data from Activity 15 with current practice (if you have time). If you can show that improvements in practice occurred during implementation, people may view your audit project more favourably, which will help with the continuation of the process.

Qualitative data

Qualitative data includes notes from interviews or observations of care and transcripts from tape and video recordings. Interpreting qualitative data is also a skilled activity and you may need to draw upon the expertise of your organisation's clinical audit staff. Morrell and Harvey (1999: 66) make the following simple practical suggestions:

- Use post-it notes to cluster comments together;
- Use different coloured highlighter pens to pick out data on different themes;
- Cluster narrative data together – either with scissors and glue or by using the cut and paste functions in word-processing software.

This next activity is about collecting data (Step 2) and analysing data (Step 3). Unless your sample is very small, it may take you some considerable time to complete. However, don't wait until you have collected all the data before you start to compare and analyse it with the standard. If you start analysing as you go along, you may identify problems with the standard, the criteria, the monitoring tool or data collection sheets. If you can address these problems quickly at the start of the analysis, you improve the confidence that can be put in your final results. On the other hand, don't change things continually throughout the process – your results will be clouded by uncertainties about what you were measuring and how.

Activity 18: Collecting and analysing data

If you haven't done any background reading on these topics, we recommend that you do it now. If you need help with specific areas, contact the clinical audit staff in your organisation.

1. Discuss the analysis and comparison of the data with the members of your clinical audit group. Has anyone any experience with these tasks, and would they be able/willing to perform them for this project? If the members of your audit group feel that interpreting the data is not something they are going to be able to do well, contact your organisation's clinical audit staff. They may be able to give you practical help, or they may

be able to offer advice on what resources are available to help you (books, videos, workshops, etc.). Agree with your clinical audit group who will interpret the results and what methods they will use to do so. If you are performing a mini-audit, and feel confident about performing the analysis and comparison, you may decide to do it yourself.

2. Before collecting the data, ensure your clinical audit group has taken the following three steps.

- Identify who will collect the data.
- Contact the members of your sample, and obtain their consent.
- If your monitoring tool is not also a data collection sheet, devise appropriate data collection sheets. If you need help, your librarian, AL set facilitator or your organisation's clinical audit staff may be able to recommend useful resources.

Now that you have done the preparation work, equip the auditors with the monitoring tool (and data collection sheet, if different from the monitoring tool). The auditors should then start collecting data from your sample. Remind the auditors that participants have the right to drop out at any point in the data collection process.

3. The auditors should pass the data collection sheets to the person responsible for comparing and analysing the data as soon as each sheet, or a batch of sheets, is completed.

The analyst should compare current practice as described by the data collection sheets with best practice as expressed by your standard. He or she should analyse the differences between current and best practice. The analyst should present a summary of the findings to the clinical audit group so that members can start trying to identify reasons for any significant variation between the standard and current practice. (There is an example of an audit summary form on p.190 of Morrell and Harvey (1999).)

Feedback

If there is a great deal of variation between your standard and current practice, investigate where the problem lies – is it with the standard or with practice? Bearing in mind that one of the DREAM criteria is 'achievable', it should be possible for the care provided to reach the standard you have set. If current practice differs a great deal from the standard set, review the standard – it may need to be revised upwards in cases of high achievement, and possibly downwards in cases of low achievement.

In the case of low achievement, you need to investigate what factors have caused it, and identify what can be done to compensate for them and to improve practice. Investigate the factors that resulted in high achievement, and consider how they can be extended to areas of low achievement. We will look at taking action to improve practice next.

Clinical audit: Phase 4 – Taking action to improve

This is a vital part of the clinical audit process. A great deal of work is involved in the previous three phases and it would be a shame to waste all that work by not taking action based on the data you have collected and analysed. Taking action to improve is the central challenge of quality improvement, as changing practice is rarely straightforward.

Morrell and Harvey (1999) suggest that this part of the audit process comprises three stages:

- feedback to participants;
- generate a team action plan and implement;
- re-audit and evaluate.

We will look at each stage in turn.

1. Feedback to participants

The data analyst provides feedback to the clinical audit group in the form of the audit summary. After discussion of the summary, members of the clinical audit group communicate the results of the data analysis process to the groups they represent. It's vital to include positive findings where the standard has been achieved or improved upon, as people are sometimes suspicious of initiatives like clinical audit and may feel that it is a management tool for highlighting poor individual performance. Patients, staff and others involved in the project are then encouraged to comment on the results. You may also find it helpful to obtain their help in interpreting the results, identifying necessary changes in practice and making action plans for improving practice.

When communicating the findings to others, consider the requirements of your audience, and bear in mind that different audiences may prefer the information to be presented in different ways. A thorough comparison and analysis presented as a lengthy report may be suitable for one audience, while for another the audit summary may do, while for another diagrammatic representations such as pie charts, etc. may be more suitable.

2. Generate a team action plan and implement

Having identified areas where current practice differs from best practice as expressed in your standard, you need to identify the problems that must be solved and any positive factors related to areas of high achievement that could be extended to areas of low achievement. Based

393

on these problems and positive factors, and on your earlier research into available evidence in the area of your audit topic, you need to identify what changes to make to improve practice and how to implement those changes. We look at these issues in 'Evaluating possible courses of action' and 'Strategies for change' below.

Evaluating possible courses of action

Interpreting the results of your audit and planning to improve practice involves choosing between possible courses of action. Techniques for doing this include:

- **Boardstorming (or Quick think).** The facilitator of your clinical audit group encourages people to explore an issue by saying whatever comes into their heads. Each point is recorded, however silly, wild or impossible it may seem. The facilitator does not allow any 'for and against' discussion or value judgements to take place. When no more ideas are forthcoming, the facilitator helps the group to look at all the ideas and engage in a 'for and against' debate. Eventually, ideas considered to be worth further exploration are identified.
- **Forcefield analysis.** This technique helps people to look at the driving and restraining forces acting on a situation. Driving forces are factors that indicate instability and an openness to change. They are positive forces for change. Restraining forces are those which promote stability and maintain the status quo, indicating resistance to change. The facilitator writes 'driving forces' at the top of a flipchart sheet, 'current situation' in the middle and 'restraining forces' at the bottom. Group members are invited to suggest the driving and restraining forces that are put on the flipchart. The forces are then analysed by the group to determine the needs and priorities to be addressed in improving supervision. See Chapter 6 of Bowman (1990: 99–114) for further information on forcefield analysis.
- **SWOT analysis.** This technique is similar to forcefield analysis in that it is a method for identifying promoters of and opponents to change. The four key dimensions are Strengths, Weaknesses, Opportunities and Threats (now often referred to as limitations). The facilitator divides the flipchart into four squares and heads each square with one of the key headings (Figure 8.4).

Group members then suggest topics or issues that should be listed under each heading. Once the lists are drawn up, group members discuss how to take advantage of strengths and opportunities, and minimise weaknesses and threats/limitations. See Chapter 4 of McGrother (1995: 12–15) for further information on SWOT analysis.

Strengths	Weaknesses
Opportunities	Threats/limitations

Figure 8.4 Grid for SWOT analysis

Activity 19: Decision making

Review a recent change that has affected you and your team. Explain the methods of boardstorming, forcefield analysis and SWOT analysis to your team (if they are unaware of them) and choose one method to analyse the change.

Analyse the change using your chosen method and make notes of any ways of improving the implementation of the change that are identified by your analysis that seem not to have been addressed in the actual implementation of the change.

Feedback

Discuss your notes with your manager, with a view to improving the implementation of the change.

Strategies for change

Instigating change may include changing attitudes, skills and relationships within the team, and knowledge and intellectual rationales for action and practice (Chin and Benne, 1985). Chin and Benne (1976) identified three theories of what may underpin responses to change:

- **Rational-empirical** – people are rational and will therefore adopt proposed changes if those changes can be rationally justified and it can be shown that they will gain from the changes.
- **Power-coercive** – change is introduced by those in power and those with less power simply comply.

- **Normative-re-educative** – this theory builds on the rational-empirical theory but allows for the fact that people generally comply with the norms of their organisation's culture. Therefore, for a change to be adopted it has to be absorbed into the organisation's culture and become the new norm.

Morrell and Harvey (1999) state that it is best to use a normative-re-educative approach to change within an improvement-based approach to clinical audit, as this approach views staff as partners in the change process and values their contributions.

A normative-re-educative model that you may find particularly helpful in implementing changes in nursing practice is Titchen's model of critical companionship. You may remember reading about this model in the 'Introduction to this textbook'. Reflective practice is also useful for implementing changes in practice and you have been reflecting on your practice as you worked through the rest of the book – using either the model we introduced in Chapter 2 or another with which you were already familiar.

Activity 20: Team action planning

With the members of your clinical audit group, discuss the findings outlined in the audit summary. Communicate these findings to the patient and professional groups involved in the audit project. Ask for their feedback and invite their participation in the interpretation and action-planning phases.

With the members of your clinical audit group, and other members of professional and patient groups who are participating, interpret the results of the data comparison and analysis and evaluate the best course of action for improving practice. Use one or more of the decision-making methods discussed above.

Identify how the change will be introduced into practice. Are there existing structures that may be used, e.g. critical companionship, clinical supervision? If not, how can such structures be introduced? Change and practice improvement are complex and often difficult issues, so you may once again need to contact your organisation's clinical audit staff for help and advice.

With the members of your clinical audit group, create a team action plan for implementing change. You may like to base it on the action plan in the 'Introduction to this textbook'. At the very least, your plan should contain:

- details of the course of action;
- names and contact details of the people responsible for each stage or task;
- timeframe for each stage or task.

Start implementing the change in accordance with your action plan.

Feedback

It's important to agree a good, clear action plan before implementing the change. A poorly thought-out action plan is unlikely to lead to effective changes in practice. At the end of the agreed timeframe, the situation should be re-audited. We will look at this next.

3. Re-audit and evaluate

When preparing to re-audit the standard, you may also wish to review:

- the available evidence;
- your monitoring tool;
- other sources of data;
- your sampling methods.

On the other hand, you don't want to change your approach too much between the audit and the re-audit, as the comparison between the two may be invalidated by your changes. The comparison should enable you to evaluate what improvements have been made and what areas require further improvement. At this point you have completed one entire audit cycle.

However, it doesn't stop there. On completing the re-auditing stage, Morrell and Harvey (1999) identify three possible further steps:

- If problems remain or new problems are identified, the group plans further action and re-audits as before.
- If they are achieving the standard, the group may elect to raise the expected level of achievement of the standard in order to aim for further improvement.
- If the standard reflects best practice, the group may set a timetable for regular re-audit and review of the standard.

Activity 21: Re-audit and beyond

Re-audit your standard, comparing your results with those from the previous audit.

With the members of your clinical audit, agree which of the three possible further steps identified above it is appropriate to take with regard to this standard.

Agree an action plan for the agreed next step, and implement it.

Feedback

Remember that clinical audit is a cyclical process. A standard can always be raised to further improve the quality of care. When best practice is achieved, it is still important to re-audit. Improvements in practice should be celebrated, and audit is a way of identifying those improvements. And there are always other topics you can audit!

Clinical audit is a very useful quality improvement tool but only if it meets certain standards itself. We look at these in Activity 22.

Activity 22: Evaluating the process of clinical audit

Use the following questions to consider the process of clinical audit in your workplace.

- Involvement of patients: are there mechanisms for involving users of the service and their families?
- Multiprofessional team building: by examining working practices, does clinical audit highlight new ways of collaborating and confirm the importance of developing patient care as a team?
- Implementing clinical practice guidelines: does your audit process involve the implementation, monitoring and evaluation of clinical guidelines?
- Support for clinical audit: are there systems, structures and staff in place in your organisation to support quality improvement initiatives?
- Integration with organisational quality: is clinical audit clearly integrated into your organisation's quality strategy and business planning agendas and linked clearly with all other quality improvements and practice development initiatives?
- Links with education and professional development: are the learning needs identified by clinical audit being met through professional training?
- The role of the purchaser in clinical audit: is there multiprofessional input to the purchasing of clinical audit, including primary care groups?
- Standards: are standards based on current evidence of best practice? Are the criteria refined using the DREAM acronym?
- Ethical issues: are issues of rigour, confidentiality and consent carefully considered when planning clinical audit initiatives?
- Links with research and development: are the standards against which practice is to be audited based on good research evidence where that evidence exists?

Feedback

If the answer to any of these questions is 'no', discuss the issue with your clinical audit group. Clinical audit can only be effective in the development of evidence-based, high-quality care if the criteria identified in this activity can be achieved.

SUMMARY

In this chapter we have looked at clinical governance and the importance of evidence-based practice. We have taken you through the clinical audit process and looked in particular at the issues surrounding setting standards and measuring outcomes in palliative care. Having completed this chapter, you should be able to:

- discuss the impact of clinical governance on the provision of palliative care within your care setting;
- explain how evidence-based practice can improve the standard of palliative care provided to patients;
- explain the process of clinical audit;
- perform a clinical audit in your workplace by:
  - defining best practice,
  - implementing best practice,
  - monitoring and comparing against best practice,
  - taking action to improve
- evaluate the process of clinical audit.

USEFUL WEBSITES

www.bournemouth.ac.uk/library/resources/nursing.html and **www.ovid. com/site/catalog/DataBase/28.jsp**
Information on the British Nursing Index. Sites accessed 13/5/08.

www.cinahl.com
Homepage of the Cumulative Index of Nursing and Allied Health Literature. Site accessed 13/5/08.

www.dh.gov.uk/en/Publicationsandstatistics/Publications/Publications PolicyAndGuidance/Browsdale/DH_4098139
The NHS Cancer Plan. Site accessed 13/5/08.

www.dh.gov.uk/en/Publicationsandstatistics/Publications/Publications PolicyAndGuidance/Browsdale/DH_4005475
You can download copies of the Department of Health publication *Essence of Care* from this website. Site accessed 13/5/08.

www2.edc.org/lastacts
Homepage of the online journal *Innovations in End-of-Life Care*. You need to register with the journal to access these pages, but registration is free. Site accessed 13/5/08.

www.elib.scot.nhs.uk
Access to evidence for journals, books and databases for NHS and related staff in Scotland. Site accessed 13/5/08.

www.healthcarecommission.org.uk/homepage.cfm
Homepage of the Healthcare Commission. Site accessed 13/5/08.

www.ncchta.org
Homepage of the Health Technology Assessment programme. Site accessed 13/5/08.

www.jr2.ox.ac.uk/cochrane
The Cochrane Pain, Palliative Care and Supportive Care (PaPaS) Collaborative Review Group. Site accessed 13/5/08.

www.medscape.com
MEDLINE homepage. Site accessed 13/5/08.

www.library.nhs.uk
Electronic library for NHS and related staff in England and Northern Ireland. Site accessed 13/5/08.

www.nhshealthquality.org
Homepage of NHS Quality Improvement Scotland. Site accessed 13/5/08.

www.nice.org.uk
Homepage of the National Institute for Clinical Excellence. Site accessed 13/5/08.

www.palliativecarescotland.org.uk
Homepage of the Scottish Partnership for Palliative Care. Site accessed 13/5/08.

www.scotland.gov.uk/library3/health/csac-00.asp
You can download *Cancer in Scotland: Action for change* from this website. Site accessed 13/5/08.

www.sign.ac.uk
Homepage of the Scottish Intercollegiate Guidelines Network. Site accessed 13/5/08.

www.wales.nhs.uk/ehl
The electronic library for NHS and related staff in Wales. Site accessed 13/5/08.

www.york.ac.uk/inst/crd
The homepage of the NHS Centre for Reviews and Dissemination. Site accessed 13/5/08.

RECOMMENDED SOURCES OF INFORMATION

Titles followed by O/P are out of print – but you may be able to find library copies.

Change/facilitation

Adair, J. (1988) *Effective teambuilding.* Aldershot: Gower.

Beer, M. (1980) *Organization change and development.* Santa Monica, CA: Goodyear Publishing Company. O/P

Binnie, A. and Titchen, A. (1999) *Freedom to practise: a study of the development of patient-centred nursing in an acute medicate unit.* Oxford: Butterworth-Heinemann.

Fretwell, J.E. (1985) *Freedom to change.* London: Royal College of Nursing. O/P

Harvey, G. (1993) *Which way to quality? A study of the implementation of four quality assurance tools.* Report no. 5. Oxford: National Institute for Nursing.

Hegyvary, S.T. (1982) *The change to primary nursing: a cross-cultural view of professional nursing practice.* St Louis: CV Mosby. O/P

Loftus-Hills, A. and Harvey, G. (2000) *A review of the role of facilitators in changing professional healthcare practice.* Oxford: Royal College of Nursing Institute.

Morison, M.J. (1992) 'Promoting the motivation to change: the role of facilitative leadership in quality assurance'. *Professional Nurse,* 7(11), pp.715–18.

Morrison, P. and Burnard, P. (1997) *Caring and communicating: the interpersonal relationship in nursing. Facilitators' manual* (2nd Ed.). Basingstoke: Macmillan.

Ottaway, R. N. (1976) 'A change strategy to implement new norms, new style and new environment in the work organization'. *Personnel Review,* 5(1), pp.13–18.

Pearson, A. (1992) *Nursing at Burford: a story of change.* London: Scutari Press. O/P

Smith, G. (1986) 'Resistance to change in geriatric care'. *International Journal of Nursing Studies,* 3(1), pp.61–70.

Titchen, A. and Binnie, A. (1993a) 'A double act: co-action researcher roles in an acute hospital setting', in *Changing nursing practice through action research.* Report no. 6. Oxford: National Institute for Nursing. O/P

Titchen, A. and Binnie, A. (1993b) 'A unified action research strategy in nursing'. *Educational Action Research,* 1(1), pp.25–33.

Titchen, A. and Binnie, A. (1993c) 'Research partnerships: collaborative action research in nursing'. *Journal of Advanced Nursing,* 18, pp.858–65.

Titchen, A. and Binnie, A. (1993d) 'Changing power relationships between nurses: a case study of early changes towards patient-centred nursing'. *Journal of Clinical Nursing,* 2, pp.219–29.

Titchen, A. and Binnie, A. (1993e) 'What am I meant to be doing?: Putting practice into theory and back again'. *Journal of Advanced Nursing,* 18, pp.1054–65.

Towell, D. (1979) 'A "social systems" approach to research and change in nursing care'. *International Journal of Nursing Studies*, 16, pp.111–21.

Towell, D. and Dartington, T. (1976) 'Encouraging innovations in hospital care'. *Journal of Advanced Nursing*, 1, pp.391–8.

Upton, T. and Brooks, B. (1995) *Managing change in the NHS*. Buckingham: Open University Press.

Clinical effectiveness

Clinical Resource and Audit Group (1992) *Clinical outcome measures: executive summary*. Edinburgh: CRAG.

Closs, S. and Cheakes, F. (1996) 'Audit or research – what is the difference?' *Journal of Clinical Nursing*, 5, pp.249–56.

Higginson, I. (1993) *Clinical audit in palliative care*. Oxford: Radcliffe Medical Press.

Scottish Office Clinical Resource Audit Group (1993) *The interface between clinical audit and management: a report of a working group set up by the Clinical Resource and Audit Group*. Edinburgh: CRAG.

Scottish Partnership for Palliative Care (2003a) *Public awareness of palliative care*. Edinburgh: SPCC. Available from: **www.palliativecare scotland.org.uk/publications/aware.pdf** (site accessed 13/5/08).

Scottish Partnership for Palliative Care (2003b) *Beyond the randomised trial: evidence and effectiveness in palliative care*. Edinburgh: SPPC. Available from: **www.palliativecarescotland.org.uk/publications/ Beyond the randomised trial.pdf** (site accessed 13/5/08).

Thompson, G. and McClement, S. (2002) 'Defining and determining quality in end of life care'. *International Journal of Palliative Nursing*, 8(6), pp.288–93.

Welsh Office (1995a) *Improving access to evidence and information: a clinical effectiveness initiative for Wales*. London: Central Office of Information.

Welsh Office (1995b) *Towards evidence based practice: a clinical effectiveness initiative for Wales*. London: Central Office of Information.

Welsh Office (1996) *Framework for the development of multi-professional clinical audit in Wales: clinical effectiveness initiative for Wales*. London: Central Office of Information.

Clinical governance

Department of Health (1998) *A first class service: quality in the new NHS*. London: HMSO. Available from: **www.dh.gov.uk/en/Publications AndStatistics/Publications/PublicationsPolicyAndGuidance/DH_ 4006902** (site accessed 13/5/08).

Royal College of Nursing (1998) *Guidance for nurses on clinical governance* (2nd Ed.). London: Royal College of Nursing.

Royal College of Nursing (2000) *Clinical governance: how nurses can get involved*. London: Royal College of Nursing.

Scottish Office Department of Health Management Executive (1998) *Clinical governance* MEL (1998)75. Scotland: SODHME.

Scottish Office Department of Health Management Executive (1997) *Designed to care: renewing the National Health Service in Scotland*. Cm. 3811 White paper. London: HMSO.

Clinical guidelines

Development of clinical guidelines

Duff, L.A., Kitson, A.L., Seers, K. and Humphris, D. (1996) 'Clinical guidelines: an introduction to their development and implementation'. *Journal of Advanced Nursing*, 23, pp.887–95.

Eccles, M., Clapp, Z., Grimshaw, J., Adams, P.C., Higgins, B., Purves, I. and Russell, I. (1996) 'Developing valid guidelines: methodological and procedural issues from the North of England evidence based guideline development project'. *Quality in Health Care*, 5, pp.44–50.

Grimshaw, J.M. and Russell, I.T. (1993) 'Achieving health gain through clinical guidelines I: Developing scientifically valid guidelines'. *Quality in Health Care*, 2, pp.243–8.

Lomas, J. (1993) 'Making clinical policy explicit: legislative policy making and lessons for developing practice guidelines'. *International Journal of Technology Assessment in Health Care*, 9, pp.11–25.

Murphy, M.K., Sanderson, C.F., Black, N.A., Askham, J., Lamping, D.L., Marteau, T. and McKee, C.M. (1998) 'Consensus development methods and their use in clinical guideline development'. *Health Technology Assessment*, 2, p.3.

Thomas, K. (2003) *Caring for the dying at home: companions on the journey*. Oxford: Radcliffe Medical Press.

Woolf, S.H. (1991) *Manual for clinical practice guideline development*. 1991 AHCPR, Washington, USA: US Department of Health and Human Services.

Woolf, S. (1996) 'Developing evidence-based clinical practice guidelines'. *Annual Review of Public Health*, 17, pp.511–38

General reading on guidelines

Clinical Resource and Audit Group (1993) *Clinical guidelines: a report by a working group set up by the Clinical Resource and Audit Group*. Edinburgh: Scottish Office.

Duff, L., Loftus-Hills, A. and Morrell, C. (2000) *Clinical guidelines for the management of venous leg ulcers: implementation guide*. London: Royal College of Nursing.

Eddy, D. (1990) 'The challenge'. *Journal of the American Medical Association*, 263, pp.287–90.

Institute for Medicine (1992) *Guidelines for clinical practice: from development to use*. Washington, DC: National Academy Press.

McClarey, M. and Duff, L. (1997) 'Making sense of clinical guidelines'. *Nursing Standard*, 12(1), pp.24–6.

McNicol, M., Layton, A. and Morgan, G. (1993) 'Team working: the key to implementing guidelines (editorial)'. *Quality in Health Care*, 2, pp.215–16.

NHS Executive (1996) *Clinical guidelines. Using clinical guidelines to improve patient care within the NHS*. London: HMSO.

Scottish Intercollegiate Guidelines Network (1995) *Clinical guidelines: criteria for appraisal for national use* (SIGN Publication No. 1). Edinburgh: SIGN.

Sheldon, T.A. (1994) 'Quality: link with effectiveness'. *Quality in Health Care*, 3(Supplement), pp.S41–S45.

Wilson, M.C., Hayward, R.S.A., Tunis, S.R., Bass, E.B. and Guyatt, G. (1995) 'Users' guides to the medical literature. VIII. How to use clinical practice guidelines. A. What are the recommendations and will they help you in caring for your patients?' *Journal of the American Medical Association*, 274(20), pp.1630–2.

Reading on using guidelines

Duff, L.A., Kitson, A.L., Seers, K. and Humphris, D. (1996) 'Clinical guidelines: an introduction to their development and implementation'. *Journal of Advanced Nursing*, 23, pp.887–95.

Grimshaw, J.M. and Russell, I.T. (1993) 'Effect of clinical guidelines on medical practice: a systematic review of rigorous evaluations'. *The Lancet*, 342, pp.1317–22.

Grimshaw, J.M. and Russell, I. (1994) 'Achieving health gain through clinical guidelines II: Ensuring guidelines change medical practice'. *Quality in Health Care*, 3, pp.45–52.

Shiffman, R.N. (1997) 'Representation of clinical practice guidelines in conventional and augmented decision tables'. *Journal of the American Medical Informatics Association*, 4(5), pp.382–93.

Thomas, L.H., McColl, E., Cullum, N., Rousseau, N., Soutter, J. and Steen, N. (1998) 'Effect of clinical guidelines in nursing, midwifery, and the therapies: a systematic review of evaluations'. *Quality in Health Care*, 7, pp.183–91.

Critical appraisal

Cochrane Collaboration (2006) *Cochrane handbook for systematic reviews of interventions 4.2.6*. Oxford: The Cochrane Library. Available from: **www.cochrane.org/resources/handbook/Handbook4.2.6Sep2006.pdf** (site accessed 13/5/08).

Goodman, C. (1993) *Literature searching and evidence interpretation for assessing health care practices*. Stockholm: SBU: Swedish Council on Technology Assessment in Health Care.

Greenhalgh, T. (1997) 'Assessing the methodological quality of published papers'. *British Medical Journal*, 315, pp.305–8.

Greenhalgh, T. (2006) *How to read a paper* (3rd Ed.). Malden: BMJ Publishing.

National Health Service Centre for Reviews and Dissemination (1996) *Undertaking systematic reviews of research on effectiveness. CRD guidelines for those carrying out or commissioning reviews*. CRD Report 4. York: University of York.

Evaluation

Beck, E.J. and Adams, S.A. (editors) (1990) *The White Paper and beyond*. Oxford: Oxford University Press. O/P.

Bergman, R. (1982) 'Evaluation of nursing care: could it make a difference?' *International Journal of Nursing Studies*, 19(2), pp.53–60.

Bergman, R. and Golander, H. (1982) 'Evaluation of care of the aged: a multi-purpose guide'. *Journal of Advanced Nursing*, 7, pp.203–10.

Bloch, D. (1975) 'Evaluation of nursing care in terms of process and outcome: issues in research and quality assurance'. *Nursing Research*, 24(4), pp.256–63.

Bond, S. and Thomas, L.H. (1991) 'Issues in measuring outcomes of nursing'. *Journal of Advanced Nursing*, 16(12), pp.1492–502.

Challis, D. (1981) 'The measurement of outcome in social care of the elderly'. *Journal of Social Policy*, 10(2), pp.179–208.

Clare, A.W. (1990) 'Some conclusions', in Hopkins, A. and Costain, D. (editors) *Measuring the outcomes of medical care*. London: Royal College of Physicians, pp.105–9. O/P

Cook, T.D. and Shadish, W.R. (1986) 'Program evaluation: the worldly science'. *Annual Review of Psychology*, 37, pp.193–232.

Crow, R. (1984) 'Criteria for evaluation'. Research paper presented at 'Nursing Research: Does it make a difference?' *Workshop of European Nurse Researchers*, April. London.

Davies, L. (1987) 'Ordinary life: does it cost more?' *Health Service Journal*, 97(5039), p.221.

Deming, W.E. (2000) *Out of the crisis* (2nd Ed.). Cambridge: MIT Press.

Donabedian, A. (1966) 'Evaluating the quality of medical care'. *Milbank Memorial Fund Quarterly*, 44, Part 2, pp.166–206.

Donabedian, A. (1980) 'The definition of quality and approaches to its assessment'. *Explorations in Quality Assessment and Monitoring*, Vol. 1. Ann Arbor: Health Administration Press. O/P.

Ellis, R. (editor) (1988) *Professional competence and quality assurance in the caring professions*. London: Chapman Hall. O/P.

Ellis, R. and Whittington, D. (1993) *Quality assurance in health care: a handbook*. London: Edward Arnold. O/P.

Ethridge, P.E. and Packard, R.W. (1976) 'An innovative approach to measurement of quality through utilisation of nursing care plans'. *Journal of Nursing Administration*, 6(1), pp.25–31.

Giovannetti, P.B., Ratner, P.A., Buchan, J., Bay, K. and Reid, D. (1992) 'Survey of nursing quality assurance programs in selected hospitals in Alberta, Canada'. *International Journal of Nursing Studies*, 29(3), pp.301–13.

Goldberg, E.M. and Connelly, N. (1982) *The effectiveness of social care for the elderly: an overview of recent and current evaluative research*. London: Heinemann Educational Books.

Guba, E.G. and Lincoln, Y.G. (1989) *Fourth generation evaluation*. Newbury Park: Sage.

Horrocks, P. (1985) 'Performance indicators'. *Health and Social Services Journal*, 94(4954), p.803.

Jennings, B.W. (1991) 'Patient outcome research: seizing the opportunity'. *Advances in Nursing Science*, 14(2), pp.59–72.

Juran, J.M. (1988) *Juran on planning for quality*. New York: The Free Press. O/P.

Kitson, A.L. (1986) 'Indicators of quality in nursing care – an alternative approach'. *Journal of Advanced Nursing*, 11(2), pp.133–44.

Kitson, A.L. (1991) *Therapeutic nursing and the hospitalised elderly*. Harrow: Scutari. O/P.

Kitson, A.L. and Harvey, G. (1991) *Bibliography of nursing quality assurance and standards of care 1932–1987*. Harrow: Scutari. O/P

Luker, K. (1981) 'An overview of evaluation research in nursing'. *Journal of Advanced Nursing*, 6, pp.87–93.

Madus, G.F., Scriven, M.S. and Stufflebeam, D.L. (1983) *Evaluation models*. Boston: Klurver-Nijhoff Publishing.

Marsland, D. and Gissane, C. (1992) 'Nursing evaluation: purposes, achievements and opportunities'. *International Journal of Nursing Studies*, 29(3), pp.231–6.

Maxwell, R.J. (1984) 'Quality assessment in health'. *British Medical Journal*, 288, pp.1470–2.

McDowell, I. and Newell, C. (2006) *Measuring health. A guide to rating scales and questionnaires* (3rd Ed.). Oxford: Oxford University Press.

Megivern, K., Halm, M.A. and Jones, G. (1992) 'Measuring patient satisfaction as an outcome of nursing care'. *Journal of Nursing Care Quality*, 6(4), pp.9–24.

Robbins, M. (1998) *Evaluating palliative care: establishing the evidence base*. Oxford: Oxford University Press.

Evidence-based practice

Bury, T. and Mead, J. (1998) *Evidence based healthcare: a guide for therapists*. Oxford: Butterworth Heinemann. O/P.

Crombie, I.K. (2007) *Pocket guide to critical appraisal* (2nd Ed.). Oxford: Blackwell.

Crump, B. and Drummond, M.F. (1993) *Evaluating clinical evidence: a handbook for managers*. London: Longman. O/P.

Dunning, M., Abi-Aad, G., Gilbert *et al.* (1998) *Turning evidence into everyday practice*. London: Kings Fund.

Entwistle, V., Watt, I.S. and Herring, J.E. (1996) *Information about health care effectiveness*. London: Kings Fund. O/P.

Greenhalgh, T. (1997) *How to read a paper: the basics of evidence based medicine*. London: BMJ Publishing.

Hope, T. (1997) *Evidence-based patient choice*. London: King's Fund.

Muir Gray, J.A. (1996) *Evidence-based health care*. Edinburgh: Churchill Livingstone. O/P.

NHSE (Anglia and Oxford Region) (2002) *The evidence-based health care open learning resource* (2nd Ed.). Available from Update Software Ltd, Summertown Pavilion, Middle Way, Oxford OX2 7LG. Tel. 01865 513902; Fax 01865 516918; e-mail **info@update.co.uk**

Policy documents

Department of Health (1995) *A policy for commissioning cancer services. A report by the expert advisor group on cancer to the Chief Medical Officers of England and Wales* (Calman-Hine report). London: HMSO.

Department of Health (1998) *A first class service: quality in the new NHS*. London: HMSO. Available from: **www.dh.gov.uk/PublicationsAnd Statistics/Publications/PublicationsPolicyAndGuidance/DH_4006902&chk=j2Tt7C** (site accessed 13/5/08).

Nursing & Midwifery Council (2004) *The NMC code: standards of conduct, performance and ethics for nurses and midwives*. London: NMC.

Questionnaires

Bell, J. (2005) *Doing your research project: a guide for first time researchers in education and social science* (4th Ed.). Maidenhead: Open University Press.

Moser, C.A. and Kalton, G. (1993) *Survey methods in social investigation* (2nd Ed.). Aldershot: Dartmouth. O/P

Oppenheim, A.N. (2000) *Questionnaire design, interviewing and attitude measurement* (new edition). London: Pinter Publishers.

Parahoo, K. (1993) 'Questionnaires: use, value and limitations'. *Nurse Researcher*, 1(2), pp.4–15.

Research instruments

Bowling, A. (2004) *Measuring health: a review of quality of life measurement scales* (3rd Ed.). Maidenhead: Open University Press.

Clamp, C.G.L. (2004) *Resources for nursing research*. London: Sage.

Frank-Stromberg, M. (1998) *Instruments for clinical nursing research*. Norwalk, CT: Appleton & Lange. O/P

McDowell, I. and Newell, C. (1996) *Measuring health: a guide to rating scales and questionnaires* (2nd Ed.). New York: Oxford University Press.

Robson, C. (2002) *Real world research* (2nd Ed.). Oxford: Blackwell Publishing Ltd.

REFERENCES

Aaronson, S.K., Ahmedzai, S., Bergman, B. *et al.* (1993) 'The European Organisation for Research and Treatment of Cancer QLQ-C30: A quality-of-life instrument for use in international clinical trials in oncology'. *Journal of the National Cancer Institute*, 85, pp.365–76.

Ahmedzai, S.H., Hunt, J. and Keeley, V. (1998) *Palliative care core standards. A multidisciplinary approach*. For Trent Hospice Audit Group, Sheffield: The University of Sheffield.

Bowman, C. (1990) *The essence of strategic management*. London: Prentice Hall.

Bruera, E. (1996) 'Quality assurance in palliative care – a growing "must"?' *Support Care Cancer*, 4, p.157.

Bruera, E., Kuehn, N., Miller, M., Selmser, P. and MacMillan, K. (1991) 'The Edmonton symptom assessment system (ESAS): a simple method for the assessment of palliative care patients'. *Journal of Palliative Care*, 7(2), pp.6–9.

Care Commission Scotland (2002) *National care standards: hospice care*. Edinburgh: HMSO.

Catterall, R.A., Cox, M., Greet, B., Sankey, J. and Griffiths, G. (1998) 'The assessment and audit of spiritual care'. *International Journal of Palliative Nursing*, 4(4), pp.162–8.

Chin, R. and Benne, K.D. (1976) 'General strategies for effecting change in human systems', in Bennis, W.G. *et al.* (editors) *The planning of change* (3rd Ed.). New York: Holt, Reinhart and Winston.

Chin, R. and Benne, K.D. (1985) 'General strategies for effecting changes in human systems', in Bennis, W.G., Benne, K.D. and Chin, R. (editors) *The planning of change* (4th Ed.). New York: Holt, Reinhart and Winston.

Clinical Outcomes Group (1993) EL(93)104 NHSME.

Cohen, S.R., Mount, B.M., Strobel, M.G. and Bui, F. (1995) 'The McGill quality of life questionnaire: a measure of quality of life appropriate for people with advanced disease. A preliminary study of validity and acceptability'. *Palliative Medicine*, 9(3), pp.207–19.

de Haes, J.C.J.M, van Knippenberg, F.C.E. and Neijt, J.P. (1990) 'Measuring psychological and physical distress in cancer patients: structure and application of the Rotterdam symptom checklist'. *British Journal of Cancer*, 62, pp.1034–8.

Department of Health (1998) *A first class service: quality in the new NHS*. London: HMSO. Available from: **www.dh.gov.uk/en/PublicationsAnd Statistics/Publications/PublicationsPolicyAndGuidance/DIL_4006902** (site accessed 13/5/08).

Department of Health (2001a) *National Service Framework for older people*. London: HMSO.

Department of Health (2001b) *Essence of care: patient-focused benchmarking for health care practitioners*. London: HMSO. Available at: **www.dh.gov.uk/en/PublicationsAndStatistics/Publications/Publications PolicyAndGuidance/DH_4005475** (site accessed 30/6/08).

Department of Health (2002) *Independent health care: national minimum standards*. London: HMSO. Available at: **www.dh.gov.uk/assetRoot/ 04/07/83/67/04078367.pdf** (site accessed 13/5/08).

Department of Health (2004) *Standards for better health*. London: HMSO. Available at: **www.dh.gov.uk/assetRoot/04/08/66/66/ 04086666.pdf** (site accessed 13/5/08).

Duff, L.A., Kitson, A.L., Seers, K. and Humphris, D. (1996) 'Clinical guidelines: an introduction to their development and implementation'. *Journal of Advanced Nursing*, 23, pp.887–95.

Duff, L., Fennessey, G. and Harvey, G. (1997) *Clinical effectiveness: embracing the challenges*. Paper given at the National Board for Northern Ireland Annual Research Conference 'Research based practice – Meeting the challenge', Nov. 1997.

Ellershaw, J.E., Peat, S.J. and Boys, L.C. (1995) 'Assessing the effectiveness of a hospital palliative care team'. *Palliative Medicine*, 9, pp.145–52.

Glickman, M. (1997) *Making palliative care better: quality improvement, multiprofessional audit and standards*. National Council for Hospice and Specialist Palliative Care Services.

Glickman, M./Working Party on Standards (1997) *Quality improvement, multiprofessional audit and standards*. Occasional Paper 12, National Council for Hospice and Specialist Palliative Care Services.

Greenhalgh (1996), cited in Higginson, I.J. (1999) 'Evidence-based palliative care?' *European Journal of Palliative Care*, 6(6), pp.188–93.

Harvey, G. (1998) 'Improving patient care: getting to grips with clinical governance'. *RCN Magazine*, Autumn 1998, pp.8–9.

Hearn, J. and Higginson, I.J. (1997) 'Outcome measures in palliative care for advanced cancer patients: a review'. *Journal of Public Health Medicine*, 19(2), pp.193–9.

Higginson, I. (1993) 'A community schedule', in Higginson, I. (editor) *Clinical audit in palliative care*. Oxford: Radcliffe Medical Press.

Higginson, I. (1998) For copies of POS, go to: **www.kcl.ac.uk/schools/ medicine/dep/3/Palliative/qat/pos.html**

Higginson, I.J. (1999) 'Evidence-based palliative care?' *European Journal of Palliative Care*, 6(6), pp.188–93.

Institute of Medicine (1992) *Guidelines for clinical practice: from development to use*. Washington, DC: National Academy Press.

Jenkinson, cited in Hearn, J. and Higginson, I.J. (1997) 'Outcome measures in palliative care for advanced cancer patients: a review'. *Journal of Public Health Medicine*, 19(2), p.193.

Kitson, A. (1990) 'Quality matters and standard setting'. *Nursing Standard*, 444, pp.32–3.

Lugton, J. and Kindlen, M. (1999) (editors) *Palliative care: the nursing role*. Edinburgh: Churchill Livingstone.

Lugton, J. and McIntyre, R. (editors) (2005) *Palliative care: the nursing role* (2nd Ed.). Edinburgh: Churchill Livingstone.

MacAdam, D.B. and Smith, M. (1987) 'An initial assessment of suffering in terminal illness'. *Palliative Medicine*, 1, pp.37–47.

Marr, H. and Giebing, H. (1994) *Quality assurance in nursing: concept, methods and case studies*. Edinburgh: Campion Press.

McCorkle, R. and Young, K. (1978) 'Development of a symptom distress scale'. *Cancer Nursing*, 101, pp.373–8.

McGrother, J. (1995) *Profiles, portfolios and how to build them*. London: Scutari Press.

Morgan, E. (1997) 'Clinical effectiveness'. *Nursing Standard*, 11(34), pp.43–50.

Morrell, C. and Harvey, G. (1999) *The clinical audit handbook: improving the quality of health care*. London: Baillière Tindall in association with the RCN.

Morris, J., Suissa, S., Sherwood, S. and Greer, D. (1986) 'Last days: a study of the quality of life of terminally ill cancer patients'. *Journal of Chronic Diseases*, 39, pp.47–62.

Mulhall, A. (1998) 'EBN notebook; nursing, research and the evidence'. *Evidence-Based Nursing*, 1(1), pp.4–6.

Munro, R. (2001) 'We can't care for the dying properly'. *Nursing Times*, 97(21), p.5.

National Institute of Clinical Effectiveness (2004) *Improving supportive and palliative care for adults with cancer*. London: NICE.

NHS QIS (2002) *Standards for specialist palliative care*. Edinburgh: NHS QIS

NICE – see National Institute for Clinical Effectiveness.

Nuffield Trust (2001) *Care of the dying in the NHS – the Buckinghamshire communiqué*. Available from the Nuffield Trust on 0207 631 8450, or at **www.nuffieldtrust.org.uk/ecomm/files/11303careofdyingbucking ham.pdf** (site accessed 13/5/08).

O'Boyle, C.A., McGee, H. and Joyce, C.R.B. (1994) 'Quality of life: assessing the individual'. *Advances in Medical Sociology*, 5, pp.159–80.

Robbins, M. (1998) *Evaluating palliative care: establishing the evidence base*. Oxford: Oxford University Press.

Royal College of Nursing (1990) *Quality patient care*. London: Royal College of Nursing.

Royal College of Nursing (1998) *Guidance for nurses on clinical governance*. London: Royal College of Nursing.

Royal College of Nursing (2000) *Clinical governance: how nurses can get involved*. London: Royal College of Nursing.

Royal College of Nursing (2003) *Clinical governance briefing sheet*. London: Royal College of Nursing. Available at: **www.rcn.org.uk/publi cations/pdf/ClinicalGovernance2003.pdf** (site accessed 13/5/08).

Sackett, D.L., Rosenberg, W.M.C., Gray, J.A.M., Haynes, R.D. and Richardson, W.S. (1996) 'Evidence based medicine. What it is and what it isn't'. *British Medical Journal*, 312, pp.71–2.

Sackett, D.L., Richardson, W.S., Rosenberg, W. and Haynes, R.B. (1997) *Evidence-based medicine*. Edinburgh: Churchill Livingstone.

Schroeder, P. (1988) 'Direction and dilemmas in nursing quality assurance'. *Nursing Clinics of North America*, 23(3), pp.657–64.

Scottish Partnership Agency for Palliative and Cancer Care (SPA) (1996) *Core standards for specialist palliative care*. Edinburgh: SPA.

Scottish Partnership for Palliative Care (SPPC) (2003a) *Beyond the randomised trial: evidence and effectiveness in palliative care*. Edinburgh: SPPC.

Scottish Partnership for Palliative Care (SPPC) (2003b) *Public awareness of palliative care*. Edinburgh: SPPC.

SPA – See Scottish Partnership Agency for Palliative and Cancer Care.

SPPC – See Scottish Partnership for Palliative Care.

Sterkenburg, C.A. and Woodward, C.A. (1996) 'A reliability and validity study of the McMaster Quality of Life Scale (MQLS) for a palliative population'. *Journal of Palliative Care*, 12(1), pp.18–25.

Abbreviations

AIDS	acquired immune deficiency syndrome
APT	adjuvant psychological therapy
CHI	Commission for Health Improvement
CNCP	chronic non-cancer pain
COAD	chronic obstructive airways disease
COPD	chronic obstructive pulmonary disease
CRF	cancer-related fatigue
CSCI	continuous subcutaneous infusion
DySSSy	The Dynamic Standard Setting System
EAPC	European Association for Palliative Care
EORTC	European Organisation for Research and Treatment of Cancer
EPDS	Edinburgh Postnatal Depression Scale
FACT-F	Functional assessment of cancer therapy – fatigue
FHP	functional health patterns
GP	general practitioner
HADS	hospital anxiety and depression scale
Hb	haemoglobin
HIV	human immunodeficiency virus
MAC	mental adjustment to cancer scale
MSHS	morphine sulphate hydrogel suppository
NHS	National Health Service
NICE	National Institute of Clinical Excellence
NMC	Nursing and Midwifery Council
NMDA	N-methyl-D-aspartate
NRS	numerical rating scale
OTFC	oral transmucosal fentanyl citrate
prn	pro re nata – as required
POS	Palliative Outcome Scale
SCQF	Scottish Credit and Qualifications Framework
SPPC	Scottish Partnership for Palliative Care
STAS	Support Team Assessment Schedule
SVCO	superior vena caval obstruction
TCA	tricyclic antidepressant
TENS	transcutaneous electrical nerve stimulation

VAS	visual analogue scale
VRS	verbal rating scale
VVAS	vertical visual analogue scale
WHO	World Health Organization
WRVS	Women's Royal Voluntary Service

Glossary

Action learning: An approach to help you to learn, from experience, how to improve your palliative care practice. The experiences are provided as you undertake the activities in the book and when you try out new skills with others in your clinical area. The book will help you to think about the effects these activities and actions have had and help you to learn from them.

Action learning set: A group of individuals who are using this book to work together over an extended period of time, carrying out some of the activities together and reflecting, evaluating and critiquing the effects of these activities and of individuals' efforts to try out new skills back in the clinical area. Set members may come from the same or different organisations.

Acute pain: An episode of pain of sudden onset, short duration and foreseeable end.

Adaptation: The process by which a patient may gradually manage to endure pain and carry on despite it, perhaps without obvious outward signs of pain.

Adjuvant analgesic: Adjuvant analgesics are drugs that are not analgesics in their own right, but can produce analgesia in certain situations; they are particularly important for pains that are relatively unresponsive to morphine.

Allodynia: Pain due to a stimulus that does not normally provoke pain.

Analgesia: Absence of pain in response to stimulation that would normally be painful.

Causalgia: A syndrome of sustained burning pain, allodynia and hyperpathia after a traumatic nerve lesion, often combined with vasomotor and sudomotor dysfunction and later trophic changes.

Central pain: Pain initiated or caused by a primary lesion or dysfunction in the central nervous system.

Chronic pain: Pain lasting for six months or more.

Co-analgesic: See adjuvant analgesic.

Critical companion: In the context of this book, an individual who can help participants on their learning journey through this book instead of, or in addition to, their action learning set.

Deep pain: Pain originating in the organs of the body, usually not as localised as superficial pain; has an aching quality.

Dysaesthesia: An unpleasant abnormal sensation whether spontaneous or evoked.

Facilitator: An individual who facilitates the setting up and the process of the action learning set and who helps action learning set members to achieve their objectives. The facilitator is not a participant.

Hyperaesthesia: Increased sensitivity to stimulation, excluding the special senses.

Hyperalgesia: An increased response to a stimulus which is normally painful.

Hyperpathia: A painful syndrome characterised by an abnormally painful reaction to a stimulus, especially a repetitive stimulus, as well as an increased threshold.

Hypoaesthesia: Decreased sensitivity to stimulation, excluding the special senses.

Hypoalgesia: Diminished pain in response to a normally painful stimulus.

Neuralgia: Pain in the distribution of a nerve or nerves.

Neuritis: Inflammation of a nerve or nerves.

Neurogenic pain: Pain initiated or caused by a primary lesion, dysfunction or transitory perturbation in the peripheral or central nervous system.

Neuropathic pain: Pain initiated or caused by a primary lesion or dysfunction in the nervous system.

Neuropathy: A disturbance of function or pathological change in a nerve.

Nociceptive pain: Pain due to the stimulation of the nociceptors in skin, bones, joints and viscera.

Nociceptor: A receptor preferentially sensitive to a noxious stimulus or to a stimulus that would become noxious if prolonged.

Nociception: Troublesome pain due to continuous stimulation of the nociceptors in skin, bones, joints and viscera; it is often indicative of ongoing tissue damage, such as osteoarthritis and chronic pancreatitis.

Noxious stimulus: A stimulus that is damaging to normal tissues.

Open learning: A method of learning which is designed to be more flexible than other more traditional methods of learning. It is self-managed and participant-centred.

Pain: An unpleasant sensory and emotional experience associated with actual or potential tissue damage or described in terms of such damage.

Pain threshold: The least experience of pain that a subject can recognise.

Pain tolerance level: The greatest level of pain that a subject is prepared to tolerate.

Paraesthesia: An abnormal sensation, whether spontaneous or evoked.

Participant: The individual who is using this book.

Peripheral neurogenic pain: Pain initiated or caused by a primary lesion, dysfunction or transitory perturbation in the peripheral nervous system.

Peripheral neuropathic pain: Pain initiated or caused by a primary lesion or dysfunction in the peripheral nervous system.

Primary nursing: Primary nursing is a work organisational design in which the authority to manage the nursing care of a small group of hospital patients, from admission to discharge, is devolved from the senior nurse in charge of the ward to a staff nurse. Primary nursing thus ensures clear lines of responsibility and accountability and guaranteed continuity of care for patients and nurses.

prn: 'pro re nata' – as required.

Professional craft knowledge: Practical 'know-how' that is tacit, intuitive and embedded in practice. It is considered so ordinary and everyday by nurses that it is usually taken for granted and is, therefore, rarely talked about. It is accrued over time, primarily through practice, and its development can be facilitated through critical companionship.

Psychogenic pain: Pain with no detectable physical cause in a patient with a history of expressing emotional problems in terms of pain.

Referred pain: Pain felt at a site other than that which has been stimulated.

Secondary analgesic: See *adjuvant analgesic*.

Somatic pain: A form of nociceptive pain, such as bone pain and pain in soft-tissue masses, is usually described by patients as aching or throbbing and is generally well localised.

Superficial Pain: Pain originating from the stimulation of the skin or mucous membranes; may be described as bright, pricking or burning, and is usually localised.

Support/discussion group: An alternative to an action learning set to help participants learn individually and in a group. Here there is no facilitator (as in an action learning set). However, the support/discussion group may appoint a facilitator from among its own members. Therefore, the facilitator is a participant. Group members may come from the same or different organisations.

Theoretical knowledge: 'Book knowledge' or research-based knowledge that is explicit, rational and talked about by communities of nurses. It is generated through scholarship and through research.

Titrate/titration: To adjust the dosage of drugs given to a patient by starting at a low level then increasing the dose until pain relief is successful.

Visceral pain: A form of nocicepive pain, described by patients as deep and aching, and is often not well localised.

Working group: A group of participants in the same organisation working through the book together to improve the practice of palliative care in their organisation.

Source: Most of the definitions relating to pain, sensation and sensitivity, and analgesia are from Merskey and Bogduk (1994: 209–14).

Index